THE WHARTONS'
BACK BOOK

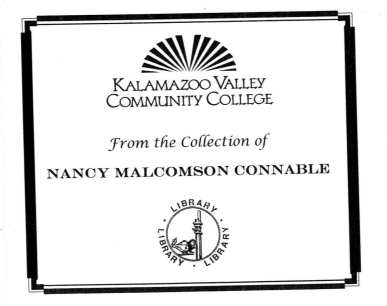

THE WHARTONS'
BACK BOOK

End back pain—now and forever—with
this simple, revolutionary program

JIM *and* PHIL WHARTON
with **Bev Browning,** *authors of* The Whartons' Stretch Book

RODALE

Notice

This book is intended as a reference volume only, not as a medical manual. The information given here is designed to help you make informed decisions about your health. It is not intended as a substitute for any treatment that may have been prescribed by your doctor. If you suspect that you have a medical problem, we urge you to seek competent medical help.

Mention of specific companies, organizations, or authorities in this book does not imply endorsement by the publisher, nor does mention of specific companies, organizations, or authorities imply that they endorse this book.

Internet addresses and telephone numbers given in this book were accurate at the time it went to press.

Some clothing provided by Mothers In Motion, Inc. (www.mothersinmotion.com)

Illustrations by Karen Kuchar
Photographs by Mitch Mandel/Rodale Images

Book design by Christina Gaugler

Library of Congress Cataloging-in-Publication Data

Wharton, Jim, date.
   The Whartons' back book : end back pain—now and forever—with this simple, revolutionary program / by Jim and Phil Wharton, with Bev Browning.
      p.   cm.
   Includes index.
   ISBN 1–57954–703–6   paperback
   1. Backache—Popular works.   I. Wharton, Phil, date.   II. Browning, Bev.   III. Title.
RD771.B217W48   2003
617.5'64—dc21   2003009402

Distributed to the book trade by St. Martin's Press

2   4   6   8   10   9   7   5   3   1   paperback

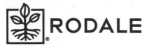

WE **INSPIRE** AND **ENABLE** PEOPLE TO IMPROVE
THEIR LIVES AND THE WORLD AROUND THEM

FOR MORE OF OUR PRODUCTS
WWW.RODALESTORE.COM
(800) 848-4735

To Robert R. Glass

Contents

.

Acknowledgments

To the people from all walks of life and ends of the world, thank you for honoring us to help you help yourselves out of pain, for giving us the gift of witnessing the extension of the healing spirit; and to the doctors, health-care professionals, and flexibility technicians who carry the torch in our mission of healing.

No book of ours can go to print without heartfelt thanks to the greatest agent and friend, Reid Boates. As he always says, "Onward!" Many, many thanks to Mariska van Aalst, our talented and tireless editor at Rodale. She's truly amazing. Kudos to Christina Gaugler, who designed *The Whartons' Back Book* to be easy to read and interesting to behold. It's a work of art transformed from typing paper.

Jim and Phil Wharton

INTRODUCTION

When your back isn't working right, nothing in your life works right. Trying to understand what has gone wrong and how to correct it has led you to this book and a unique opportunity to explore injury not as a *patient*, but as an *athlete*.

"Athlete?" you're thinking. "I'm not an athlete."

Yes, you are! We all are athletes. If you're living in a body and using it every day to create your life and your work, you're an athlete in need of optimal health, strength, flexibility, balance, and more.

Seeing yourself as an athlete affords you a unique perspective. You see yourself not as a helpless victim, but as a person on a mission to take control. You approach getting well with energy that comes into focus only when you reach for the best in yourself. Use this book, and you'll not only relieve and prevent pain—you'll find yourself stronger and more fit than when your back problems began, secure in the knowledge that they won't happen again. Together, we'll get you there.

WE'VE BEEN WHERE YOU ARE TODAY

Are you in pain? Struggling with a chronic injury? Or do you just want to relieve stiffness, a lack of mo-bility, or a surprising twinge that comes and goes, taking your breath and your confidence with it?

We can help.

Your success is personal to us, because we began our careers with trying to solve a back problem. When Phil developed scoliosis in college, we learned what would become the Active-Isolated Stretching and Strengthening program. Using this method not only relieved his pain but entirely *reversed* his condition, preventing the need for surgery or an immobilizing brace. (For his complete story, see page 6 in chapter 1.) Today, we are a father-and-son training team that travels the world, helping relieve the back pain of hundreds of high-profile athletes, performers, and other luminaries. Now, we want to help you, too!

We started our practice nearly 20 years ago, out of a small office in New York City. Our practice grew by whispers, behind the scenes of some of the largest arenas and venues in the world. Soon, we were training and rehabilitating professional athletes, Broadway dancers, famous musicians, and Hollywood actors with roles that were physically challenging. We were especially delighted when, during the 1992 Olympic Games in Barcelona, Spain, the athletes with whom we worked brought home 13 gold medals. (If we were our own country, we would have placed third in the world!)

Quietly, discreetly, our reputations as "The Mechanics" spread, on account of our reported ability to fine-tune a high-performance body or "fix" one when things go wrong. All this, with nothing more than a flat surface, a length of rope, and the Active-Isolated method.

What's our secret? Well, over the years, we've certainly learned a lot about physiology and the inherent talents and changing moods of the human body. We can tell you what is the best move to do when, and why, and we can help you coax your body into position. But the truth is, while we may be helpful, we're not miracle workers—the Active-Isolated method is. We've seen, beyond a doubt, that the same training method that unlocks and relieves the pain of Olympic medalists, hulking NFL football players, and delicate ballerinas can and *will* work for everyone who's ready to take control. And that means *you!*

REVOLUTIONARY TRAINING AND REHABILITATION

With this book, we tailor our trademark Active-Isolated method specifically to help prevent and cure back pain. You'll learn a quick, easy method that can help get you out of pain immediately and help you strengthen your back so that pain will be a thing of the past. In the process, you'll also enjoy better circulation and mobility, enriched sleep, lowered stress, and increased energy. You'll do more and hurt less.

By giving your back new life, you'll get your own life back.

First, we want to help you understand the anatomy of your back. Ever notice how when your knee goes out, your back acts up 2 days later? We'll trace those seemingly mystical links and explain how your back is really the epicenter of all sensation in your body.

From medical and biomechanical standpoints, we'll review some of the things that can go wrong with your back, and why. Then we'll advise you on professional care available for diagnosis, treatment and rehabilitation, and the results you can expect.

The core of the book is a training program of your own. With your physician's permission and using our signature systems of Active-Isolated Stretching and Strengthening, you can improve not only your back but also your entire fitness level.

Later in the book, we'll also cover some of the situations and conditions that can lead to back pain, and we'll give you complete strategies for preventing and relieving pain in those key moments—*exactly* when and how you need them.

Throughout the book, you'll read about the experiences of some of our favorite clients—all of whom have found relief with this very same program. (Please note: We've changed some of our clients' names and personal details to protect their privacy.)

With the Active-Isolated method, even the smallest efforts will yield surprising, even revolutionary results. You'll feel better from the very first time you try these exercises. Your healthy back—flexible, strong, and pain-free—is waiting for you, athlete. Let's get started!

Part 1

The Pain-Free Back

Chapter 1

A NEW WAY TO THINK ABOUT YOUR BACK

If you suffer with back pain, you aren't alone. You're one of an estimated 60 to 80 percent of all American adults (about 65 million people) who are complaining of back pain—particularly lower-back pain—at any given time. Back problems constitute one of the most costly ailments in our country, accounting for billions of dollars in medical care and lost wages annually.

As sympathetic as we are, we're also convinced that most of these problems are absolutely preventable. And once they manifest, they can be easily treated in their early stages, before they become debilitating and expensive. Even when they become extreme, surgery might not be the only answer.

Sound crazy? Believe it. We've seen the proof, hundreds of times. And we're going to show you how a simple, do-it-yourself method has helped hundreds of our clients prevent, diminish, or completely obliterate their back pain, quickly, easily, and often forever.

What it will take is a shift in your thinking. We know that when your back isn't working right, nothing in your life works right. Your attempts to understand what's happening and to control your pain have led you to us. Now we're here to help you seize this opportunity to, as we said earlier, explore your injury not as a *patient*, but as an *athlete*.

We think it's very interesting that our elite athletes never think of back injury as "injury." Although almost all are very knowledgeable in anatomy and biomechanics and are certainly well-informed about every aspect of the pain they're suffering, they never define the injury at all. They see it merely as a mistake in training or performance. Perhaps it's even a wake-up call.

Well, here is your wake-up call. You can control your own pain. You can rehabilitate your body. You can even learn to "PREhabilitate" your back, to prevent pain from ever striking again. Just listen to the stories of your fellow athletes.

BANISHING PAIN ON STAGE AND ON THE COURT

Take this case, for instance: Lauren Bacall, a beautiful actress here in New York City, had just completed an arduous run on Broadway when she consulted us about back pain that had resulted from the demands made on her by the performances. Rather than succumb to the pain and retreat to her bed, she was already working out at La Palestra, one of the best gyms in New York City, to try to bring her body back into alignment. We examined her and realized that a knee irritation, which had been with her for some time, was causing her to favor her opposite leg. Because she was compensating, she had thrown her back into an imbalance, and pain and weakness followed.

We pointed out to Lauren that performing on stage is no different from performing in an Olympic arena. Both are athletic and require the same training and preparation. She smiled. She already knew. We were on the same wavelength.

We worked out with her and taught her the same techniques that we'll show you in chapter 4. We got her out of pain very quickly, but warned her as seriously as we could, "You have homework to do now—will you do it?"

She said, "I like the sound of that. Absolutely."

We said, "We're going to give you this stretch rope to assist you if you promise to do the work."

She said, "If I'm now considered an athlete, I'll do the work, but you have to get me a serious warmup suit."

We laughed. She did the work. We got her the suit.

The point is that this graceful actress knew that her body is her gift and her responsibility. When her back was in pain, she didn't cave in. She headed straight for the gym and eventually to us. She didn't fixate on the injury. She used it as a wake-up call. As a result, she's doing better than ever. Still active and energetic, and still very beautiful.

We'll give you another example: We were invited to the New York Knicks preseason training to teach the team quick routines to prepare and recover quickly. The Knicks were facing an 81-game season, and there was some concern about keeping everyone healthy and on the court.

Over a series of visits to their training center, we got to know the players pretty well. They're great guys who responded appreciatively to our care. But one player was particularly interested: Patrick Ewing.

Patrick admitted that he'd been suffering with back pain for a couple of years. We suspected that it had stemmed from a slight knee injury (just like Lauren), so we designed an intensive personal program for him and got right to work. We started first with flexibility and strengthening, concentrating on his knee. When we straightened that problem out, Patrick reported that his back stopped hurting. He was willing to do the work, even when he couldn't quite make the direct connection between the imbalances caused by his knee and the pain in his back.

He didn't give up. He's not about injury—he's about winning. He used the work to become a better athlete. He used the opportunity to take performance to the next level.

NEW ATTITUDE, NEW YOU

As we've discussed, athletes view injuries as mistakes and opportunities: Their bodies have pointed out mistakes and have given them opportunities to make corrections and rocket their performances to the next level.

Nonathletes, on the other hand, sometimes fixate on their injuries, regarding them as unfortunate circumstances. In an effort to avoid further pain, they may allow the injury to limit their activity, sometimes to the point that life itself winds down to nearly nothing. Sadly, the approaches between athlete and nonathlete are 180 degrees off each other. But they shouldn't be.

We want you to think like an athlete. We want you to see a back problem as an opportunity. So much suffering and surgery might be prevented if you are willing to switch your mindset. You *are* an athlete. You might not play on a professional ball team or dance in musicals or compete in the Olympics, but if you use your body to live, work, play, and love, then you are an athlete. You deserve to be flexible, strong, fit, healthy . . . and pain-free. You deserve to reclaim your life.

Your success is personal to us, because we began our careers with trying to solve a back problem. Let us tell you the story of how an injury turned out to be the opportunity of a lifetime. Our story.

In high school, Phil was an up-and-coming track athlete who averaged 35 miles of running per week and took summers off to rest and recover from the pounding his body took during the school year. Hard work paid off when Phil was accepted to the University of Florida to run with the prestigious Florida Track Team, the team that developed stars like Frank Shorter, Jack Bacheler, John Parker, Margaret Tolbert, and Marty Liquori. It was a dream come true that would soon turn into a nightmare.

When Phil ramped up his running to 80 miles per week and all but eliminated the rest cycle, things suddenly started going very wrong. At first, he felt a twinge in his hip. Then an ache in his back. Day by day, "discomfort"—at first easily explained and even ignored—turned uglier.

It didn't take long for every step that he ran to fire a jolting, searing pain up his spine. The pain would plague him even after he stepped off the track. Days of suffering in the classroom were followed by sessions of having to stand up in the library as he studied and sleepless nights spent tossing and turning to find comfortable positions.

His whole life started coming unraveled. Like most people trying to solve back problems, he and his coaches tried every protocol they thought might bring relief, from massage and rest to chiropractics and medications, and everything in between. The team physicians at the University of Florida finally diagnosed him with scoliosis, curvature of the spine, and suggested implanting rods on either side of his spine to straighten it. They also informed him that if he didn't stop running, they could practically guarantee that his disability was going to get a whole lot worse. He might even suffer permanent nerve damage or paralysis.

Implanting the rods would mean that his running career would be over anyhow, which the surgeons thought would be a small price to pay for the relief he would get. But the surgeons didn't understand the heart of a runner. Running was Phil's life. It filled him with joy and defined him as a person. Period. There had to be another way.

Randy Brower, a trainer who worked with the Florida Track Team, had one more suggestion, even though it was a long shot. He directed Phil to Aaron Mattes, a well-respected kinesiologist with a clinic only a few hours away in Sarasota. Despairing but still looking for a nonsurgical solution, we took Randy's advice and made an appointment. Within a couple of days, we drove down the coast to meet with Aaron. He did a muscle-by-muscle evaluation of Phil's body and matter-of-factly pointed out areas that were weak and imbalanced.

Weak and imbalanced?! Heresy! Impossible! Phil was a front-runner for the mighty Florida Track Team, an athlete who prided himself on his strong, lean, highly trained, high-performance body. Aaron wasn't impressed at all. He flatly informed us that he thought the scoliosis had nothing to do with any deformity of Phil's spine. It had everything to do with Phil's being out of balance on one side and drawing his spine out of alignment and into curvature. In fact, *he* was causing the problem.

Before Phil could catapult from his initial shock into righteous indignation and outrage, Aaron told us that he thought he could help. And he did. After one session with Aaron, Phil felt measurable relief. Against overwhelming odds, we had found the answer. We were believers.

We both were intrigued by Aaron's approach, for it combined all that we understood about physics with our knowledge of the biomechanics of running. Everything Aaron said made a lot of sense. Besides, we had nothing to lose and everything to gain by following his advice.

Together, we embarked on a year of hard work to get Phil out of pain and back onto the track. Phil worked with Active-Isolated Stretching and Strengthening exercises 6 days a week for the full year; he was a man on a mission. Once a week, the two of us would travel to Aaron's clinic in Sarasota for an evaluation to check progress and finely tune the workouts.

Here's the happy ending: Phil corrected the imbalances and strengthened the weaknesses. His spine straightened, and his pain disappeared. He returned to running—this time 100 miles per week—with no problem.

Today, 20 years later, he trains every day without injury and competes on the world-class level in the 26.2-mile marathon. Not only did we find a solution to Phil's back problem that would actually improve his performance, we eventually became students of Aaron Mattes. It meant starting all over and going back to school for both of us, but the sacrifices of an abrupt about-face would be worth the effort.

We embarked on a long, long journey that would change the course of our lives and the world of sports forever. Today, we train and rehabilitate athletes all over the world. Our clinic in New York City is a small, unassuming haven on the Upper West Side just off Central Park in Manhattan. But don't let "small, unassuming" fool you. Our clinic looks like a public relations junket for the finest athletes and entertainers in the world. Among unrecognizable faces are those of NBA basketball players, Kenyan runners, Italian soccer players, and Olympic swimmers chatting with famous actors and Broadway dancers. The air is definitely international and charged with the high energy of people who reach for the best in themselves. All are there for one of two reasons: Either they're injured and need fast, effective rehab, or they're preparing to do something that will make unfamiliar demands on their bodies, and they need to be trained to achieve the next level.

We want you to have those same opportunities. We want to open the doors of our clinic to you through the pages of this book. We want to get you to stop thinking like a patient with a bad back and start thinking like an athlete who needs rehabilitation or requires training to take performance to the next level.

HOW TO USE THE BOOK

This book is divided into the following six parts:

1. The Pain-Free Back
2. Try PREhab, Not Rehab
3. Stopping the Pain
4. Protecting Your Back As Your Body Changes
5. Stress and Slumber
6. Pain-Free Solutions for Everyday Situations

How you use the book depends on why you're reading it. If you're reading it to prevent back problems, you'll be particularly interested in training like an athlete to become as strong and flexible as you can. You'll benefit from the general information in part 1 and the PREhab program in part 2.

PREhab (as opposed to rehab) is a term we coined when we found our early practice dominated by rehabilitating athletes who had made basic biomechanical mistakes with catastrophic consequences. After treating the thousandth injury, we decided to step into athletes' lives earlier—*before* they got hurt. Now we design PREhabilitation programs, so we have to do less rehabilitation.

We'd rather work this way, of course, but it's not always possible. If you're reading the book because you're already suffering with back problems, in part 3, we'll help you design your own at-home rehab program. We call it your Get-Out-of-Pain-Free-Plan. If that doesn't do the trick, we'll help you make decisions about the right professional help. After you're well, and with your physician's blessing, you can continue with training to make sure you'll stay out of trouble for a lifetime.

We understand that no back exists in a perfect, unstrained world, so in parts 4, 5, and 6, we'll give you advice for dozens of situations in which you may become injured, feel pain, or aggravate old injuries. You'll know the best way to prepare for these situations, and you'll learn "quick release" moves to help get you out of those painful seize-ups that can instantly immobilize you, those moments that can make you want to lie down on the floor and never get up. We've been there, and we're here to help.

ACTIVE-ISOLATED? WHAT DOES THAT MEAN?

When we say that our method is called "Active-Isolated," what does that mean, exactly? We'll explain more later, but, essentially, you'll be encouraging your muscles to function in the way nature intended.

You see, muscles work in opposite pairs. Every time one contracts, a companion muscle must relax.

Try it yourself: Make a fist and flex your elbow to bend your arm up. Your biceps, the muscle on the front side of your upper arm, contracts to bring your fist up. At that very same moment, your triceps muscle, at the back side of your upper arm, is completely relaxed. It needed to let go and elongate so that your biceps could shorten.

This simple principle underlies all of the Active-Isolated work. You isolate a specific muscle or groups of muscles and activate, or "fire," them one at a time in a prescribed sequence. As you do this, the opposite muscles will relax for a good stretch, allowing a greater range of motion and a fuller, more complete workout of the muscle fibers from one end to the other. For the same principle on the flip side, during an Active-Isolated Strengthening move, you'll relax one muscle so that the opposite muscle can fire for the lift.

How is this different from conventional methods? Mother Nature designed the muscles in the body to be helpful to each other. When one is weak, fatigued, cramped, or struggling, your body automatically recruits volunteers—other muscles that can kick in to get the job done. So let's say that you're trying to do a situp, but your abdominal muscles aren't very strong. What happens? Your body recruits other volunteer muscles to assist—probably ones in your hip—and those weaker ab muscles get shut out, stay weak, and get progressively weaker as time goes on.

What if the goal had been to strengthen that weak muscle, instead of just doing the situp? What if the goal had been to stretch a weak muscle, instead of getting your nose to your knee? This is what Active-Isolated work is all about.

The goal of your Wharton workout is to isolate a muscle or a muscle group, so your body will not be able to recruit others against your wishes. You activate the targeted area only, so *you* are in control of which muscles you stretch or strengthen. And because you'll be targeting specific muscles, the moves are small and gentle—perfect for helping you to get out of pain and back to full function.

You're probably eager to get going. But before you begin, you need to get a good understanding of the raw materials we'll be working with. Behold, the amazing mechanics of your spine.

A CLOSER LOOK AT THE INNER WORKINGS OF THE SPINE

The spine is a fascinating, miraculous system, but on the days it seems most painful, it can be hard to imagine that it's anything but a source of agony. But let's review the many ways that the spine helps you get through your day.

- It keeps you upright so that you don't collapse on the ground in a heap (no small thing!).
- It houses and protects the spinal cord and nerve roots that communicate with your brain and then transmit messages to every part of your body—from the top of your head to the tips of your toes, and to many major internal organs in between—and back again.
- It is the base of attachment for connective tissue like tendons (which attach muscle to bone) and ligaments (which attach bone to bone).
- It is also the base of attachment for muscles. In fact, a *lot* of muscles attach to the spine.
- It directly supports your head, shoulders, and chest.
- It connects your upper body to your lower body.
- It has sensors and compensation systems that keep your weight distributed properly so that you can balance.
- The individual vertebrae produce red blood cells in the marrow and store minerals.
- Its flexibility allows you to bend forward and backward and to both sides. It will rotate your upper half from side to side while your lower half stays still, and the other way around.

■ It can and will combine any of the movements above. (Here you thought it was just a source of excruciating pain!)

Composed of 33 bones (vertebrae) all working in concert, the spine's structure is really an amazing feat of biomechanical architecture in five parts.

1. Your neck
2. Your midback
3. Your lower back
4. Your sacrum
5. Your coccyx

Let's take a look at these five areas, as well as some other amazingly well-designed parts of the spine.

THE FIVE PARTS OF THE SPINE

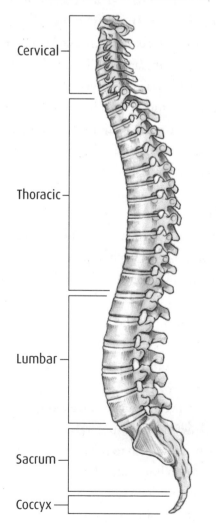

Cervical

Thoracic

Lumbar

Sacrum

Coccyx

Your Neck

Yes, your neck *is* your back; it's the part that holds your head on.

This is the cervical spine, made up of seven vertebrae. The medical shorthand for this is C1 through C7, meaning cervical vertebra number 1 through cervical vertebra number 7.

The upper bones C1 and C2 are unique among all the other vertebrae, because they are in charge of head and neck rotation. C1, a ring of bone that supports the skull, is called the atlas, named after the mythical Greek god who supported the weight of the world on his shoulders. C2 is called the axis, because its function is literally that. It has a little blunt knob on the top that projects up into a hole in the atlas, allowing the neck to pivot. They are supported by special ligaments.

The cervical spine is highly mobile and busy all the time. The pressure of the weight of your head and the constant turning and bending of your head and neck lead sometimes to wear and tear. This is why neck pain and problems are common.

Typical concerns: One of the problems that manifests in the cervical spine is locked neck. The symptoms are that the neck is contracted to either side and it seems to be locked into position.

Another clue to the condition is that one shoulder is cocked up or carried too high, as though the body is unbalanced. The smallest movement is not only painful but also impossible. It doesn't take long for that tension in the neck to cause a throbbing tension headache. Typically, the cervical spinal muscles are constricted and stressed, causing the spasm that reveals itself through pain and immobility.

Another malady of the cervical spine is frozen shoulder. Even though the shoulder is located beside the cervical spine and would seem to be unrelated, restriction of the cervical spine can most certainly cause muscles on each side to lock down, too.

The frozen shoulder is a loss of range of motion in the shoulder joint. Clients describe it as a knot of congestion, pain in the upper back, a feeling that their shoulder blades are being drawn together. Frequently, the shoulder is not only locked up but also rolled forward in constriction.

When the cervical spine is contracted, the pectoralis major muscles in the upper chest fatigue and draw the shoulder forward, causing the upper back to struggle to maintain upright posture and function. Then trapezius and rhomboid muscles in the upper back short out, and all muscles in the upper chest and upper back tighten to protect themselves. It's a war of muscles. It's a vicious cycle. The tighter the front, the tighter the back. The tighter the back, the tighter the front. The result is pain, fatigue, and a shoulder that seems to be frozen.

Getting the muscles to release is a matter of restoring circulation and range of motion, and keeping them flexible and strong enough to make sure that the structural integrity of the shoulder will be protected.

Thankfully, both of these painful situations can be completely avoided with flexibility and strengthening exercises found in chapter 4.

Your Midback

The longest designation of the spine is distinguished as the part of your spine that supports all your ribs, except the lower two (the "floating ribs" that are fused to ribs above them rather than to vertebrae). It runs from below your cervical spine to your waist behind your chest. The upper part, between your shoulder blades, is typically the place where you carry all your tension.

The midback is known as the thoracic spine, made up of 12 vertebrae. The medical shorthand for this is T1 through T12, meaning thoracic vertebra number 1 through thoracic vertebra number 12. The thoracic spine has a very limited range of motion because the ribs provide added support and the formation of each vertebra is designed to lock into place.

Typical concerns: The thoracic spine is particularly vulnerable to that knot of tension that almost everyone has carried between the shoulder blades.

This knot can cause a specific point of pain that we've heard described as "feeling like I've been hit with a rock," which is a spasm of the deeper muscles in the back that feels tender to the touch.

The knot can occur from tension over a long period of time, during which adhesions or scar tissue can actually set into the muscle fibers and cause problems. Or it can occur in an instant, such as when a sprinter clenches her fists, tightens her back, and explodes off the starting block. When the body perceives that a muscle is injured instantly or over time, it builds a natural splint by creating a spasm to immobilize the area and protect it from further harm.

If you want a spasm between your shoulder blades to release, you have to convince the body that there is no injury. You have to relax the muscles and restore circulation and range of motion. We'll tell you how on page 252 in chapter 12.

Another complaint we get in our clinic is for nonspecific backache in the thoracic region. General though this pain may be, it can throb. Intermittent or chronic, the pain can intensify with every breath because the ribs are connected at the thoracic spine and their expansions and contractions can irritate a back in trouble. It's just an ache that saps the energy and fun right out of life. The major stabilizing muscles in the thoracic spine can weaken over time in the battle to "brake" us, or hold us up against gravity. Preventing nonspecific backache is a simple matter of getting strong and flexible. You have to get moving.

Your Lower Back

This notorious problem area, which runs from right below your lowest rib all the way to the top of your pelvis, is called the lumbar spine and is where strains most often cause pain.

The lumbar spine is made up of five vertebrae. The medical shorthand for this is L1 through L5, meaning lumbar vertebra number 1 through lumbar vertebra number 5.

The lumbar vertebrae bear much of your weight and take most of the stress of movement. They are the largest and flattest of all the vertebrae, but that doesn't always protect them from injury, fatigue, and imbalance.

Typical concerns: When we see a client with one hip hiked up, we know that the lumbar spine is involved. As long as the pelvis is level and everything is working well, the body can move easily to the side. But when the body has a tight psoas—the primary hip flexor that helps us stand erect, which originates from L1 to L5, passes through the pelvis, and attaches to the femur (thighbone)—it pulls the pelvis forward and down, so the other erector muscles must struggle to compensate. When they tighten and fatigue, they can hike one hip up. The result is pain and fatigue caused by muscles trying to take up the slack and make up for immobility.

Interesting fact: We're born with shortened psoas and quadriceps to hold us in the fetal position. Crawling is our first attempt to elongate these two muscles so that we can stand erect. When you learned to stand and walk, you were successful at elongating them, but both muscles have a tendency to attempt to return to this shortening. Lumbar spine pain and imbalance are clear warnings that you have work to do.

The most common complaint we hear is lower-back pain. It comes in all shapes and sizes: dull or sharp, chronic or intermittent. A confluence of muscles and connective tissue forms a band across your back just over your hipbone. When the lower back is injured or the muscles tighten, it causes pain, weakness, and dysfunction. We attack this problem from the back *and* the front. Not only do we restore range of motion and strength to stabilize the lumbar spine, but we work on the abdominal muscles that support the back. If you suffer from lower-back pain and your physician has ruled out injury, disease, or dysfunction that must be medically treated, then getting fit can eliminate lower-back pain.

Your Sacrum

The sacrum is where your spine joins your pelvis down to your tailbone. This set of wide bones forms a sort of solid inverted triangle. Made up of five fused vertebrae, the sacral spine's medical shorthand is S1 through S5.

Typical concerns: Because the sacrum is fused, it's rarely the source of problems, but occasionally we see people with piriformis syndrome. This is an acute inflammation of the sciatic nerve, a nerve that is actually woven through the bands of the inner fibers of the gluteal muscles—the muscles that run from the sacral spine through the buttocks. When the buttocks are bruised or weakened from sitting, the hip rotators beneath them can swell or spasm to compress that sciatic nerve. The result is a pain that shoots down the sacrum, through the buttocks, and into the back of the leg. Releasing the nerve is a matter of relaxing the stranglehold of the muscles with Active-Isolated Stretching.

Your Coccyx

Pronounced "COX-six," this is your tailbone. If the sacrum is an inverted triangle, the coccyx forms the point at the bottom.

The coccyx is made up of four vertebrae. No medical shorthand exists for the individual bones, because the coccyx encases no spinal cord and is generally thought of as one unit. If you break your tailbone, it doesn't matter which of the bones broke. You only know you landed on it, it hurts like the dickens, and there's no way to put it in a cast.

Typical concerns: Because the coccyx is a relatively simple structure, the only injuries we ever see are bruising and fracturing. The coccyx completes the spine and certainly contributes to the shape of the body, but it is insignificant in terms of muscles and connective tissue that could be injured and cause dysfunction in related structures. When the coccyx is bruised or fractured, we merely advise our clients to protect it with padding on seats and to exercise extra care and attention to activities that might further injure the bones. Ice and painkillers are the only other things that might help.

Your Vertebrae

Each vertebra is shaped in a different way so that when they're stacked together, they interlock like 3-D puzzle pieces to protect the delicate spinal cord that runs up through their open centers. The interlocking positions must be perfect so that the spine can move but the cord is kept safe and secure without disruptions. The whole spine is held together by ligaments that allow the spine to bend and twist in a perfect balance of strength and mobility.

Although each vertebra is different, they all have a few things in common. Each is a rounded body with a hole in the center called a foramen, through which the spinal cord runs. Most have bony processes coming off them—one at the rear and one on each side—that look a little like wings and act as a type of brakes that stop the spine from moving too far backward or too far to each side. Going too far would impinge or damage the spinal cord, so nature has designed this physical limit for each vertebra.

SIDE VIEW OF VERTEBRAE

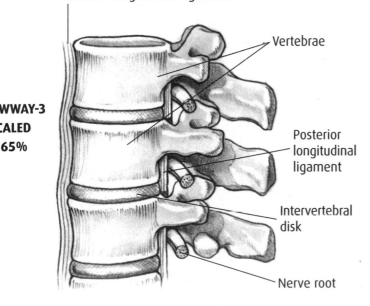

Anterior longitudinal ligament

Vertebrae

Posterior longitudinal ligament

Intervertebral disk

Nerve root

NEWWAY-3
SCALED
165%

Your Disks

In between each vertebra is a type of joint called a facet. Within each facet is an intervertebral disk, a sort of cushion that allows movement without rubbing the bones against each other.

Disks are like jelly doughnuts, crispy on the outside and soft on the inside. With a fibrous outer lining and a gelatinous inner core, these disks act as spinal shock absorbers and account for about 20 percent of the height of the spine.

Sometimes a disk can be injured or ruptured. Because the disk itself has few nerves and no blood supply of its own, it has no way to repair itself. When the disk is injured, a cascade of horrors can be set into motion, making life miserable. Vertebrae rub together. Nerves can be pinched or inflamed by leaking inflammatory proteins, sending pain shooting all over the place and disrupting normal function in muscles and organs. Even though the disk itself can't feel pain, inflammation and pain can be rampant nearly everywhere else.

Disks get hammered every day. Subject to this wear and tear, they're the first to succumb to a lifetime of work and the first to show signs of aging. At birth, the disks are 80 percent water, but as life goes on, they dehydrate and deteriorate, becoming less supple. Some of the jelly in our doughnuts dries out. For this reason, people get shorter as they age, and less supple. The good news is that as we age, there are fewer inflammatory proteins in the disks, so disk pain becomes pretty rare after age 60.

Your Nerves and Nerve Roots

Running through the center of the spinal column is the spinal cord, starting at your brain and ending at the bottom of your lumbar spine in a bundle of nerves that looks a little like a horse's tail. For this reason, it's called the cauda equina (Latin for "horse's tail").

These nerves are responsible for your leg muscle function, your ability to feel sensation all the way down to your toes, and your bladder, intestinal, and genital function. That's why an injury in your lumbar region will radiate pain through your butt to your legs. In severe injury, physicians will even look at disruption in the bladder, intestines, and bowels as clues to locate the injury and determine its severity.

At each disk from the cauda equina up, a pair of nerve roots branch off from the spinal cord through a little opening in the vertebrae. These nerves transmit information from the brain through the spinal cord and out to the body and back again.

STABILITY IS A MATTER OF STRENGTH AND FLEXIBILITY

The spine is a dynamic system designed to move. If it were meant to be completely stable, it would be a solid column of one thick bone with a hole bored through it for your spinal column. But that's not the way it works. Stability means that the spine lets you move the way you're supposed to and stops you from moving the way you shouldn't.

When you straighten your spine and stand fully erect, your back muscles are not the only ones involved. You are also contracting opposing muscles at the same time: the abdominals and the erector spinae, which runs up and down the spine. These oppositional forces balance each other and give you extra support. If you stand up and tighten up, front and back, you will notice how your back is rigid and erect.

Muscles are pivotal in holding everything together and are attached to every segmental level. The stronger the muscle, the better the support. Even muscles some distance from the spine itself can affect stability. For example, abdominal muscles are pivotal in holding the spine in place, although they're nowhere near it. But since they are attached to the sternum, the rib cage, and the pelvis, contracting the abdominals results in flexion, or lateral bending, of the spine.

Keeping your spine and back in good working order isn't magic—it's smart planning. It's focused, efficient training. It's about enjoying the benefits of being an athlete rather than the miseries of a patient. If you follow our program, you will become:

- **Lean,** so your spine doesn't have to support and balance excess pounds.
- **Flexible,** so your spine can move within full range of motion and keep blood flowing and muscles firing properly.
- **Strong** throughout your entire body, so your spine can handle the loads you put on it in bending forward, backward, and sideways, in rotation, and in combination of all of these.
- **Balanced** throughout your body, so your back isn't called upon to compensate for weakened or shortened muscles.
- **Healthy,** so disease and deficiencies will not weaken your bones or impede you from activity.
- **Cardiovascularly strong,** so endurance is not a problem, and you can oxygenate your blood and maximize your body's ability to remove metabolic waste.
- **Smart,** so you'll avoid putting yourself and your back into situations where it can become stressed, overly fatigued, or injured.

Too many people suffer needlessly. Don't be one of them.

Although some back problems result from accident, disease, or congenital deformity and will require medical intervention and surgery, *most* back problems are entirely preventable. Some back injuries start out small but eventually get out of hand until they, too, will require medical intervention and surgery. And *most* of these are entirely preventable.

What we're telling you is that back pain might not be your fate. And surgery might not be your future.

It's up to you. You're in control. Make that leap. Stop thinking of yourself as a patient with a back problem—and start thinking of yourself as one of our athletes in training. You have the opportunity to correct a problem and get out of pain and, in doing so, become stronger, more flexible, and more fit than you thought possible.

THE PAIN-FREE BACK

Trust us—we've seen it happen with our clients, hundreds of times. Join us and become more flexible, vital, and pain-free than you've ever dreamed possible.

BEFORE YOU BEGIN

Before you begin our program, make sure that your physician says it's all right. In fact, please take this book to him or her to get the green light. Even if you've been under care for a while, you might be surprised at the encouragement you'll get. Long ago, back pain meant bed rest, but recent studies have shown that bed rest isn't the right answer for most back problems. In fact, it can make things worse. Moving is the order of the day, especially if the movement is Active-Isolated Stretching and Strengthening.

We have designed a personal workout program that will give you real results in your first session. You'll feel better immediately, and you'll feel progressively stronger and more flexible and have less pain for the duration of the 18 weeks of the program and beyond.

The Active-Isolated Stretching and Strengthening program contains three components of a comprehensive workout.

- Active-Isolated Stretching
- Active-Isolated Strengthening
- Cardio Training

We'll begin with Active-Isolated Stretching. When we're working with new clients, we always compare Active-Isolated Stretching to the process of busting up a logjam: Loggers move one log in the river and then another, and, pretty soon, things just start to flow. Active-Isolated Stretching is very quick and gentle, so rather than strain an injured back, it relaxes it while it restores range of motion and gets things moving again. That's how we'll start off.

When you're ready, we'll introduce Active-Isolated Strengthening, so you can slowly and gently become stronger and stronger.

And then when your body is really functioning, we'll introduce you to cardio training—primarily walking—to get your heart pumping and increase your endurance.

You'll go at your own pace. We will coach you through each exercise individually and then teach you to put them all together into three 6-week cycles that will take you from "beginner" to "advanced." Once you have mastered the exercises, you'll have them combined into a routine blocked on one simple page for quick reference. You can work out without flipping pages. (We'll go into more detail in chapter 4, where you'll find your workout and the log you'll keep to track your progress.)

You tailor the workout to your personal goals. It costs nearly nothing. There's really no special equipment required other than a stretch rope and a set of ankle weights. There's no special clothing except a pair of comfortable shoes to walk in (and surely you already own a pair!). It's easy, fast, and fun.

Are you ready, athlete? Prepare to be amazed by how quickly, easily, and comfortably you can completely rejuvenate your back, your body, and your health.

YOUR BODY IS READY
AND WILLING TO GET WELL

We work with athletes every day, and we never cease to be stunned and touched by the miracle of the human body. It works hard—through a series of nearly heroic compensations—to overcome every abuse and neglect. And through it all, your body is constantly trying to bring itself back to healing and to perfect function and form. Fortunately, your body is forgiving of mistakes and responds dramatically, even gratefully, to training. That's the good news. The great news is that it's never too late to put exercise into your life or to fine-tune an already good training program.

Chapter 2

POSTURE AND PRESSURES
ALL THE WAY DOWN YOUR SPINE

We always tell our clients that, while the rest of the body's parts may be on call, the back is always on duty. Always.

Unlike the bodies of most other mammals, the human body was designed to stand upright, with the hands and arms free and the face oriented toward the front. In fact, almost all of our movement—from our sight to the reach of our arms to the way our knees and hips bend to propel us forward—is directed to the front of our bodies.

With all this forward movement, we need a stabilizing force to keep us from falling on our faces. The back's job is to hold us upright and throw the brakes on to keep us from wiping out. You might assume that such a stabilizing system of bone and muscle would be tight and rigid—but it is quite fluid. Starting at the pelvis, the spine is continually adjusting, moving, stabilizing, and balancing against gravity so that we can move in an astonishing assortment of ways. Mastering the best ways to protect your posture from unnecessary pressure will help you make the most of this vibrant system for the long haul.

SITTING, STANDING, WALKING

Since the dawn of time, mothers have chanted a universal mantra, "Stand up straight!" They couldn't be more *wrong*. In fact, straight is not the point. Being flexible and strong is the point. The spine is dynamic and always in motion, facilitating the countless positions and movements we're capable of.

Gordon Gow is a Canadian kinesiologist who builds the weight equipment we use with our clients all over the world. One evening, when we were discussing spinal dynamics, he introduced us to a simple yet graphic representation of the spine, which showed how it works in relation to posture. He balanced a broomstick by placing the end of the handle in his palm with the bristle end in the air. As it swayed from side to side and threatened to topple, he moved his palm swiftly from side to side to keep it in balance. He explained that this is the way a spine works in concert with the pelvis. The palm represents the pelvis—free-floating and serving as a sort of gyroscope for maintaining equilibrium—and the broomstick represents the spine.

In the early 1900s, physiologists set the standard for good posture by describing an alignment that was optimal for anatomical function. And, frankly, they did a pretty good job. Human bodies have not changed much in the last 100 years—but, my, how we use them has. We have gone from a society of standing, walking, dirt-digging, corn-harvesting, butter-churning, stickball-playing, washboard-scrubbing people to a group of office-dwelling, car-driving, keyboard-tapping, television-watching sitters. And we pay a heavy toll for all this inactivity in terms of dysfunction and pain.

It doesn't have to be that way. We are certainly capable of managing our bodies as nature designed them. But first, we have to know what nature had in mind.

When you stand in perfect alignment with perfect posture, your earlobes line up directly over your shoulders. Your shoulders line up directly over the points where your femurs (thighbones) connect to your pelvis. Those points on your pelvis line up directly over the midpoints between the fronts and backs of your knees. And your knees line up directly over your anklebones.

Few people have perfect posture. The good news is that minor postural anomalies are not necessarily associated with pain and dysfunction. The older we get, however, the more likely they are to become problematic to some degree.

SLUFF OFF THAT SLOUCH

Slouching is standing or sitting with a rounded upper back, a chest that caves in, and shoulders that are rolled forward. Nearly everything we do requires that we face forward, reach forward, bend forward, and move forward. When combined with gravity, these activities make slouching seem like the natural result of a life lived in front of you.

When the muscles in the back of your upper body are weaker than those in the front, you can't help slouching. Remember, muscles work in opposition to each other. One flexes while the other extends. One contracts while the other relaxes. So when the muscles in your back (rhomboids and trapezius) are weak, the muscles in the front overwork and develop more strongly. They pull you forward because your back isn't strong enough to hold you back.

When you're slouched, you force neck muscles to overwork to hold your face up. And you compress internal organs, including your lungs. You are not able to draw a full breath if your chest is compressed. If your slouch is pronounced, you can develop a hunchback—not good at all.

We make you this promise: If you'll do the flexibility and strengthening exercises we've outlined for you in chapter 4, you'll balance the strength and flexibility of the important muscles that hold you upright against the strength of those that pull you forward. Also, once you've done the test in "How Do You Line Up?" on page 18 and you know what your trouble spots are, we would ask you to make a conscious effort to align your spine as you stand until you get used to the fun and ease of moving properly.

SITTING PRETTY

When most of us sit, we tend to sort of settle into a puddle. If the chair has a back, all the better. We lean back and in and curl up into relaxation. We roll our shoulders forward, stressing the upper back and caving in our chest muscles. This posture might feel fine for a little while, but if you're in for the long haul, you're in trouble.

Let's start with a refresher course in gravity, the force of pull from "out there" straight to the center of the earth. Gravity is constant, anchoring you to the ground, from straight up to straight down. When you're standing, the forces of gravity run through the top of your head and are absorbed and dissipated through your hips, knees, ankles, and feet. But when you're sitting in perfect posture, those same forces run through the top of your head and are stopped at your butt, absorbed directly by your lower back and sacrum. That can be pretty tough on the body, but it gets worse. When you curl up or swing your leg over the arm of the chair, then the body part that absorbs that same force of gravity will change, placing an odd strain on your back as it fights to keep you in balance.

Notice how you are sitting right now. Imagine

gravity as a force in a line from "out there" straight to the center of the earth. If your spine isn't in alignment with your butt, where are the forces exerting themselves and which muscles in your back must compensate to hold you up in balance? Isn't it an amazing coincidence that these same muscles are the ones that always seem to be fatigued and strained?

Short of moving to the International Space Station, we can do nothing about the force of gravity—it's inevitable. When we're sitting, we are confining our bodies to small spaces. For the best result, sit with your fanny planted evenly on the seat. Put your feet flat on the floor, with your knees bent at 90-degree angles. We're designed to sit this way, but we weren't designed to sit as long as most of us do now.

To maintain a seated posture, it's necessary to get that gravitational pressure relieved from time to time so that your back can rest. We encourage squirming and shifting in your seat. But better than this, you should take short, frequent breaks—say one every hour.

All you have to do is stand up and move a little. Take a few deep breaths and imagine that you have a helium balloon lifting your head off your shoulders. Tighten your abdominals and elongate your spine from the base of your sacrum all the way up. We call this "resetting." Think of the compression on your spine that's caused by sitting as being a logjam. If you can move even one little log, you can get things moving. Every small thing helps. Move and reset. And plan to do it again in an hour.

STANDING TALL

For many with back pain, everything feels better and more relaxed when they're standing with body weight distributed and their spines in alignment. But no one starts out standing—standing is a matter of lifting your body upright from another position, and this can be problematic. Just as we would coach an athlete to move from one position to another efficiently and powerfully, we're going to tell you how to manage these transitions safely so that you can spare your back and avoid injury.

Rolling out of bed: Lie on your back and tighten your abdominals. Roll to one side and push yourself up using your elbow, while at the same time pushing down with your opposite hand. Pivoting at the hip, drop your feet over the edge of the bed; your feet act as counterweights. Scoot your hips to the edge. Look around and get oriented. Keeping your feet spaced under your hips, put one foot in front of the other. Put your hands on the bed. Contract the abdominals. Push up with your hands until your back knee is locked. Now you're standing.

Getting up off the floor: If you're on the floor, roll over to the crawl position. Then rise up to your knees. Rock your buttocks back toward your heels. Bring up one knee until your foot is flat on the floor.

Put the toes of your back foot on the floor. Put your hand on the same side, on your knee. Put the other hand on the floor. Rock back a little more and find your balance until you can rise. Use your hands for support and lift with your glutes. Now you're standing.

Rising from your chair: Keeping your feet spaced under your hips, put one foot in front of the other. Put your hands on the seat beside your hips or on the arms of the chair. Flex your trunk forward slightly. Contract the abdominals. Push up with your hands and glutes until your back knee is locked. Now you're standing.

Getting out of your car: Open the door, pivot on your buttocks until you're facing sideways, and swing your feet out of the car. Reach over your head with one hand and hold the door frame to pull yourself forward. Reach down with your other hand and place it firmly on the seat to push off. Now you're standing.

WALKING UPRIGHT

Like all of us, you *think* you know how to walk. You've been walking since you were a toddler. Like many things you learned when you were in diapers, however, you probably missed some of the finer points.

Take a Load Off Your Back

All postures and body positions place different loads on the lumbar spine, which has to support the pressure of the forces. If you're looking to get the load off your back, consider these positions. They're listed from the least amount of pressure to the most.

- Lying flat on your back
- Lying on your side
- Standing and relaxed

- Sitting in a chair
- Standing and bending forward from the hips
- Sitting in a chair and bending forward from the hips
- Standing and bending forward from the hips while bearing weight
- Sitting in a chair and bending forward from the hips while bearing weight (astonishingly, up to 300 times the pressure of lying flat on your back!)

One evening we got into a debate with a running coach about the choreography of simple walking in prelude to the running gait. She argued rather credibly that walking is nothing more than catching yourself from falling in a series of self-rescues that move you forward. She theorized that a walker leans forward in the direction she wants to go, and, at the point of imbalance, she has two choices: either fall on her face or thrust one leg forward and catch herself. Once she's on that outthrust leg, she passes her torso over the top of it and then faces the choices again: flat on her face or throw her other leg out there.

She made the point by grabbing Jim by the front of his T-shirt and pulling him forward. "Make a choice!" she challenged. Always interested in exploring anatomical nuances, Jim toppled forward and then at the last minute caught himself by doing exactly what she thought he would do. He thrust his leg out and caught himself. Our coach friend grinned in triumph and continued to pull him forward. "Make a choice!" she repeated. Jim saved himself again from bodily harm by taking another imposed step. Before he knew it, he was halfway across the floor, step by step, with the front of his stretched-out T-shirt clenched in the fist of our smug friend. This was walking as she had observed it—and basically as most people do it. But it's not right.

Walking is not so much a matter of constantly losing and regaining equilibrium, of pulling yourself forward through space by catching yourself over each leg, but more a function of being pushed. That push comes primarily from your butt (gluteal muscles).

Before you teach yourself the correct way to walk, take a few steps as you normally would so that you'll remember how it felt. Now, the next step you take will open a whole new world of power and balance, because we're going to teach you to walk properly. Here's how walking should work.

1. Stand with your left foot forward. Contract your abdominals, and clench your right glute to lift your pelvis slightly forward and up.

2. Your left arm, the opposite to the walking leg, swings to mirror the move to balance you and help you move forward.

3. The hip flexors—the muscles that lift your thigh slightly to elevate and swing your leg—finish what the glute starts.

4. Your calf will help by working with your hamstrings to extend your knee and propel you forward.

5. You have just passed your torso and center of gravity over your supporting leg.

6. Your right foot should now hit the ground at midfoot, not at your heel.

7. Your arch will flatten slightly under the weight, but it is designed to spring back into shape to cushion the impact and give your step a little momentum as your ankle muscles stabilize your foot.

8. The forces of impact from that step translate right up into your knee.

9. Your knee doesn't spring, but it absorbs shock through muscles in the inner and outer thigh all the way to the hip.

Your right step is complete. At this moment, engage your left glute to lift your pelvis slightly forward and up, and start the next step with your left leg.

The point we're trying to make is that this walking gait is distinctively different from what we have traditionally thought biomechanically efficient. The power in this gait, for both walking and running, is in your butt. By pushing from behind with your glute, rather than drawing forward by raising your thigh from your hip flexors and extending your knee to get your foot out before you fall on your face, you're aiding your natural postural alignment and keeping the strain off your back.

By the way, our running coach friend didn't take long to figure out why our runners were beating hers. We had switched the power source and dominated the field. Of course, now that she knows this, her runners are fast catching up to ours. Darn.

SQUATTING FOR REST

As we've already told you, one of the reasons that our backs are stressed is that we humans sit too much. The forces that translate down our spines and through our buttocks when they're planted in chairs are enormous. We sit to rest, but sitting can tire our backs even more, compressing vertebrae, fatiguing muscles, and straining connective tissues.

We were designed to rest and relax from standing long before chairs were invented. Though you wouldn't know it in this country, we were designed to squat for rest. In fact, when we're working in Japan and Kenya, we observe a lot of people at rest by squatting, and we're happy to join them. Squatting relaxes your posture and elongates your spine like little else. For this reason, squatting is also a wonderful way to test how functionally flexible your back is. Only the flexible and fit can squat comfortably.

It's probably been a long time since you've tried to squat, so it will likely take a little practice, particularly if you're inflexible or carrying a few extra pounds. Squat only if you have healthy knees, because squatting requires them to support your weight on the way down and puts them into complete flexion while you're down, which can lead to strain. Also, what goes down must come up, so you also have to be strong enough to make that happen. There's nothing more depressing than getting into an impressive squat and then having to roll over onto the floor before you can wench yourself up.

Try it for a minute or two initially, to see how adept you are at straightening up. As you get stronger legs, you'll be able to stay down longer, but don't push it at first. If you start the squat and things don't seem to be going well—either you feel weak or something hurts—quit immediately and get yourself back up. But presuming all is going well, this is what a good squat looks like.

1. Stand with your feet shoulder-width apart. Bend your knees and flex your trunk forward.
2. Put your hands out in front of you and lean forward.
3. Keep bending your knees until your hands touch the ground.
4. Continue to bend your knees as you lower your buttocks toward the floor.
5. You're all the way down when the backs of your thighs and the backs of your calves touch. Once you've mastered this position, your heels should be flat on the floor.
6. Hold your arms forward to counterbalance.

We call this the "complete collapse" phase. In other places in the world, people happily maintain the squat for long periods of time, but in our Western culture, we are accustomed to sitting in chairs and have abandoned one of the really great postures. In our clinic, we use it to test function in the back and to quickly stretch out. It's fun if you're in shape.

Squatting isn't for everyone, particularly if you're out of practice, but if you are able, we encourage you to join many cultures in the world and rediscover resting your back the way nature intended it to be. If you can master the squat, you'll have yourself a wonderful way to rest. Your spine will elongate, and your back muscles will relax.

Chapter 3

TRACING PAIN'S MYSTICAL LINKS

The late astronomer Carl Sagan said, "We are all made of star stuff." We think he's right—especially when we're talking about the back.

Each one of us is a universe, a perfectly calibrated, interwoven system. These bodies of ours are always thinking, even on the cellular level. Yet, when we feel pain, we usually point to the specific location of the pain and say, "Here it is. This is the injury." But that exact spot may not necessarily indicate where the injury really originated.

An injury or an imbalance in one place can trigger pain or discomfort someplace else entirely. Why? Because in this integrated organism, all parts work together, and every part is related to every other part. When we focus on one aspect, such as a "contained" pain, we're forgetting that each of us is a whole system, perfect and miraculous, and that if one part of the system is disrupted, compressed, or stressed, it affects everything else in the body.

Your body is only as strong and healthy as the weakest link in your system. It's constantly fighting against weakness to help you achieve perfection (or as close as you can get). Muscles recruit other muscles to compensate and counterbalance, whether you're moving or not. This shifting and balancing can create a whole litany of other complaints, which can camouflage the origins of back pain. Because the origins can be so elusive, back pain can seem a touch more mysterious than other injuries and aches, but there's usually a very simple answer. Solving the mystery just takes a little detective work.

LABELING THE PAIN

Whether you've had it for a long time or it suddenly strikes you, back pain can be specifically pinpointed or be so general and widespread that you can't spot the exact site. Sometimes you can move a certain way, and it disappears altogether. When you move another way, it shoots all over again. A back problem can even cause pain somewhere else in the body.

One type of back pain, radicular pain, is a deep, steady pain that radiates from the spine and can run all the way to your foot. Sometimes it's accompanied by weakness, loss of function, tingling, or numbness. Radicular pain usually results from inflammation of a spinal nerve root.

Referred pain is a dull ache that tends to travel around and is maddeningly inconsistent. Sometimes it hurts badly; sometimes it's not that bad. Referred pain starts in your lower back and radiates into the groin, buttocks, and thighs.

The reason pain travels to and from your spine is

CASE STUDY: JILL NICKLAUS

When we met Jill, she was a principal dancer in the then-longest-running play on Broadway, *Cats*. She sometimes did two arduous, high-energy performances a day. She came to us with terrible back pain. Like most professional dancers, Jill is hypermobile—meaning that she's as flexible as a rubber band. And she's strong in all the muscles she uses to dance. But that's not all of them. Her quads, glutes, and abductors (outer thighs) were extremely tight and compromised. All the lateral muscles in her hip and trunk were contracted and tight. Her lower abs and inner and outer thighs were extremely strong, but her lower back was weak. Over time Jill had developed a series of compensations that had shorted her out. The other problem is that the stage on which she performed was raked—meaning, slanted toward the audience. Dancing day after day on an uneven surface had thrown one side of her body out of balance.

How Jill Got Out of Pain: In Jill's case, flexibility was less the issue than strength. Getting her out of pain was a matter of working fast to keep her on stage and giving her very light, small strengthening exercises to bring her back muscles up to par with her legs. We worked on glutes, lower abs, and abductors (to put them into balance with her adductors). We did modified leg raises, using a pillow to take the strain off her back. We worked on her neck for flexibility but emphasized strength for her upper back—trapezius and rhomboid muscles. We stabilized her from all angles.

We trained her personal therapist to work with her three times a week with Active-Isolated Strengthening and Stretching. Her back let go. She was pain-free, strong, and balanced within 4 weeks. Like any smart athlete, Jill realized that pain had been her friend. It had given her ample warning that she needed to balance muscles to become a better dancer. A cat might have nine lives, but a Broadway dancer has only one. Jill made sure she could enjoy hers.

---

that your spinal column is the conduit through which all messages are sent from the brain to the body and from the body to the brain. The area is rich in nerves and is linked everywhere, which makes it an excellent communications center. Too bad some of the messages are really bad news.

PAIN COULD BE A BLOCK IN YOUR ENERGY

We don't want to get all mystical on you, but even the most skeptical among us will admit that there's more to the universe than we can see. We think so, and, if we hadn't before, our experiences with our clients would have certainly changed our mindset. And we doubt that we're alone.

Several years ago, the Dalai Lama's personal physician was invited to a prestigious hospital here in New York City to diagnose a patient. This Tibetan physician was offered the use of the finest imaging and diagnostic equipment in the world. Every lab test was at his fingertips. He politely declined and quietly approached the bedside. He examined the patient with *his* tools: his hands.

The doctor scanned and checked pulses—triggers of energy that run through meridians, which are channels of energy, or "chi" (life force), just below the skin surface. This procedure is standard in Chinese medicine and is used here in the United States by practitioners of acupuncture. An experienced physician or practitioner can detect blockages in energy and relate them directly to the source of injury or imbalance.

The Tibetan physician worked for a few minutes and then gave his medical opinion—which turned out to be identical to the diagnosis determined earlier by New York physicians with equipment and lab work. If the patient had been under the Tibetan physician's care, the doctor would have unblocked the energy with acupuncture, by inserting small needles to stimulate the point of block called the gateway. Or he simply might have applied stimulating pressure with his hand. Either way, these methods have been practiced for thousands of years, and they seem to work. And with all the medical mysteries that still remain, who are we to say it doesn't?

PAIN CAN ALSO BE EMOTIONAL

We know that pain is largely a matter of perception, so as long as most of it has to do with judgment, it stands to reason that pain can not only be affected by thoughts and feelings but also be *caused* by thoughts and feelings. The human mind is capable of producing extreme pain. How many times have you flinched when getting an injection, and the needle was still behind the back of the smirking nurse?

We don't understand how, but we know this to be true: The body remembers pain, fear, and sorrow, and stores them. On an obvious level, you can observe this yourself. Walk into a restaurant and watch people for a few minutes. Without effort, you'll be able to pick out those people who are sad or afraid or are in some sort of pain. When we do deep-muscle massage or happen to agitate certain trigger points in a client, we sometimes accidentally unlock a muscle memory, where the body is storing emotion. It is not uncommon for the client to break the peaceful silence and comfort of a massage with an outburst of uncontrollable weeping.

Many is the time that we've had to stop and comfort. And although we are not qualified counselors, we are the solitary witnesses to the body's release of a long-forgotten hurt, so we take the time to draw our clients into conversation. What just happened? What did you remember? What has caused you this much pain? Inevitably, the story is one of an incident so horrific that the mind suppressed it—or hid it somewhere in the body. When we release it, it doesn't go away, but it's better.

Such a trigger point in your back could be causing you to tense up and experience pain. Or maybe it's not one of these hidden memories, but, rather, carrying the figurative weight of the world on your shoulders has turned into literal slouching, slumping, and hurting.

Getting to the bottom of emotional pain or disruptions in your energy are, no doubt, very worthy endeavors. But short of getting you on our table or into the hands of a Tibetan physician, we really can't help you there. What we can do is help you connect the dots behind your own pain, narrow down where it's coming from, and help you chart a course for a new universe of pain-free living.

READING THE BODY'S MAP

If you're suffering generalized back pain, you have to find the source of the pain before you can correct it. Surprisingly, the source of generalized back pain is seldom in the back. But where do you start looking for clues to the source?

The body is a unique flowchart, a sort of intricate spiderweb of connected systems. As we have explained, all muscles work in pairs, and the pairs work in teams to get you to move. When one muscle shorts out, it creates a point of tension and fatigue somewhere beyond itself. First, its companion muscle will strain. And when the pair is not doing its job, other muscles struggle to compensate. Eventually, a second short-out and a second compensation occur, setting off a chain reaction.

When we see unexplained pain or an overuse injury in the body, we start tracing it backward to look for clues to the source of the problem. We ask, "Why did this happen? What weak link in the chain caused this to short out?" Very little is ever as it appears to be.

Really nailing down the origin of a back injury is important for a number of reasons. Soothing an injury is not enough if the source of the problem—the weak link—is not treated and corrected, because that weak link will continue to cause trouble and pain. Massages

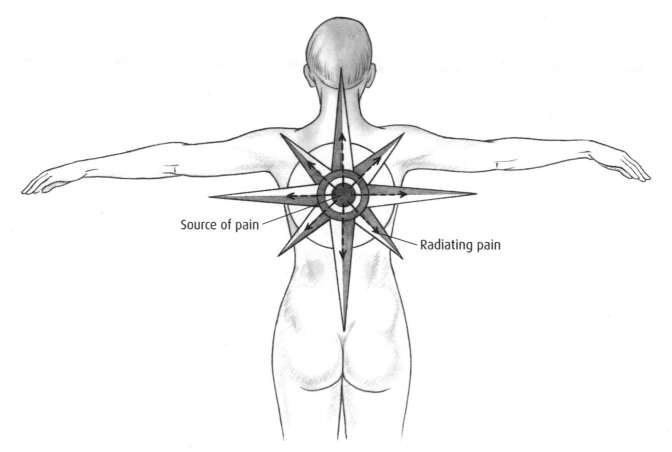

Source of pain

Radiating pain

and chiropractic adjustments can provide your back some relief, but the relief might not last long. Treating the problem without correcting the cause is a surefire guarantee that you'll be back in pain shortly.

When we are tracing an injury to its source, we put a mental dot on the source of pain and imagine lines radiating out from this point, from north to south and from east to west. Then we fill in northwest, southwest, northeast, and southeast. The result is an imaginary star-shaped compass with its center on the injury.

From a back injury, most of the weak links are to the south, most likely below the pelvis. If the pain is on the right, the weak links are probably on your left. If the pain is on the left, the weak links are probably on your right. In the case of the upper back, neck, and shoulders, their weak links are sometimes revealed when you look for clues to both the east and west.

Starting at the point of your back pain, test your

muscles and joints one at a time by isolating them and activating them with the simple exercises in this book. (See chapter 4.) Test how flexible and strong each area is individually. When you find a muscle that seems weaker than those surrounding it, or you have very little range of motion in one position, you might have the culprit.

Still, keep going. Keep testing down the line, moving on to the next set of muscles and the next joint. Often you'll find yourself going from the point of pain in your back, right through your buttocks, down your thigh, past your knee, through your ankle, and right to the bottom of your foot. It's important to keep going until you pass over the "last" weak muscle and inflexible joint in the line.

Once you've figured out exactly where your weak link is, make a point during your exercise sessions to focus on strengthening and unlocking from that point *up* to the injury in your back.

STANDING ON YOUR OWN WEAK LINKS: YOUR FEET

One of our favorite songs begins, "The foot bone's connected to the anklebone; the anklebone's connected to the shinbone; the shinbone's connected to the kneebone . . ." (You get the picture.) We sing this to our baffled clients who can't believe that a fallen arch can cause a back spasm.

When one of our clients comes in with back pain, we begin by whipping his shoes off. Why such interest in the foot when the back is in pain? Believe it or not, one of the biggest culprits in back pain is the flat foot. When the arch has "fallen" and rocked the ankle inward, the flat foot basically has ensured that the body will be unable to absorb shock.

The arch is the shock absorber that takes the weight and pressure from each footstrike and compresses to translate this vertical force into horizontal force, evenly distributed and gentle. When shock absorption is gone, it sets up a ripple effect that ends in the back. Let's watch.

1. Ideally, when your foot rolls forward through your step, the compressed arch springs back into position to give you a little push off for your next step. But when the arch is flattened, the ankle rolls to the inside.
2. Without the support of the ankle, the whole leg rotates toward the midline of the body. When the ankle and lower leg are rolled inward, the knee is thrown out of alignment. The stabilizer and cushion for the knee is the medial meniscus, a pad on the inside of the upper kneecap. Over time, strain from the imbalance imposed by the ankle compromises the medial meniscus.
3. Without full function of the medial meniscus, your knee loses its ability to stabilize and cushion, and the joint becomes stressed. Eventually, the pressure will blow out the anterior cruciate ligament, the attachment that holds the bones in your thigh to the bones in your shin through your knee.
4. As the knee is the juncture between your lower and upper leg, it's the joint responsible for moving the body forward. When the anterior cruciate ligament is compromised and becomes lax, pain, irritation, and weakness make a proper gait impossible.
5. As we move up the chain from the weak link, we see that if the knee can't create a proper gait, the hip muscles take over in a series of compensations. The quadriceps and hamstrings contract to protect the knee. But they're not designed to move the leg forward and do the knee's job. So they, too, become fatigued and weakened.
6. Continuing up the chain, when the quadriceps and hamstrings are compromised, the hip flexors take over to try and help lift the leg up from the thigh so that you can move forward.
7. Outer and inner thigh muscles struggle to stabilize the pelvis, which will have to rotate now to move that leg forward.
8. Underneath the glutes in the buttocks, six deep rotators, which are involved with internal and external rotation of the hip, finally fatigue and lose function.
9. If we go one step further up the chain, we find the lower back kicking in to stabilize the pelvis. And, suddenly, you guessed it—you have back pain.

(You know, just an aside, in reflexology and compression massage, the trigger point for the spine is in the foot. Coincidence, you think?)

Sometimes, the culprit isn't all the way down in the feet. You could have a weak muscle somewhere up the line—like quadriceps—that's causing the back pain. But the best way to start checking for weakness and imbalance is to track it through the chain, from the back downward.

HAS A WEAK LINK THROWN YOU OUT OF BALANCE?

Therapists and trainers often used to blame simple leg-length discrepancy for pain in the back. An athlete

Case Study: Wanda Panfil

Poland's Wanda Panfil was one of the greatest marathon runners in the world, and one of the nicest people. She has won the Boston Marathon, the New York City Marathon, and the World Championships. But marathon training and running are brutal, and Wanda had to balance on that fine line between "enough miles" and "too many miles." At one point in her career, she made the mistake of crossing that line. She developed chronic lower-back pain, not realizing that she was causing it by imbalances.

She kept treating the lower-back pain, but her lower-back pain was never the problem. She allowed the injury to evolve into a serious hip injury that shot straight to her back and became so severe that she was nearly shut down.

How Wanda Got Out Of Pain: She flew to New York, where we worked intensively for 3 days. Our clinic was packed with a group of therapists, trainers, and her coach and support staff. Everyone was there to assist us and to take care of Wanda.

We opened the session with a gentle flexibility work-out to assess her ranges of motion and spot the areas of inflexibility and tension. At the same time, we were able to slightly increase the range of motion of her joints and release tension. Then we started all over again, this time with gently increased intensity. As we were stretching an external hip rotator, we heard a loud "pop" in her hip joint. Startled, Wanda's handlers panicked, but the therapists and trainers grinned. With some translating and gesturing, we were able to explain that she had just released an adhesion—an area of a sort of "scar tissue" in muscles that had locked up her hip. Soft tissue that had been stuck was suddenly loose again. With the release of the adhesion, we were able to make real progress in stretching her entire body and rebalancing muscles that had been compensating for the adhesion.

We added strengthening to Wanda's program so that muscles that had become weakened with the injury could get strong enough to work properly. Her rehabilitation extended beyond those days in our clinic, but she felt better immediately and had the discipline and motivation to build on that small success.

was evaluated by lying flat on a table with an observer at the foot of the table. The observer took both of the athlete's feet in his hands, pressed the ankles together, eyeballed the soles of the feet, and finally declared, "You're out of whack. Your left anklebone is a full inch below your right one. Your left leg definitely is longer." Then the athlete would go out and get a 1-inch lift for the right shoe so that both legs could be even.

This apparent leg-length discrepancy probably was caused not by a leg bone that was longer, but by an imbalance in the muscles and tendons of the pelvis, the foundation of the body. And the source of this imbalance might surprise you. A tight hamstring at the back of one thigh can jack up the opposite side of the pelvis. A tight iliotibial band in the knee on one side could jack up the other side of the pelvis.

When the lower extremities are in balance and the pelvis is free-floating and flexible, the leg-length discrepancy may mysteriously disappear. All you have to do is follow the injury from your back to the source and correct the problems all the way down the line with stretching and strengthening.

If your back hurts and you suspect that the pain might be the result of a weak link somewhere down the line, remember that your pelvis is the foundation of the body. It's the fulcrum that connects and balances your lower extremities against your upper body and your back. If your back is in pain above the foundation, it's possible that the culprit is below, throwing your pelvis out of kilter and straining your back. The only way to find out is to check for imbalance. Here's how.

1. First, ask a friend to help you. It's important that you feel comfortable with her, because relaxation is a big part of this process.
2. Lie on your back on a flat surface with your legs together and have your partner press down with the palms of her hands on your hipbones, one hand on the left and one hand on the right.
3. Your partner should rock you back and forth, pressing left, right, left, right, until you are relaxed. It should take only a minute.
4. Now have your partner look down to see if your anklebones are even. (If they're not, you'll be tempted to think that you have a leg-length difference, but 8 or 9 times out of 10 it's from tight muscles in lower extremities that have unbalanced your pelvis, and jacked one leg up, causing it to appear to be shorter.)
5. Do a full Active-Isolated Stretching routine (see page 38), and repeat the exercise.

Now if your anklebones are even or closer, the good news is that you don't have a leg-length discrepancy. The bad news is that somewhere between your back and your feet, you have an imbalance caused by muscles and connective tissues that have been compromised, weakened, and tightened in their efforts to compensate. You now have a great opportunity to do some work to get that back out of pain.

PUTTING THE MAP TO WORK

Let's look at the experience of one of our clients, Gene Pressman. When we met Gene, he owned Barneys, a clothing-store chain based in New York City. He's a hard-charging, high-energy businessman. He decided that he wanted to run the New York City Marathon and came to us to help him put together a training program.

Since marathons are our passion, we were only too pleased to jump right in. We put him on a precise schedule. We worked with him in our clinic and sometimes in his gym at Barneys. We sometimes accompanied him on long runs in Rockefeller Park near his home in Westchester. A warm friendship developed. Gene worked hard, and it paid off. He competed in the marathon and did very well. We didn't see him for a while.

Then one day he phoned to say that his back shorted out. He was in exhausting pain. He wondered if we could take a look at it. In conversation in our clinic, Gene disclosed that he had suffered a knee injury in a skiing accident that had resulted in surgery but that his physician had not really stressed rehab much, so Gene went about his business, thinking everything was all right.

Bingo. His knee had been weakened and sore from surgery, so he favored the other leg. He limped. It didn't take much time for this imbalance to translate right up to his back.

Limping had weakened the muscles below the injured knee. In fact, the damage had gone all the way to his foot. The arch had given way from stress and could no longer absorb shock. So with each step, the shock was translating all the way up through his ankle to his knee.

In Gene's case, the fallen arch had fatigued and strained his ankle, and his ankle had further aggravated his knee, which had weakened his adductors, the muscles on the insides of his thighs. In fact, when we laid Gene on his side, his adductors were so weak that he couldn't lift his lower leg straight up to his upper leg. His abductors, the muscles on the outsides of his thighs, were so weak that he was unable to stabilize his pelvis.

And it got worse. Instead of using his glutes when he walked, he was using his hip flexors, muscles at the base of the torso that can lift the thighs straight up with each step but are not intended to

CASE STUDY: ART MONK

Art is a retired football player. Most of his long career was spent with the Washington Redskins. For more than 11 years, he held the record for most consecutive passes caught as a wide receiver in the NFL. Later he played with the New York Jets. We worked with him often and considered it a privilege. His stretch rope went with him, wherever he went. Since retiring, he's played on many all-star teams in exhibition games. He's a wonderful guy and still a great athlete.

While competing, Art came into the clinic complaining of back pain. When we examined him closely, we identified weak adductor muscles on the insides of his thighs. As a wide receiver who did strength training, Art was shocked when we isolated the muscles and asked him to lift a weight, using only those muscles, and he couldn't lift one-quarter of the weight he could heft in the Jets' training room with equipment.

There's a big difference between working out on a machine that allows you to recruit other muscles to get a lift done and working out an isolated muscle. We explained that when a muscle is weakened, other muscles are recruited to compensate. This compensation stemming from weakened muscles—his adductors—had fatigued other muscles that were constantly recruited, specifically those in his hips and pelvis. This was shorting out his back.

In the course of testing, we also determined that Art's lower abdominals were weak. (That's a difficult thing to tell a wide receiver.) Also, he wasn't as flexible as he should have been. Many of us equate flexibility with being noodlelike and tightness with being strong. But the problem is that muscles that are weakened and stressed tighten up. They present the illusion of being powerful, but aren't.

A muscle that can't elongate and contract fully can't be strengthened from end to end, because a bundle at the insertion points at either end will never be engaged. This vulnerable spot requires other muscles to be recruited to get the job done, causing more weakness and tightness. A vicious cycle, true even of Art Monk.

How Art Got Out Of Pain: We started Art with stretching, so we could get full range of motion and retrain his muscles to work from end to end without recruiting help from compensating muscles. When he was flexible, we added strength training, isolating and activating muscles one by one. We were able to strengthen the adductors and lower abdominals, balance the muscles, and voilà! His pelvis no longer had to compensate, and it stabilized. And his back stopped hurting.

Art accomplished this in a 3-week cycle. Fast results like Art's are possible because smaller muscles like the adductors and lower abdominals take less time to strengthen. A little time yields amazing results.

---

support walking exclusively. From the point of pain in his back, we could easily trace backward to the glutes, hip flexors, abductors, adductors, knee, lower leg, ankle, and arch. The knee started it. The limp aggravated it. The arch finished it. And the back felt it.

Gene's recovery started with three simple exercises to strengthen his ankles and arch. We're going to give them to you in detail here, because we'll mention them a couple of times later in case studies, and we want you to know what they are.

1. To strengthen his ankles, we put an ankle weight in the toe of a long tube sock and tied the sock around his ankle, threading the weighted end of the sock between his big toe and the toe next to it (like a flip-flop) and letting it dangle. He sat upright on the edge of one of our tables with the weight just above the floor. We put a rolled towel under his knee to take the strain off his kneecap. He extended his ankle and pointed his toes toward the floor. From this starting position, he brought his foot straight up, leading with his toes. The little weight provided resistance. He angled his foot to the inside and lifted in a sweep, leading with his toes. He lowered the weight to the starting position and then angled his foot to the outside and lifted in a sweep, leading with his toes. He did 10 on each side.

2. To strengthen his ankle evertors and invertors (the muscles that turn the ankle outward and inward), we simply laid him on his side and wrapped a single ankle weight around both of his feet under the arches and over the tops. He relaxed his feet and let them hang off the table. Then, without moving his legs, he lifted both feet from the ankles up toward the ceiling. He did 10 repetitions on each side.

3. To strengthen his arches, we put a towel on the floor, vertically in front of Gene, and had him sit in a chair at the edge of it. He worked with one foot at a time without moving his heel, contracting all his toes to bunch the towel up and draw the far edge toward him in a series of "grips." When he was finished, we straightened the towel out and placed it horizontally in front of him. He put his foot on it. He started with his little toe and, without moving his heel, contracted all his toes to bunch the towel up and sweep it toward the midline of his body in a series of 10 contractions. This strengthened his supinators, the muscles in the ankle that turn the forefoot inward. Finally, we straightened the towel and had him lead with his big toe and, without moving his heel, sweep the towel to the outside of his body. This strengthened his pronators, the muscles in the ankle that turn the forefoot outward.

For Gene, getting well was a matter of getting back to basics. In addition to these three small exercises, we reintroduced Gene to all the stretching and strengthening exercises you'll find in this book—the same ones he had used to train for a successful marathon. We put special emphasis on redeveloping his glutes to get them refiring. This instantly took stress off his back. We redeveloped the sacrospinalis, a band of muscles in the lower back at the top of the pelvis. We concentrated on his abdominals so that they would kick in to support his lower back.

The irritation in his back was so severe from compensation that we had to modify all the stretching and strengthening exercises. He worked out with very small movements, gently and lightly executed, and he used pillows to support his body and take the pressure off his joints.

Although he felt better after the first session, it took 6 weeks to get him fully well. Now he's free from back pain and back into a regular training program, but the moral of his story is that he is a solid athlete who got derailed by a deceptively small injury. By tracing back the mystical links, we were able to get him out on the trails again. The same detective methods can work for you.

Part 2

Try PREhab, Not Rehab

Chapter 4

THE WHARTONS' ACTIVE-ISOLATED PLAN FOR FLEXIBLE, STRONG, PAIN-FREE BACKS

We've spent a great deal of our careers repairing injured athletes. Unless the athletes' injuries are the result of accidents, they're usually the products of mistakes in training or performance. We consider the need for intense rehabilitation to be tragic—usually, the injury could have been prevented if the person had been better trained and prepared. Instead of doing rehab, we would much rather do PREhab—that is, help our athletes prepare properly so that injuries never happen.

These same principles can help you in everyday life. It's tough out there. You make extraordinary demands on your body every day. And you're going to live a long time, so your body has to adapt to your changing lifestyles and activities—and hold up through it all. You have to be prepared, just as a professional athlete has to be.

If you don't suffer from chronic back problems and never want to, you have added incentive. By doing our program, you'll get all the benefit of exercise—and the satisfying security of knowing that you've headed problems off at the pass. With PREhab, your fit, lean, and healthy body will have you living life more fully and powerfully than you thought possible.

If you do suffer from chronic back problems and your physician has ruled out disease, injury, and genetic anomalies, *re*hab may be in order. It may be time for you to take some action, literally. Get moving. Gone are the days when you'd be relegated to your bed for days on end. In fact, research tells us that bed rest for a bad back is bad advice—you'll probably get better faster if you move.

Maximum function in your back is, most often, a matter of being lean, flexible, strong, balanced, and healthy. With our program, you have the simple tools you need to achieve revolutionary results in less than 30 minutes a day. Trust us—this investment in yourself can pay huge dividends. Within days of beginning our program, our clients report feeling more energetic, having greater range of motion, and even experiencing relief from chronic pain. And now it's your turn—let's get started!

THE PRINCIPLES OF ACTIVE-ISOLATED TRAINING

The foundation of our programs is flexibility—specifically, Active-Isolated Stretching—and this is where we'll begin. It's impossible to overestimate the importance of being flexible. When your joints are able to move through their full ranges of motion, your body moves the way it was designed: completely, easily, painlessly, and efficiently. You may have forgotten the joy of living in such a body, but you're about to rediscover that freedom.

The principles of "Active-Isolated" are remarkably simple. As we've explained, muscles work in pairs of opposites. When one muscle lengthens, the opposite muscle shortens to make movement happen. If you want that one to lengthen or stretch, you have to relax it, but that muscle can't relax if it's working. That's where the *opposite* muscles come in. When you fire, engage, and activate those muscles, they shorten. Then, the muscles you intend to stretch are *relaxed* because they are isolated. As a result, they get stretched very efficiently and precisely.

Let's look at an example. Picture a runner preparing to do laps at the track. He throws his heel up on the bench, straightens his knee, bends over, takes hold of his ankle, and pulls himself "nose to toes." He can't quite get there because he's not warmed up yet, so he bounces, trying to go lower with every bounce.

You've seen it. You've probably even done it. Our runner was doing the hamstring stretch—or was he? With his leg up and his knee straight, his quadriceps (the muscle group in the front of his thigh) is totally relaxed. Those muscles are ready to be stretched. The hamstrings (the muscle group in the back of his thigh, opposing the relaxed quads) are activated and firing. In fact, they're tightening up to protect themselves from being overly stretched and ripped. And they're contracting to help our well-intentioned runner hold his body in balance as he teeters from his heel on the bench. From his upper back all the way down to his ankle, every muscle behind him is firing, tightening,

activating, protecting, recoiling, working. Not stretching. And most muscles in front of him are relaxed and ready for a stretch that will never happen.

So let's flip our thinking upside down and get this right. If you want to stretch the hamstrings, you have to relax them by firing the opposite muscles—the quads. This is Active-Isolated Stretching.

We have expanded the principles of Active-Isolated Stretching to Active-Isolated Strengthening exercises. The principles are identical, but the focus of your intention is opposite. In Active-Isolated Strengthening, when one muscle lengthens and stretches in relaxation, the opposite muscle shortens to make that movement possible. That shortened muscle is working and being *activated*. (If you add a weight, then it's lifting.) At the same time, the opposite, relaxing muscle is *isolated* and stretched.

A COMPLETE BACK PROGRAM

We have designed a program that will give you real results immediately. In contrast to other programs that can take weeks to see results, the benefits of these exercises start to kick in after your first session. From the first day, you'll understand why the deceptively simple principles of Active-Isolated Stretching and Strengthening have revolutionized the world of sports performance.

The program contains three components of a comprehensive workout.

- Active-Isolated Stretching
- Active-Isolated Strengthening
- Cardio Training

We will coach you through each exercise individually and then teach you to put them all together into three cycles, or phases, that will take you from "beginner" through "intermediate" to "advanced." The three cycles allow us to adjust workout patterns so that you can progress steadily and safely. You'll see results that will amaze you, especially when we start combining workout components for maximum benefit in minimum time.

The first component of the program is Active-

Isolated Stretching. In our program, you'll start as a beginner, no matter how fit you are. You'll determine your own starting point, depending on how tight your joints are when you start. Within one session, you'll feel your joints begin to unlock, allowing you a measure of freedom of movement within your body that you may not have felt in a long time. As your program progresses, you will improve significantly from the first workout, but at your own pace. You'll feel more relaxed as your joints move through their full ranges of motion the way they were intended. Your circulation will improve. You'll sleep better. You'll feel better.

Once we have you moving, we'll add some weight lifting with Active-Isolated Strengthening, to give your muscles strength and tone. You'll start with weights that feel right for you and advance when you're ready. You'll build the muscles that will support and protect your back from future pain and injury. Within a few sessions, you'll feel power and real energy kick in.

When you're strong and moving easily, we'll add a walking program to burn calories, boost your cardiovascular system, and give you back your stamina. At this point in the program, we consider you an "advanced" athlete, meaning that you've mastered the same tools that have helped dozens of Olympians keep their backs healthy and strong.

When to Throw the Brakes on a Workout

Athletes describe working out as "effort." No doubt about it, effort can be uncomfortable. You'll learn to live with that, and even like it. But there are signals that your workout must cease immediately and you need to take action without hesitation.

1. **Discomfort in any degree of severity in the upper body: chest, arms, neck, and jaw**
   The symptoms of a heart attack are described as an ache, burn, tightness, pressure, a sensation of fullness, or an overwhelming sense of unexplained dread. The sensations can be very subtle—don't dismiss them. Dial 911 for an ambulance, take an aspirin, and lie down immediately.

2. **Faintness, dizziness, light-headedness, or nausea**
   Feeling faint or light-headed is a signal that your brain isn't getting enough blood and oxygen. You have two immediate problems: You have to prevent blacking out and falling on your face, and you have to figure out what's happening. You don't have a lot of time—stop whatever you're doing and "go to ground." Lie down and get your feet higher than your head. Often, lying down will relieve the symptoms.

If you can't get recovered while lying down, dial 911. Even if the symptoms go away and you're able to go on with your day, tell your physician as soon as possible.

3. **Shortness of breath, effort, wheezing, or inability to recover to easy breathing within 5 minutes**
   When you start an exercise program, or you work out harder than usual, breathing a little hard is perfectly normal. If you're panting and gasping so hard that you can't speak or control your breath, stop and settle down. If, after 5 minutes of rest, you still can't catch your breath, dial 911 for an ambulance, take an aspirin, and lie down.

4. **Pain in your back, bones, or joints during or after exercise**
   Nothing should hurt in these workouts. Muscle aches and slight discomfort as you push yourself from level to level are normal, but *not* pain in your back, bones, and joints. Pain is nature's way of telling you that something is very wrong. We always pay attention to pain and react quickly. If it hurts, stop. Take a few days off, lower the intensity of the exercise, and try it again. If it still hurts, see your physician.

THE TOOLS YOU'LL NEED

Two reasons that Active-Isolated workouts are so popular? They're simple, and they're fast. They fit right into a tight space and a tighter schedule. You don't need a special gym; all the exercises can be done almost anywhere. Here's what you'll need.

- A bed or enough open floor space to lie down and extend your arms out to your sides
- A sturdy chair
- An 8-foot stretch rope, narrow enough in diameter to wrap around your hand
- A set of ankle weights (see page 63 for information on choosing weights)

With the most effective workout system in the world in your hands, you'll even have the time to get it done. You'll need only 30 minutes a day for the first two of the three 6-week cycles. In the last 6-week cycle, when we add walking to your program, you'll enjoy an extra 20 to 30 minutes of "me" time, 2 or 3 days a week. By the time you get to that last 6 weeks, you'll be so excited about your revitalized body that you'll be bounding down the street.

We're here to coach you—we'll teach you each exercise, one at a time. Once you've mastered the exercises, you'll be able to use the at-a-glance pages, starting on page 98, for quick reference.

YOUR WHARTON JUMP START

You're about to embark on a program that's identical to the one we use to train elite athletes. It's the one we use ourselves. We're going to show you how to unlock your joints, strengthen your muscles, and increase your stamina using principles that take advantage of the way your body was designed. This is fitness the way nature intended it. Simple. Fun. Fast. And revolutionary. But before we begin, here are a few thoughts about getting your program off to the best start possible.

First get your physician's approval. There are times when fitness programs should be approached with caution, and having a back injury tops that list. Take this book to your physician and,

together, outline the best plan for your situation.

Just begin. Getting started on a fitness program is really pretty simple. Forget having to start on a Monday. Forget having to forge through a list of things that you have to complete first. Forget waiting for your best friend to get ready so that you can do it together. Forget having to lose 10 pounds first. Starting an exercise program begins with a decision to do it. Now.

Make an appointment. Until you are comfortable with integrating workouts into your daily life, we urge you to block out the time each day on a calendar, as though you were scheduling an appointment that you must keep. Before you know it, you'll be looking forward to the time that is yours.

Swap activities. We have some of our new clients keep time logs for a few days, so they can examine exactly how they're spending time. Only after the schedule is on paper in 15-minute increments can they see blocks of time that could be easily traded for a workout. Sometimes, the trade-off involves a bit of sacrifice, but, more often than not, it's a matter of tightening up some inefficiencies to free an hour to train. Watch a little less television. Read on the stationary bike instead of in your recliner. Get up ½ hour earlier. Resign from a chat room.

Get your clothes and equipment together. All your good intentions will fall to the wayside if you realize that you can't lift a weight because you forgot to get one. Get it all together before you start.

Start slowly and progress gradually. One of the greatest myths in training is that it has to hurt in order for it to be doing you any good. That little catchphrase, "Go for the burn!" has ruined a generation of good trainers and hapless clients.

Athletes describe a good workout not as "pain," but as "effort." You know you're working when you're pushing a little. Anything beyond this is risking injury. When your workout no longer challenges you and is so easy that you're not putting any effort into it, then it's time to slightly increase weight, time, or duration. We'll show you how.

Exercise between meals. If you're planning a no-holds-barred workout, wait a couple of hours after eating. After you've eaten, your body puts its energy and blood supply into digesting food in your stomach. If you divert that energy and blood supply into large muscles, then you inhibit your body's ability to digest. A common reaction is vomiting. We don't know about you, but we think nothing spoils a good workout like throwing up.

Adjust your workout to suit the weather and time of day. Working out raises your metabolism and your body temperature, so dress to stay cool. But keep your common sense: If you're going for a brisk walk, don't wear shorts in a snowstorm. When in doubt, wear layers of clothing that you can peel off. Also, be mindful of your safety. Changing light conditions alter your depth perception, and a path that looks flat at 7:00 in the morning might look like tossed rubble at noon.

We're often asked, "When is the best time of day to work out?" Our answer is, "Any time you can." Although some literature suggests that working out right before bedtime revs you up so that sleeping is difficult, we do it every night and sleep fine. In fact, we rely heavily on exercise to diffuse the stresses of the day and relax us right before bed.

One caution about early-morning workouts: Please be careful about rocketing right into a hard cardio workout. Going from zero to 60 is hard on the heart. Warm up first and start slowly.

Divide your workout for convenience. Research assures us that two or three short workouts can be as beneficial as one longer one, as long as all the workouts are equal in intensity. If you don't have time to get it all done in one workout, divide it into two or three parts and save some of it for later.

Keep a record of your workouts. You'll find a personal workout log on page 97. Make photocopies of it for your personal use. Keeping a log helps you stay on track and gives you a clear picture of your progress.

Do your exercises in order. The workouts are specifically organized to warm up and unlock muscles and then engage them when they're ready to fire. Don't skip around; follow the sequence of exercises presented in the Stretching and Strengthening programs in the order specified.

Don't rush a move or a release. In both stretching and strengthening, bring a movement to its conclusion. Extend all the way out, hold, and flex all the way back as far as you can go. If you cut a movement short, you'll deprive all the muscle fibers of participating, and they'll actually become weaker.

Rather than rock and roll, think of this as a waltz. We break our clients of their gym music habits—pounding, driving rhythms are good for excitement but bad for pacing—by having them sing "Itsy Bitsy Spider" as they move, until they can adjust to a slower, more effective pace.

Know your own limits. How will you know that

The 21-Day Guarantee

If it's been a while since you've worked out, we know that starting can sometimes feel overwhelming. But we know that you *will* succeed with the Active-Isolated program, even if you've bailed out of others in the past.

Here's why: You're going to feel better from your first workout, and you'll feel even better every day. You'll be stronger and more flexible and will have more stamina. You'll be able to move with energy

and power. That relief and freedom from pain will probably be more than enough to keep you going.

Researchers also tell us that it takes 21 days for a habit to take hold. If you stay on track for only 21 days, you'll have made working out a habit—an integral, joyful, and important part of your life. You'll already have seen amazing results and will be well on your way to the body that you deserve.

If I Stretch, Will I Tear?

No. You can stretch a muscle 1.6 times its length, but the joints of your body have limited ranges of motion to keep you from flopping all over the place. Also, nature designed you to have a built-in range-limit detector—it's called *pain*.

As you approach the limit of your range of motion in a stretch, you experience the sensation of tightness, followed by discomfort, then pain. In fact, your joints have sensors that signal your body to draw back from being overly stretched, in order to prevent tearing. That's why the first sensation is tightness: The muscle is contracting back to protect itself. (While it's true that you can stretch a muscle until it tears, this is due to trauma and will not happen during a normal Active-Isolated Stretching workout.)

So how flexible can you expect to be? It depends on where you start. Some people were born flexible and have remained so all their lives. And some of us started out with flexibility, but lost it as we aged. No matter how flexible you are right now, you'll see tremendous gains as you work out.

---

you're working hard enough to make it count? We've organized the individual exercises to contain guidelines. Stretches (or flexes) require a little tug of the rope at the end of each move. Strengthening exercises (or lifts) are a matter of judgment on your part. The lifts should take effort, but not pain and extreme exertion.

If you poop out, cut back. If you get midway through a workout and decide that you can't do more, quit. Do as much as you can and be proud of it. Don't worry. You'll soon build up to the point where you can handle the whole workout.

There are days when even the thought of working out seems totally overwhelming. The question to answer is, "Am I really too tired to work out, or do I just think I am?" If you're too tired, bag the workout. If you're not sure, start the workout and see how you feel after 5 to 10 minutes. Remember that working out can energize you when your energy is low. Once you get moving, you might feel better and discover that the workout is no problem. If you don't feel more energized, cut the workout short.

If it hurts, stop immediately. As you progress, you'll learn to distinguish between the discomfort of exertion and real pain. Until you know the difference, treat all pain the same. It's a message from your body that you're doing (or are about to do) damage and you need to back off. If backing off alleviates the pain immediately, you might test the exercise again, only with less weight (if you're lifting) or fewer repetitions. If the pain is acute or persists, see your physician.

Remember to breathe. Don't hold your breath. To time exercise naturally, exhale as you stretch and inhale as you return to the neutral position of each stretch.

THE ACTIVE-ISOLATED STRETCHING ROUTINE FOR BACKS

Where's the best place to do your Active-Isolated Stretching routine? We like to stretch on the floor or on a bed. Anywhere is all right. (In the beginning, we advise picking a place close to a large mirror, where you can check your form.) You'll be sitting and lying down, so you want to be as comfortable as possible. Extend that feeling into your dress—wear loose-fitting, comfortable clothing. And stash a bottle of water so that it's within easy reach. You're ready to begin!

Please note: We've included the complete series here. Please see page 98 for an easy, at-a-glance reference to the exact exercises you'll do each day of the program.

TRY PREHAB, NOT REHAB

1. SINGLE-LEG PELVIC TILTS

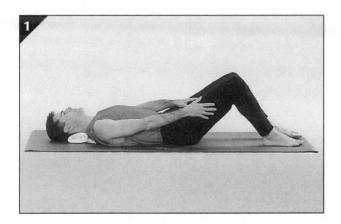

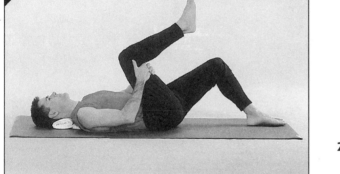

Active Muscles You Contract: Abdominals and muscles from the fronts of your hips down the fronts of your thighs

Isolated Muscles You Stretch: Lower back and buttocks

Hold Each Stretch: 2 seconds

Reps: 10 right, 10 left

1. Lie on your back on a flat surface. Tuck a rolled towel or small pillow under your neck and head. Bend your nonexercising knee to relax your back and keep the pressure off. Bend your exercising leg at the knee as well, as shown, and reach down to weave your fingers together behind your knee to support your leg and provide a little assistance toward the end of the stretch. If you can't reach all the way to your knee, hold the back of your thigh as close to your knee as you can.

2. Using your abdominals and hip flexors (muscles along the fronts of your hips), and leading with your knee toward your shoulder, lift your exercising leg toward your chest as far as you can. At the end of your stretch, gently assist with your hands, but don't force it. Add the slightest pressure, extending the range of the stretch just a little more. Hold for 2 seconds and then relax in preparation for the next stretch.

2. DOUBLE-LEG PELVIC TILTS

Active Muscles You Contract: Abdominals and muscles from the fronts of your hips down the fronts of your thighs

Isolated Muscles You Stretch: Lower back and buttocks

Hold Each Stretch: 2 seconds

Reps: 10

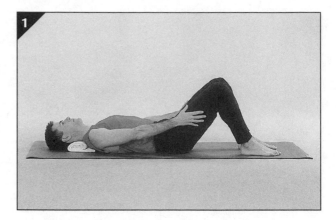

1. Lie down on your back on a flat surface. Tuck a rolled towel or small pillow under your neck and head. To relax your back, bend both knees and place your feet flat on the surface on which you are lying. Reach down and place one hand behind each knee to support your legs and provide a little assistance toward the end of the stretch. If you can't reach all the way to your knees, hold the backs of your thighs as close to your knees as you can. Keep your knees bent and relaxed.

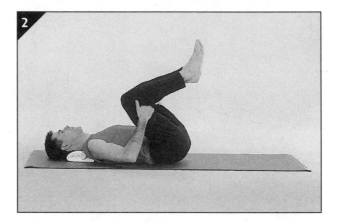

2. Using your abdominals and quadriceps, lift your legs toward your chest as far as you can. At the end of your stretch, gently assist with your hands, but don't force it. Add the slightest pressure, extending the range of the stretch just a little more. Hold for 2 seconds and then relax in preparation for the next stretch.

TRY PREHAB, NOT REHAB

3. BENT-LEG HAMSTRINGS

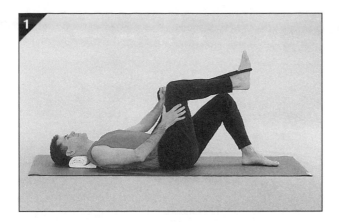

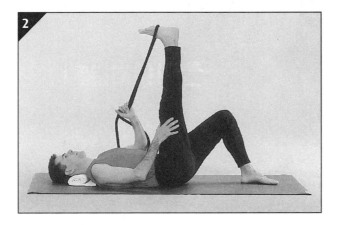

Active Muscles You Contract: Muscles in the fronts of your thighs

Isolated Muscles You Stretch: Large muscles in the backs of your thighs, just behind your knees

Hold Each Stretch: 2 seconds

Reps: 10 right, 10 left

1. Lie down on your back on a flat surface. Tuck a rolled towel or small pillow under your neck and head. To relax your back, bend both knees and place your feet flat on the surface on which you are lying. Take your rope and hold the ends together so that it forms a loop. Slip the foot of your exercising leg into the loop, positioning the loop in the arch between your heel and the ball of your foot. Take out the slack and snug it up.

   Keeping your knee bent and relaxed, lift your exercising leg up until your thigh is perpendicular to the surface and your lower leg is parallel, as shown. Hold the ends of the rope in one hand and put enough tension on the loop to keep it from slipping away from the bottom of your foot. Put the other hand on top of the thigh of your exercising leg to stabilize it.

2. Straighten your leg by contracting your quadriceps until your knee is locked. When you're very skilled, the bottom of your foot will be aimed at the ceiling, but this takes practice, so settle for an angle that is comfortable at first. Eventually, you'll achieve "perpendicular" and beyond. At the end of your stretch, gently assist with your rope, but don't force it. Add the slightest pressure, extending the range of the stretch just a little more. Hold for 2 seconds and then relax in preparation for the next stretch.

4. STRAIGHT-LEG HAMSTRINGS

Active Muscles You Contract: Muscles from the fronts of your hips down the fronts of your thighs

Isolated Muscles You Stretch: Large muscles in the backs of your thighs

Hold Each Stretch: 2 seconds

Reps: 10 right, 10 left

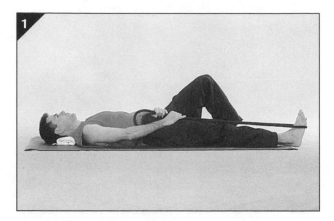

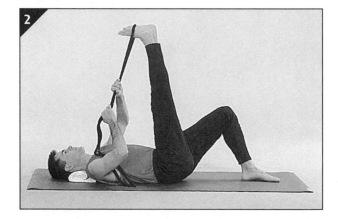

1. Lie down on your back on a flat surface. Tuck a rolled towel or small pillow under your neck and head. Your exercising leg should be straight out. Your nonexercising leg should be bent at the knee, with your foot flat on the surface on which you're lying. Take your rope and hold the ends together so that it forms a loop. Slip the foot of your exercising leg into the loop, positioning the loop in the arch between your heel and the ball of your foot. Take out the slack and snug it up. Lock your knee.

2. From your hip and using your quadriceps, aim the bottom of your foot toward the ceiling and lift your leg straight up as far as you can. Grasp the ends of the rope (to maintain tension so the loop won't slip off your foot) with both hands and "climb" up the rope, quickly hand over hand as your leg lifts. When you're very skilled, the bottom of your foot will be aimed at the ceiling, but this takes practice, so settle for an angle that is comfortable at first. Eventually, you'll achieve "perpendicular" and beyond. At the end of your stretch, gently assist with your rope, but don't force it. Add the slightest pressure, extending the range of the stretch just a little more. Hold for 2 seconds and then relax in preparation for the next stretch.

TRY PREHAB, NOT REHAB

5. HIP ADDUCTORS

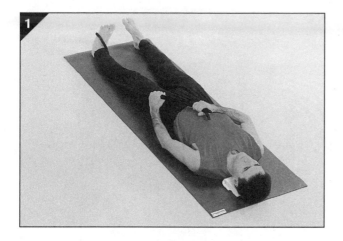

Active Muscles You Contract: Muscles on the outsides of your thighs, muscles in the middle of your buttocks, and muscles that cross over your front thighs

Isolated Muscles You Stretch: Muscles on the insides of your thighs

Hold Each Stretch: 2 seconds

Reps: 10 right, 10 left

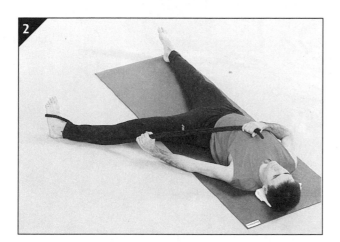

1. Lie down on your back on a flat surface with both legs extended straight out. Tuck a rolled towel or small pillow under your neck and head. Take your rope and hold the ends together so that it forms a loop. Slip the foot of your exercising leg into the loop, positioning the loop in the arch between your heel and the ball of your foot. Wrap the rope around the inside of the ankle so that the ends of the rope are on the outside. Lock your knee.

   Lift your heel slightly off the floor so that you can move your leg without dragging your foot. Take the slack out of your rope and snug it up. Rotate your nonexercising leg inward slightly, as shown, to stabilize your body.

2. From your hip and using your abductors (muscles on the outside of your thigh), extend your leg out from the side of your body, leading with your heel. Keep slight tension on the rope. Slide the same-side hand down the rope and hold the top of the rope with the hand on the opposite side. At the end of your stretch, gently assist with your rope, but don't force it. Add the slightest pressure, extending the range of the stretch just a little more. Hold for 2 seconds and then relax in preparation for the next stretch.

6. HIP ABDUCTORS

Active Muscles You Contract: Muscles on the insides of your thighs

Isolated Muscles You Stretch: Muscles on the outsides of your thighs and hips

Hold Each Stretch: 2 seconds

Reps: 10 right, 10 left

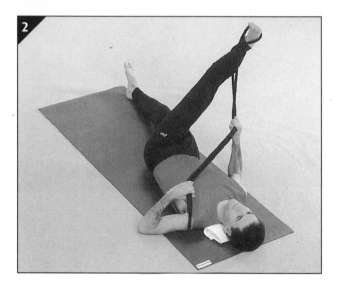

1. Lie down on your back on a flat surface with both legs extended straight out. Tuck a rolled towel or small pillow under your neck and head. Take your rope and hold the ends together so that it forms a loop. Slip the foot of your exercising leg into the loop, positioning the loop in the arch between your heel and the ball of your foot. Wrap the rope around the outside of the ankle so that the ends of the rope are on the inside. Lock your knee.

   Rotate your nonexercising leg inward slightly and rotate your exercising leg outward slightly. They end up both pointing in the same direction, as shown. Take the slack out of your rope and snug it up.

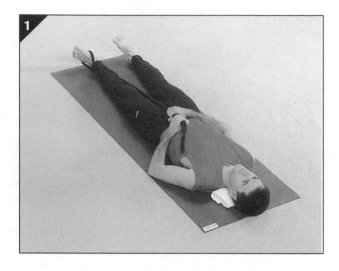

2. From your groin and using your adductors (muscles on the inside of your thigh), sweep your exercising leg across the midline of your body, leading with your heel, just above your nonexercising leg. Remember to keep your knee locked. Keep slight tension on the rope. At the end of your stretch, gently assist with your rope, but don't force it. Add the slightest pressure, extending the range of the stretch just a little more. Hold for 2 seconds and then relax in preparation for the next stretch.

7. PSOAS

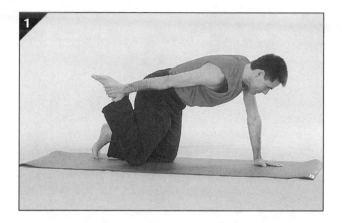

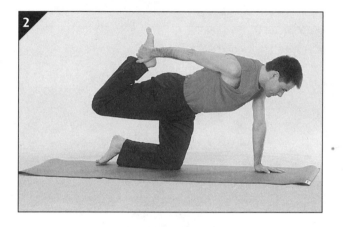

Active Muscles You Contract: Muscles in your buttocks and the backs of your thighs

Isolated Muscles You Stretch: Muscles in your groin and the fronts of your upper thighs

Hold Each Stretch: 2 seconds

Reps: 10 right, 10 left

1. Get on your hands and knees. With the knee bent, extend your exercising leg until your foot is off the floor. Bring that foot up behind you until you can reach back with your hand and grasp your ankle. Get a firm grasp, but don't strain your back. If you can't reach your ankle, settle for your shin. In time, the ankle will be within reach.

2. Using your hamstrings and gluteal muscles, lift your exercising leg up until your thigh is parallel to the ground or horizontal to your body. Be careful not to arch your back. Go as far as you can. At the end of your stretch, gently assist with your hand, but don't force it. Add the slightest pressure, extending the range of the stretch just a little more. Hold for 2 seconds and then relax in preparation for the next stretch.

8. QUADRICEPS

Active Muscles You Contract: Muscles in your buttocks and the backs of your thighs

Isolated Muscles You Stretch: Muscles in the fronts of your thighs

Hold Each Stretch: 2 seconds

Reps: 10 right, 10 left

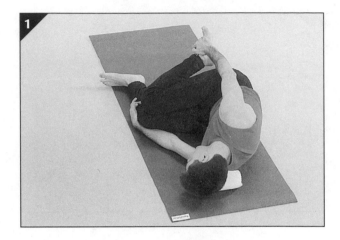

1. Lie on your side on a flat surface with your knees curled up against your chest in a fetal position. Support your neck and keep it relaxed by resting your head on the surface or on a rolled towel or small pillow. You will be exercising the thigh of your top leg. Slide your bottom arm under the thigh of your bottom leg and lock your elbow around the back of your knee. Tighten your abdominal muscles to keep you from rolling.

   Reach down with your upper hand and grasp the ankle of your upper leg, as shown. If you are unable to bend your knee sufficiently in order for you to reach your ankle with your hand, simply wrap the rope around your ankle, take out the slack, and hold the rope in your hand. Keep your knee bent and your leg parallel to the surface on which you are lying.

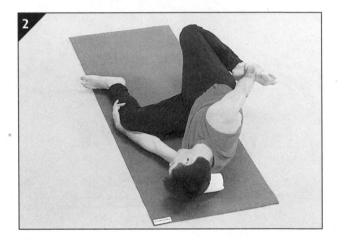

2. Contract your hamstrings and gluteal muscles and extend that upper leg back as far as you can. At the end of your stretch, gently assist with your hand or rope (if using), but don't force it. Add the slightest pressure, extending the range of the stretch just a little more. Hold for 2 seconds and then relax in preparation for the next stretch. You will have to roll over to do 10 repetitions of this stretch on the other side.

9. GLUTEALS

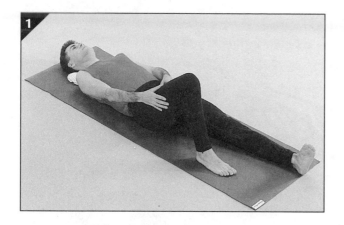

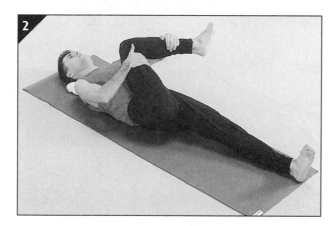

Active Muscles You Contract: Abdominals and muscles from the fronts of your hips down the fronts of your thighs

Isolated Muscles You Stretch: Muscles in your lower back that rotate your torso, the muscles that rotate your hips, and buttocks

Hold Each Stretch: 2 seconds

Reps: 10 right, 10 left

1. Lie flat on your back on a flat surface with both legs extended straight out. Tuck a rolled towel or small pillow under your neck and head. Rotate your nonexercising leg toward the midline of your body by pointing your toes inward to stabilize your hips. Bend the knee of your exercising leg.

2. Using your abdominal muscles and hip flexors (muscles along the fronts of your hips), lift your bent knee toward the opposite shoulder. Keep your lower back flat on the surface so that you can feel the stretch in your hip. As soon as you can reach your rising knee, place your hand on the outside of your knee and gently guide the stretch.

   If you want a deeper stretch of the gluteus, you can grasp the outside of your shin with your opposite hand, as shown, and press your heel toward the floor as your knee nears your shoulder. Be careful that you do not irritate your knee. And be sure that you don't lift one side of your pelvis off the surface. At the end of your stretch, gently assist with your hand, but don't force it. Add the slightest pressure, extending the range of the stretch just a little more. Hold for 2 seconds and then relax in preparation for the next stretch.

10. PIRIFORMIS

Active Muscles You Contract: Lower abdominal muscles, the muscles in your hips that rotate your legs, and the muscles on the insides and fronts of your thighs

Isolated Muscles You Stretch: The piriformis muscle that lies underneath the big muscle in your buttock

Hold Each Stretch: 2 seconds

Reps: 10 right, 10 left

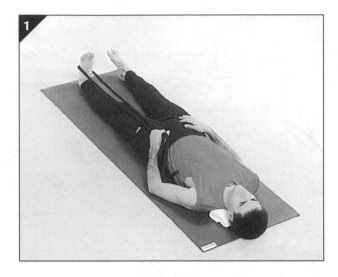

1. Lie down on your back on a flat surface with both legs extended. Tuck a rolled towel or small pillow under your neck and head. Take your rope and hold the ends together so that it forms a loop. Slip the foot of your exercising leg into the loop, positioning the loop in the arch between your heel and the ball of your foot. Take out the slack and snug it up. Lock the knee of your exercising leg so that your leg is straight. If you're uncomfortable, relax your knee very slightly.

2. From your hip and using your quadriceps and hip flexors (muscles along the fronts of your hips), lift your leg straight up until it is perpendicular to your body, or as close as you can get it. Use the rope to lift your leg by drawing up the ends of the rope with both hands, in a hand-over-hand maneuver. Aim the bottom of your foot toward the ceiling.

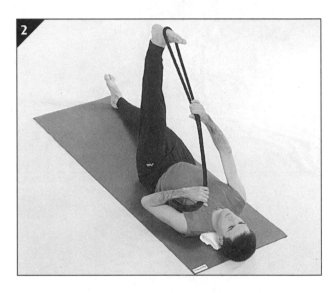

3. When your leg is in position, grasp the rope with the hand opposite your exercising leg. Keep the loop snug. Extend your other hand (the one on the same side as your exercising leg) straight out to stabilize your body and keep you from rolling. Contract your adductors (muscles on the inside of your thigh) and lower abdominals to bring your leg across your body and straight down to the surface until your hip begins to roll up. Keep slight tension on the rope. At the end of your stretch, gently assist with your rope, but don't force it. Add the slightest pressure, extending the range of the stretch just a little more. Hold for 2 seconds and then relax in preparation for the next stretch.

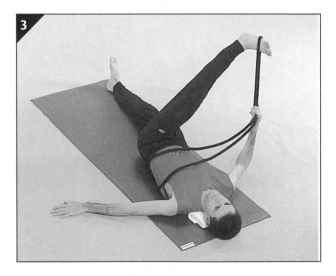

11. TRUNK EXTENSORS

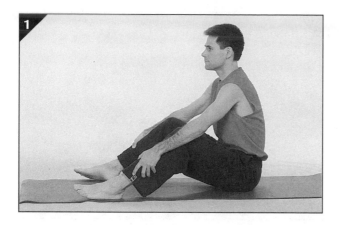

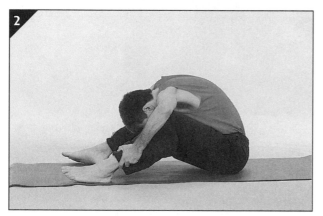

Active Muscles You Contract: Abdominals

Isolated Muscles You Stretch: Muscles that run from your pelvis to the base of your skull along the spine, and the lower-back muscles below your belt line

Hold Each Stretch: 2 seconds

Reps: 10

1. Sit on a flat surface with your back straight, your knees bent, your toes pointed slightly up, and your feet resting on your heels, as shown.

2. Tuck your chin down, contract your abdominal muscles, bend at your hips, and pull your torso forward and down as far as you can go. Grasp the sides of the lower legs with your hands to gently assist at the end of each stretch, but don't force it. Add the slightest pressure, extending the range of the stretch just a little more. Hold for 2 seconds and then relax in preparation for the next stretch. (For a deeper lower-back stretch, or if your hamstrings are tight, bring your heels closer to your body and repeat the exercise.)

12. THORACIC-LUMBAR ROTATORS

Active Muscles You Contract: Abdominals, the muscles on the sides of your chest, and the thoracic-lumbar rotators on the side opposite the exercising side

Isolated Muscles You Stretch: Muscles that run from your pelvis to the base of your skull along the spine; the stabilizing, rotating, and balancing muscles in your back and sides; and the lower-back muscles below your belt line

Hold Each Stretch: 2 seconds

Reps: 10 right, 10 left

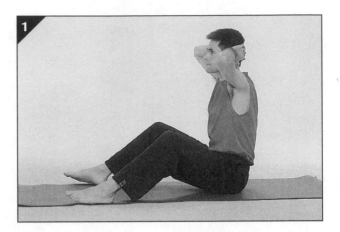

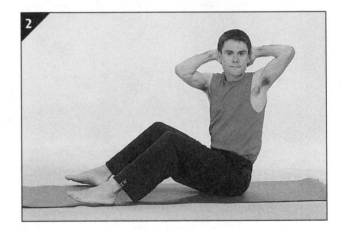

1. Sit on a flat surface with your back straight, your knees bent, your toes pointed slightly up, and your feet resting on your heels, as shown. Lock your hands by lacing your fingers together behind your head with your elbows out. Tuck your chin down.

2. Contract your entire abdomen, including the muscles in your side, and the opposite thoracic-lumbar rotator muscles to rotate your upper body in one direction until you have rotated as far as you can go. Do this four or five times until you feel loosened up.

3. When you're ready, rotate one more time, hold and then flex your body forward, leading toward the surface with your elbow. Hold for 2 seconds. Return to an upright position. Relax in preparation for the next stretch. Work one side at a time, completing all repetitions before beginning the opposite side. Note: There is no way to assist this stretch with gentle pressure at the end without the help of a workout partner, but gravity and momentum do help a little.

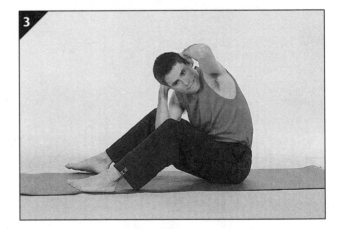

13. TRUNK LATERAL FLEXORS

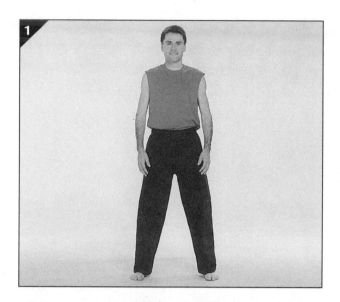

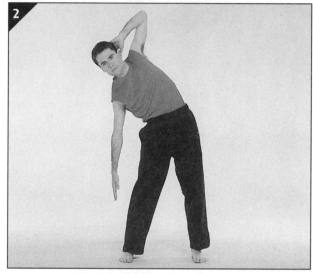

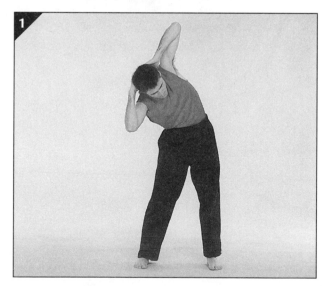

Active Muscles You Contract: Abdominals, the muscles on the sides of your chest, and the thoracic-lumbar rotators on the side opposite the exercising side

Isolated Muscles You Stretch: Muscles in your back along the spine and the muscles in the sides of your trunk opposite the exercising side

Hold Each Stretch: 2 seconds

Reps: 10 right, 10 left

1. Stand straight with both arms relaxed at your sides, as shown. Raise one arm, placing your hand behind your head with your elbow pointed away from your body.

2. Bend at the waist and point your elbow to the ceiling. Hold for 2 seconds. Return to the upright position and then relax in preparation for the next stretch. Work one side at a time, completing all repetitions before beginning the opposite side. Note: There is no way to assist this stretch with gentle pressure at the end without the help of a workout partner, but gravity and momentum do help a little.

MODIFICATION

1. This stretch can be modified by placing both hands behind your head. Lean slightly forward or backward before bending at the waist and lowering your elbow toward the floor.

14. SHOULDER CIRCUMDUCTION

Active Muscles You Contract: Shoulders

Isolated Muscles You Stretch: No muscles are specifically isolated. This is a tension reliever and a way to warm up. It increases circulation in your shoulder joints, which are anatomically complex but have a surprisingly limited blood supply.

Hold Each Stretch: Technically, there is no stretch here.

Reps: 10 clockwise, 10 counterclockwise

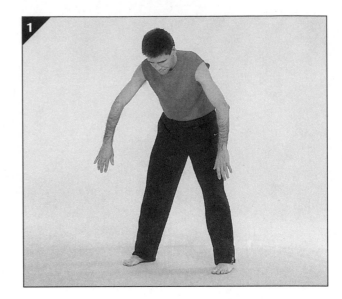

1. Stand and bend forward at the waist. Allow your arms to dangle loosely from your shoulders. Relax as completely as you can. Bend your knees slightly to keep tension out of your back. Move your arms in small circles, allowing the entire arm, from shoulder to fingertip, to circle. Move your arms in a clockwise rotation, and then counterclockwise. Start with small circles, moving to larger circles. Stay relaxed and keep your abdominal muscles tight.

15. PECTORALIS MAJORS

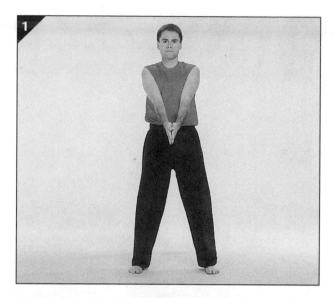

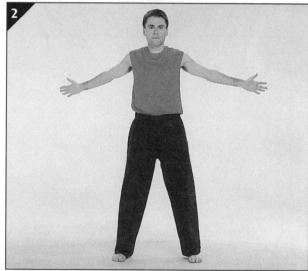

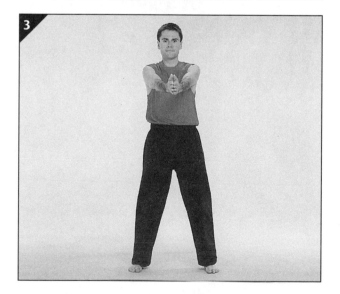

Active Muscles You Contract: Backs of your shoulders and the area between your shoulder blades

Isolated Muscles You Stretch: Muscles in your chest and shoulders

Hold Each Stretch: 2 seconds

Reps: 10

1. Stand on a flat surface with your feet slightly apart and your knees relaxed. Straighten your arms, palms facing forward with elbows locked, with your pinkie finger next to your thigh. Swing your arms forward so that your fingertips touch, as shown. Inhale.

2. Use the muscles in the backs of your shoulders and between your shoulder blades to swing your arms straight back until they can go no farther. Exhale.

3. This stretch is done in progressive stages, with each swing a little higher than the one before it.

16. ANTERIOR DELTOIDS

Active Muscles You Contract: Backs of your shoulders, the triceps, and the posterior deltoids (the muscles on the backs of your shoulders)

Isolated Muscles You Stretch: Upper arms and fronts of your shoulders

Hold Each Stretch: 2 seconds

Reps: 10

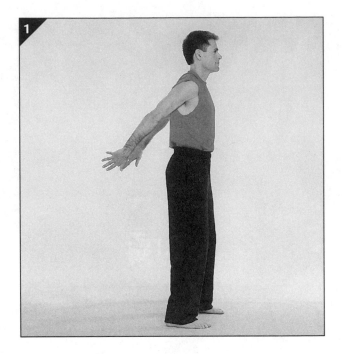

1. Stand with your feet slightly apart on a flat surface and dangle your arms loosely by your sides. You'll be working both sides simultaneously. Swing your arms straight back, as shown, keeping your elbows locked and palms facing each other. Loosen up with about 10 gentle repetitions. For a deeper stretch, touch your fingertips together behind your back. Keep your elbows locked and raise your arms slightly, leading with your hands, to achieve the stretch. Hold for 2 seconds and then relax in preparation for the next stretch.

TRY PREHAB, NOT REHAB

17. SHOULDER INTERNAL ROTATORS

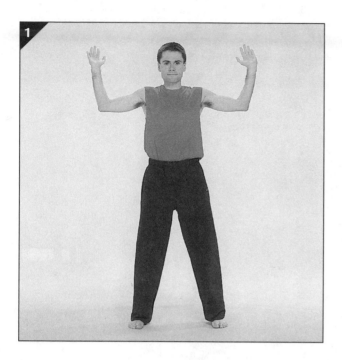

Active Muscles You Contract: External rotator muscles in the backs of your shoulders

Isolated Muscles You Stretch: Internal rotator muscles in your shoulders

Hold Each Stretch: 2 seconds

Reps: 10

1. Stand on a flat surface with your feet slightly apart. You'll be working both shoulders simultaneously. Raise arms out to the sides so that your elbows are level with your shoulders and your upper arms are up, fingertips pointed to the ceiling, palms forward. Your elbows should be at 90-degree angles, still level with your shoulders. This is your starting position. Hold and lock the angles of your elbows. Rotate your shoulders so that your forearms and hands move up and back until they have passed behind your head. Go as far as you can. Push the stretch gently at the end. Hold for 2 seconds and then relax in preparation for the next stretch.

18. SHOULDER EXTERNAL ROTATORS

Active Muscles You Contract: Internal rotator muscles in your shoulders

Isolated Muscles You Stretch: External rotator muscles in the backs of your shoulders

Hold Each Stretch: 2 seconds

Reps: 10

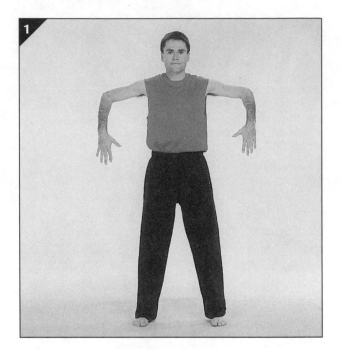

1. Stand on a flat surface with your feet slightly apart. You'll be working both shoulders simultaneously. Raise your arms out to the sides so that your elbows are level with your shoulders and your upper arms are down, fingertips pointed to the floor, palms backward. Your elbows should be at 90-degree angles, still level with your shoulders. Hold and lock the angles of your elbows, and rotate your arms down and back until your forearms and hands are behind the midpoint of your body. Palms should be facing behind. Go as far as you can. Push the stretch gently at the end. Hold for 2 seconds and then relax in preparation for the next stretch.

TRY PREHAB, NOT REHAB

19. ROTATOR CUFF 1

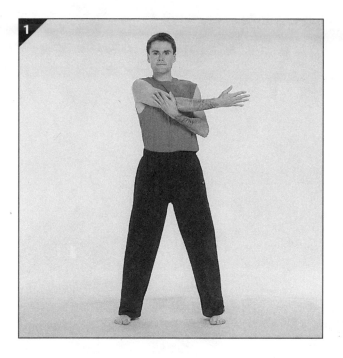

Active Muscles You Contract: Muscles in the fronts of your shoulders and your chest

Isolated Muscles You Stretch: External shoulder rotators, commonly called the rotator cuff

Hold Each Stretch: 2 seconds

Reps: 10 right, 10 left

1. Stand on a flat surface with your feet slightly apart and your arms relaxed at your sides. Lift one arm straight up until it is level with your shoulder. Lock your elbow. Pass your arm straight across your chest toward your opposite shoulder. Keep your torso stationary and relaxed, and be sure that you don't hike up the stretching shoulder. Go as far as you can. Assist the stretch gently at the end with your opposite hand at the elbow, as shown. Hold for 2 seconds and then relax in preparation for the next stretch.

20. ROTATOR CUFF 2

Active Muscles You Contract: Muscles in the fronts of your shoulders

Isolated Muscles You Stretch: External shoulder rotators—commonly called the rotator cuffs—and the muscles below your shoulder blades

Hold Each Stretch: 2 seconds

Reps: 10 right, 10 left

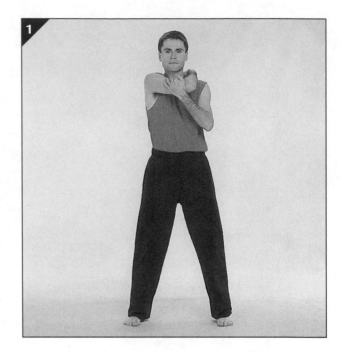

1. Stand on a flat surface with your feet slightly apart and your arms relaxed at your sides. Lift one arm with your elbow bent. Pass that arm straight across your chest toward your opposite shoulder. Keep your torso stationary and relaxed. Stretch until your hand reaches down your back or as far as it can go. Assist the stretch gently at the end with your opposite hand at your elbow, as shown. Hold for 2 seconds and then relax in preparation for the next stretch.

TRY PREHAB, NOT REHAB

21. FORWARD ELEVATORS OF THE SHOULDER

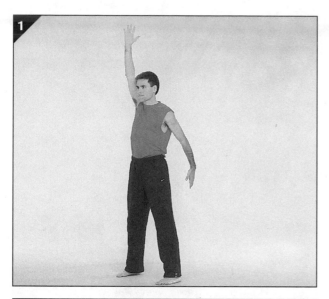

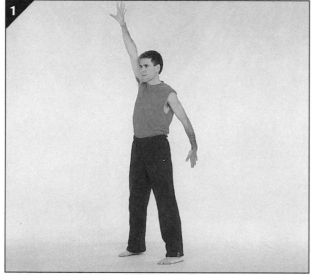

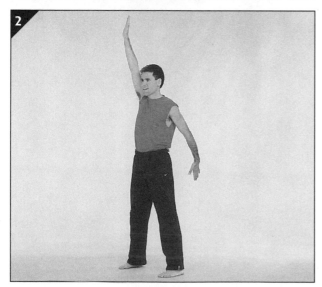

Active Muscles You Contract: Muscles in your shoulders

Isolated Muscles You Stretch: Muscles in your shoulders

Hold Each Stretch: 2 seconds

Reps: 10 right, 10 left (in opposition)

1. Stand on a flat surface with your feet slightly apart and your arms relaxed by your sides. Raise one arm, with your elbow locked straight, above your head. Working in opposition with equal resistance, straighten and extend your nonexercising arm behind you, as shown. Palms of your hands should face in toward the center line of your body. (We call this stretch "the tin soldier" because it looks like an exaggerated marching form.) Do several repetitions with palms in, then move on to the modifications.

MODIFICATION

1. Do the exercise above, with your exercising palm facing backward.

2. Do the exercise above, with your exercising palm facing forward.

   Stretch your shoulders in opposition until you can go no farther. Push the two stretches gently at the end with a little effort and momentum. Hold for 2 seconds and then relax in preparation for the next stretches.

22. SIDE ELEVATORS OF THE SHOULDER

Active Muscles You Contract: Muscles in your shoulders

Isolated Muscles You Stretch: Muscles in your shoulders

Hold Each Stretch: 2 seconds

Reps: 10 right, 10 left

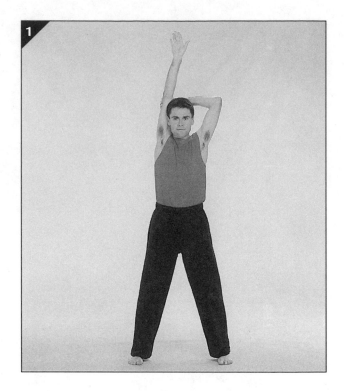

1. Stand on a flat surface with your feet slightly apart and arms by your sides. Relax your knees and tighten your abdominals for stability. (There is temptation to cock your hip to compensate for a momentary imbalance. Resist.) With your elbow straightened and locked, and the palm of your hand facing forward, raise your exercising arm above and behind your head. With your nonexercising hand, reach over and grasp your exercising arm between your elbow and shoulder, as shown, and gently assist the stretch until you feel the pull in your back beneath your shoulder blade. Learn to bring your arm straight over and back without having to nod your head to get it out of the way. Hold for 2 seconds and then relax in preparation for the next stretches.

23. NECK EXTENSORS

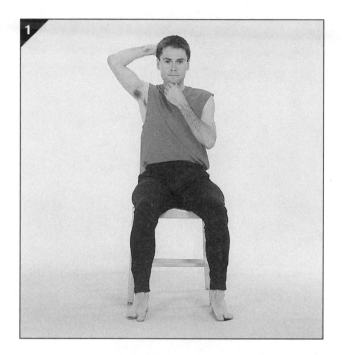

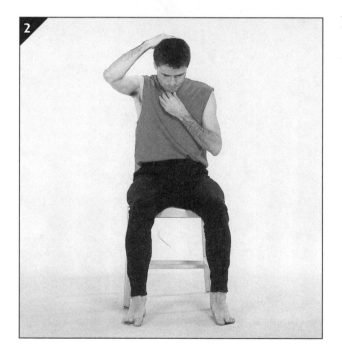

Active Muscles You Contract: Muscles in the front of your neck

Isolated Muscles You Stretch: Muscles in the back of your neck

Hold Each Stretch: 2 seconds

Reps: 10

1. Sit in a chair with your back straight and your feet flat on the floor. Face forward. Place one hand on the back of your head and one hand on your chin to assist the stretch.

2. Tuck your chin down and gently roll your head forward until your chin meets your chest. Keep your shoulders completely relaxed and keep your torso straight. Resist the urge to roll your entire body down. You want the stretch in your neck only. You can gently assist the end of the movement by pressing your head forward and down with your hand at the back of your head. Be very careful not to strain your neck. Hold for 2 seconds and then relax in preparation for the next stretch.

24. NECK LATERAL FLEXORS

Active Muscles You Contract: Muscles in the opposite sides of your neck

Isolated Muscles You Stretch: Muscles in the sides of your neck

Hold Each Stretch: 2 seconds

Reps: 10 right, 10 left

1. Sit in a chair with your back straight and your feet flat on the floor. Face forward.

2. Cock your head to one side by bringing your ear straight down toward the top of your shoulder. Keep your shoulders down and relaxed and your torso still. As you lower, reach up and over the top of your head with the hand on the same side, place your fingertips lightly on the side of your head over your ear, and pull your head gently down toward your shoulder to assist the end of the stretch. Be very careful not to strain your neck. Hold for 2 seconds and then relax in preparation for the next stretch.

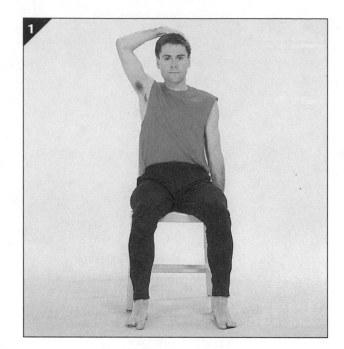

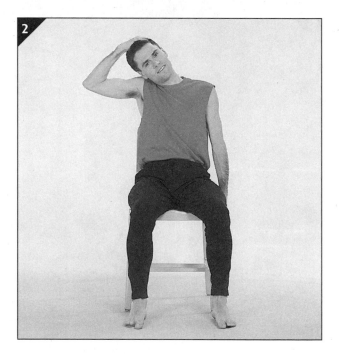

TRY PREHAB, NOT REHAB

THE ACTIVE-ISOLATED STRENGTHENING ROUTINE FOR BACKS

You already understand the principles of Active-Isolated Stretching. Now it's time to apply those principles to strengthening your muscles. Using small amounts of weight and the resistance of your own body to work out, you isolate specific muscles or groups of muscles and "fire" them one at a time in a specific sequence. By bolstering weakened muscles, you'll relieve the strain on other, compensating muscles; help remedy current aches; and prevent back pain in the future.

As we discussed earlier, muscles work in pairs. When you fire one muscle, the opposite muscle will relax. When one is fatigued or struggling, your body automatically deploys other muscles to kick in and assist. The irony of this is that you might be able to get the job done—lift something—but still have a weak muscle, because all the *real* work was done by other recruited muscles. When you work out using conventional methods, there's no accommodation for this phenomenon. That's what's different about Active-Isolated Strengthening: You actually strengthen a specific muscle, instead of just lifting a weight. By isolating the targeted muscles, your body cannot recruit help, so the intended muscle is truly strengthened, precisely and efficiently.

As with the stretching routines, you should always work out in comfortable clothing that allows you to move freely and keeps you cool. We suggest shorts and a T-shirt. Wear nonskid shoes or go barefoot. Keep your trusty bottle of water by your side, and find two small towels or pillows to use during your workouts.

You'll also need two ankle weights. In order to select a beginning weight, first lift a 1-pound weight. If it's too light, move to a 2-pounder. Continue moving up until you find a weight that's fairly easy to lift but still gets your attention. Try it on both your wrist and ankle, because you're going to use the same weight on both.

Don't be a hero. Don't overestimate your ability just because the number is smaller than you think worthy. Don't buy a weight that you can "grow into" or "work up to." You have to be able to work with the weight *right now*. Remember that the weight will be attached to one of your limbs, which will provide even more weight to lift when the time comes. You'll work with this weight until your strength increases. When this weight no longer feels heavy, go back to the store and move up to the next denomination, looking for the same sensation you had with the first weight. (Some stores even allow a trade-in.)

For the first week, do one set of each exercise. If the exercise calls for the use of weights, start with 1-pound weights. In the beginning, your single set will teach your body to repattern your neurological pathways. When that set becomes easy, add another set. When *that* set is easy, add more weight (if applicable), in 1-pound increments. As always, if you need to do so, rest between sets.

25. QUADRICEPS—KNEE EXTENSORS

Muscles You Strengthen: The four muscles that form the strongest in the body—the "quad" group in the top of your thigh from under your knee to your hipbone

The Basic Lift: Extend your knee

Pace of Lifting: Up slowly, pause, down slowly

Equipment: Rolled towel or small pillow, ankle weights

Reps: 10 right, 10 left

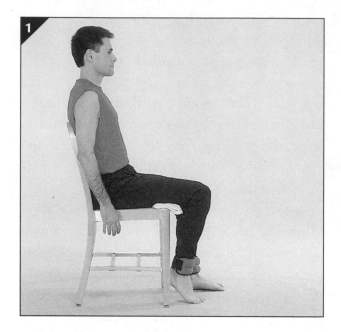

1. Fasten a weight around each of your ankles. Sit on a chair with your back straight and your feet flat on the floor. Tuck a rolled towel or a small pillow under the back of the knee of your exercising leg, as shown, to take the pressure off your back. Your foot should dangle above the floor slightly. Tighten your abdominal muscles to stabilize your torso.

2. Flex your toes up. Extend your leg straight out. Lock your knee. Contract the medial head of the vastus medialis—the insertion of the small muscle at the top of the kneecap on the inside of your thigh. Pause and return slowly to the starting position in preparation for the next rep. There is no need to rest between repetitions. Keep it going. Work one leg at a time for the full 10 reps.

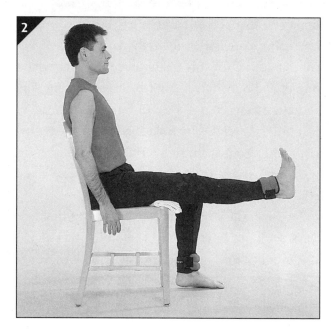

TRY PREHAB, NOT REHAB

26. QUADRICEPS—HIP FLEXORS

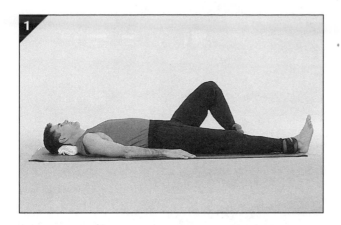

Muscles You Strengthen: Muscles in the top of your thighs from under your knee to the front of your hip

The Basic Lift: Flex your hip

Pace of Lifting: Up slowly, pause, down slowly

Equipment: Rolled towel or small pillow, ankle weights

Reps: 12 right, 12 left

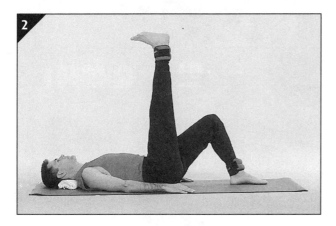

This exercise has three distinct positions. Because the positions of these lifts are similar, it's efficient to combine them. Notice that there are 12 reps for each leg. Here's how we want you to manage each set so that all muscles are worked. Put ankle weights on both ankles. Right leg: front, inside, outside. Left leg: front, inside, outside. Repeat the sequence four times to work out both sets of hip flexors and quads.

1. **Front:** Lie on your back on flat surface. Tuck a rolled towel or small pillow under your neck and head. Bend your nonexercising leg at the knee and place your foot flat on the surface to keep pressure off your back. Straighten your exercising leg by extending your knee. Lock your knee. Keep your foot relaxed.

2. Lifting from your hip and using your quadriceps to power the move, bring your leg straight up toward your head as far as you can. (With practice you should be able to bring your leg to perpendicular to your body.) Aim the bottom of your foot toward the ceiling. Pause and return slowly to the starting position in preparation for the next rep. There is no need to rest between repetitions. Keep it going for 12, then move on to the inside exercise.

(continued)

3. Inside: Then, without adjusting your basic position, rotate your exercising leg from your hip by pointing your toes to the outside. Keep your knee locked. From your hip and contracting your front and inner thigh muscles, lift your leg straight up toward your head as far as you can. Aim your foot toward the ceiling. This isolates the muscles on the inside of your upper thigh. Pause and return slowly to the starting position in preparation for the next rep. There is no need to rest between repetitions. Move on to the outside exercise.

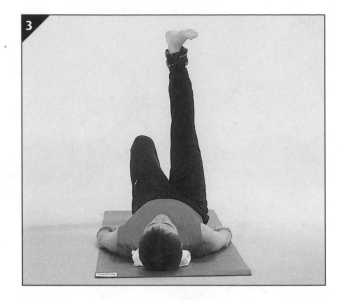

4. Outside: Hold your basic position, but rotate your exercising leg from your hip by pointing your toes to the inside. Keep your knee locked. From your hip and contracting your front and outer thigh muscles, lift your leg straight up toward your head as far as you can. Aim your foot toward the ceiling. This isolates the muscles on the outside of your upper thigh. Pause and return slowly to the starting position in preparation for the next rep. There is no need to rest between repetitions. Then change legs and move through the three variations again.

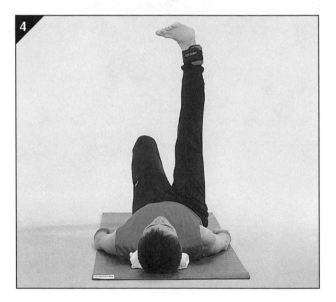

TRY PREHAB, NOT REHAB

27. HAMSTRINGS

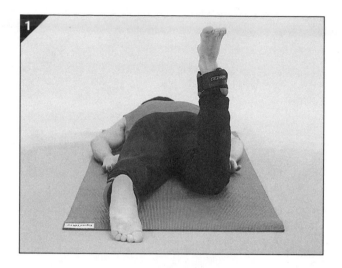

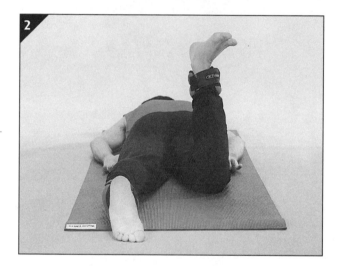

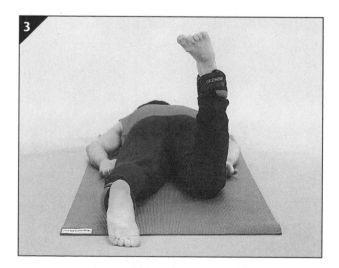

Muscles You Strengthen: Muscles in the rear of your thighs from behind your knee to your buttocks

The Basic Lift: Flex your knee

Pace of Lifting: Up slowly, pause, down slowly

Equipment: Ankle weights

Reps: 12 right, 12 left

This exercise has three distinct but similar positions, so it's efficient to combine them. Here's how to manage each set. Put ankle weights on both ankles. Right leg: back, inside, outside. Left leg: back, inside, outside. Repeat the sequence four times (totaling 12 reps for each leg).

1. **Straight Up and Back:** Lie on your stomach on a flat surface. Flex your knee by contracting your hamstrings, bringing your foot toward your buttocks. Keep your hips flat on the surface and your foot straight. This isolates the muscles in the middle of the rear thigh. Pause and return slowly to the starting position in preparation for the next rep. There is no need to rest between repetitions.

2. **Inside:** Without adjusting your body position, rotate your exercising foot out. Bring your foot toward your buttocks by contracting your hamstring muscles. Keep your hips flat and your foot turned out. This isolates the muscles on the inside of the rear thigh. Pause and return slowly to the starting position in preparation for the next rep. There is no need to rest between repetitions.

3. **Outside:** Without adjusting your body position, rotate your exercising foot in. Bring your foot toward your buttocks by contracting your hamstring muscles. Keep your hips flat and your foot turned in. This isolates the muscles on the outside of the rear thigh. Pause and return slowly to the starting position in preparation for the next rep.

28. HIP EXTENSORS/HAMSTRINGS

Muscles You Strengthen: Muscles in the rear of your thighs that attach to the head of your gluteals at the fold of your buttocks

The Basic Lift: Extend your hip

Pace of Lifting: Up slowly, pause, down slowly

Equipment: Ankle weights

Reps: 10 right, 10 left

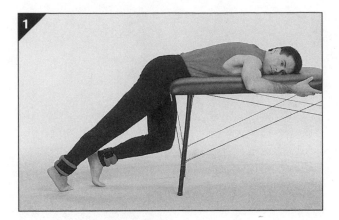

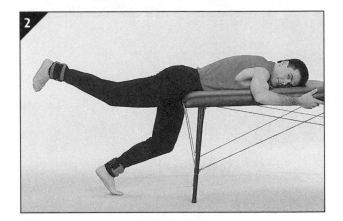

1. Put ankle weights around both ankles. Lean forward over a workout table or high bed with your hips poised right at the edge, your abdomen flat on the surface, and your feet flat on the floor.

   Bend your nonexercising leg to a 90-degree angle and let it relax. You should feel balanced and stable, but the leg should not support your weight. Straighten your exercising leg, extend it out behind you, and rotate it in from the hip, as shown.

2. With your foot turned inward and your knee straight, lift your exercising leg toward the ceiling, leading with your heel, until you feel the muscles in your buttocks engage, but not beyond parallel with your back and hips. Pause, lower your leg, and return slowly to the starting position in preparation for the next rep. There is no need to rest between repetitions. Keep it going. Work one leg at a time for the full 10 reps.

29. HIP ABDUCTORS

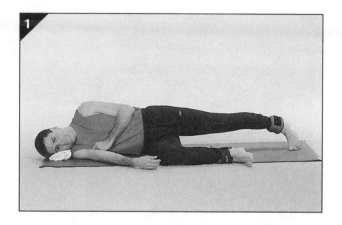

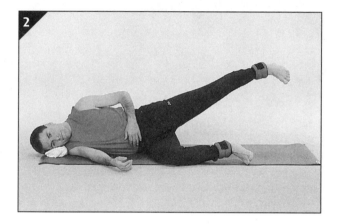

Muscles You Strengthen: Muscles in the top of your thighs from the top of your knee to your groin

The Basic Lift: Lying on your side, lift your leg toward the ceiling

Pace of Lifting: Up slowly, pause, down slowly

Equipment: Rolled towel or small pillow, ankle weights

Reps: 10 right, 10 left

1. Lie on your side on a flat surface with both legs extended and your body straight. Get comfortable by tucking a rolled towel or small pillow under your neck and head. Fasten weights on both ankles, but work only one leg at a time. Bend the knee of your bottom (nonexercising) leg 90 degrees toward your chest to take the pressure off your back and keep you from rolling. Keep the knee of your top (exercising) leg straight.

2. Lift your foot straight up toward the ceiling, leading with your heel. This keeps your leg internally rotated. When you have gone as far as you can go, pause, lower your leg, and return slowly to the starting position in preparation for the next rep. Be careful not to slam your toes to the floor. There is no need to rest between repetitions. Keep it going. Work one leg at a time for the full 10 reps.

30. HIP ADDUCTORS

Muscles You Strengthen: Muscles in the insides of your thighs from your knee to the top of your groin area

The Basic Lift: Lying on your side, lift your inner thigh toward midline

Pace of Lifting: Up slowly, pause, down slowly

Equipment: Rolled towel or small pillow; ankle weights; coffee table, chair, or some other stable surface of moderate height next to which you can lie

Reps: 10 right, 10 left

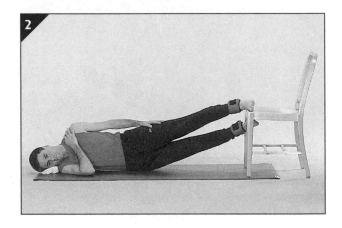

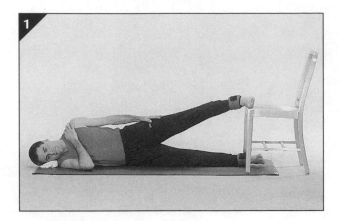

1. Lie on your side on a flat surface with both knees straight and legs extended straight out. Get comfortable by tucking a rolled towel or small pillow under your neck and head. Fasten the weights around both ankles. Your bottom leg will be your exercising leg until you roll over. Lift your top leg and rest your foot or ankle on a low, stable surface such as a chair. Your top leg should be approximately at a 45-degree angle to the floor. Contract your abdominals to keep from rolling and to stabilize your torso.

2. Contract your inner thigh muscles to bring your exercising leg up to meet your top leg. Keep your knee locked. Pause, lower your leg, and return slowly to the starting position in preparation for the next rep. There is no need to rest between repetitions. Keep it going. Work one leg at a time for the full 10 reps and then roll over.

31. GLUTEALS

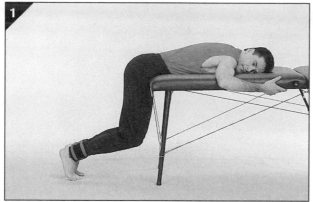

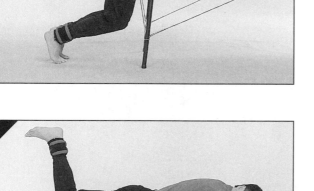

Muscles You Strengthen: Buttocks

The Basic Lift: Bend your knee and extend your hip

Pace of Lifting: Up slowly, pause, down slowly

Equipment: Ankle weights

Reps: 10 right, 10 left

1. Put the ankle weights around both ankles. Lean forward over a workout table or bed with your hips poised right at the edge, your abdomen flat on the surface, and your feet flat on the floor. Bend your nonexercising leg to a 90-degree angle and let it relax. You should feel balanced and stable, but the leg should not support your weight or serve as a brace. Bend your exercising leg to 90 degrees, as shown, and let it do all the work. Hold the angle.

2. Lift your leg up, leading with the foot and your heel aimed toward the ceiling, until you feel your gluteals engage. You should be able to get your thigh parallel with your hips. Pause, lower your leg, and return slowly to the starting position in preparation for the next rep. There is no need to rest between repetitions. Keep it going. Work one leg at a time for the full 10 reps.

32. HIP EXTERNAL ROTATORS

Muscles You Strengthen: Deep muscles in your buttocks that externally rotate your hips

The Basic Lift: From a seated position, rotate your hips internally and rotate your thighbone externally (or laterally)

Pace of Lifting: Up slowly, pause, down slowly (This is a strengthening stretch.)

Equipment: Rolled towel, ankle weights, stretch rope

Reps: 10 right, 10 left

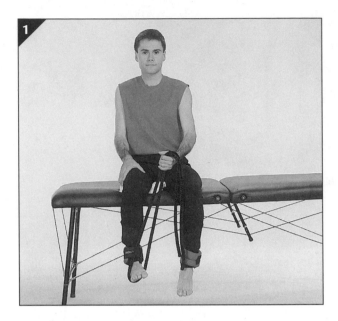

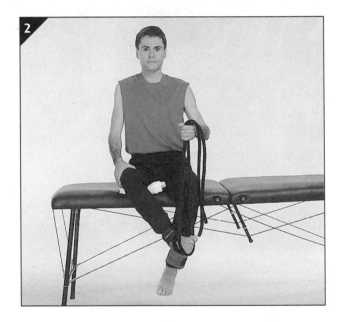

1. Sit on a bed or table with the backs of your knees at the edge and your lower legs relaxed and dangling. Fasten the weights around both ankles. Place a rolled towel under the knee of your exercising leg to take the strain off. Loop your rope around the arch of the foot of your exercising leg with the loose ends to the inside. Hold the rope with the hand on the opposite side of your body and gently lift up to remove slack and snug it up. Place your other hand (on the same side as your exercising leg) on the top of your thigh just above the knee. Squeeze and press your thumb on the inside to stabilize your leg and to assist in the rotation. Keep the nonexercising leg relaxed.

2. Rotate your lower exercising leg toward the midline of your body, leading with your foot like a pendulum. Go as far as you can. At the end of the move, assist by pulling upward on the rope to extend your range of motion. Pause. (Added benefit: You'll get a good Active-Isolated stretch.) Relax the tension on the rope and slowly return to the starting position in preparation for the next rep. There is no need to rest between repetitions. Keep it going. Work one leg at a time for the full 10 reps.

33. HIP INTERNAL ROTATORS

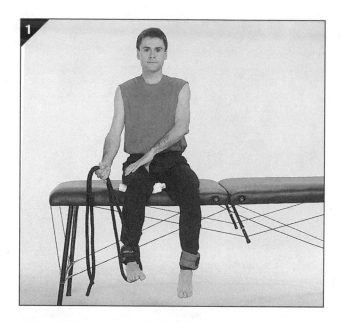

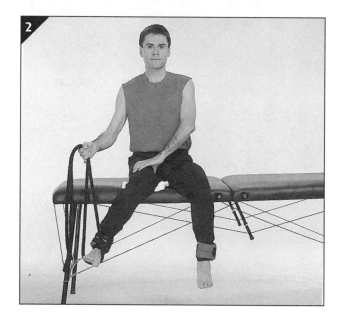

Muscles You Strengthen: Deep muscles in your buttocks that internally rotate your hips

The Basic Lift: From a seated position, rotate your hips externally and rotate your thighbone internally (or medially)

Pace of Lifting: Up slowly, pause, down slowly (This is a strengthening stretch.)

Equipment: Rolled towel, ankle weights, stretch rope

Reps: 10 right, 10 left

1. Sit on a bed or table with the backs of your knees at the edge and your lower legs relaxed and dangling. Fasten the weights around both ankles. Place a rolled towel under the knee of your exercising leg to take the strain off. Loop your rope around the arch of the foot of your exercising leg with the loose ends to the outside. Hold the rope with the hand on the same side of your body and gently lift up to remove slack and snug it up. Place your other hand (on the opposite side as your exercising leg) on the top of your thigh just above the knee. Squeeze and press your thumb on the inside to stabilize your leg and to assist in the rotation. Keep your nonexercising leg relaxed.

2. Rotate your lower exercising leg away the midline of your body, leading with your foot like a pendulum. Go as far as you can. At the end of the move, assist by pulling upward on the rope to extend your range of motion. Pause. (Added benefit: You'll get a good Active-Isolated stretch.) Relax the tension on the rope and slowly return to the starting position in preparation for the next rep. There is no need to rest between reps. Keep it going. Work one leg at a time for the full 10 reps.

34. SACROSPINALIS

Muscles You Strengthen: Lower back

The Basic Lift: Extend both hips with straight legs

Pace of Lifting: Up slowly, pause, down slowly

Equipment: Ankle weights, rolled towel

Reps: 10, right and left simultaneously

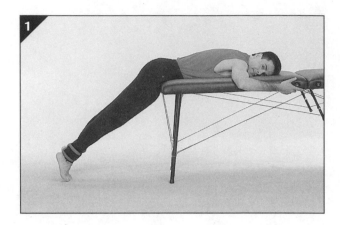

1. Put your feet together and fasten one ankle weight around each of them. Bend over a bed or table with your pelvis at the edge, your abdomen on the surface, and your feet on the floor. Grip the edge of the table to stabilize your body. Straighten your legs. Lock your knees.

2. Leading with your heels, lift your legs toward the ceiling until you feel the muscles in your buttocks (gluteals) engage. Lift as far as you can go. Pause. Slowly return to the starting position in preparation for the next rep. There is no need to rest between repetitions. Keep it going. Work both legs for the full 10 reps.

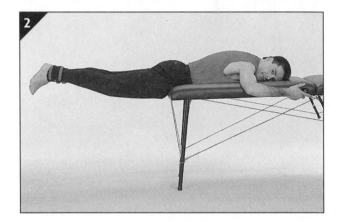

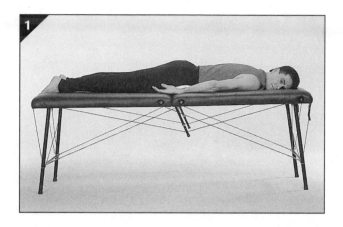

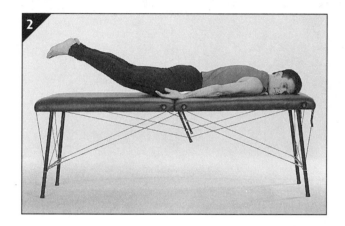

MODIFICATION

1. **Note:** If you're a beginner and your back is not yet strong, place a rolled towel or a pillow under your hips to take pressure off your back. Lie on your abdomen on a surface that supports your entire body, from the top of your head to the tips of your toes. Use no ankle weights. Place your arms against your body at your sides. Relax everything above your waist. Straighten your legs and point your toes. Lock your knees.

2. Lift your legs gently off the surface until you feel the muscles in your buttocks (gluteals) engage. Don't use your back. Keep it relaxed. Lift as far as you're able without discomfort. Pause. Slowly return to the starting position in preparation for the next rep. There is no need to rest between repetitions. Keep it going. Work both legs simultaneously for the full 10 reps.

35. UPPER ABDOMINALS

Muscles You Strengthen: Muscles in your upper abdomen

The Basic Lift: Flex your trunk with bent knees

Pace of Lifting: Up slowly, pause, down slowly

Equipment: Heavy furniture or a companion to hold your feet down. When you are advanced, you can hold an ankle weight in your hands against your chest to add more resistance.

Reps: 10

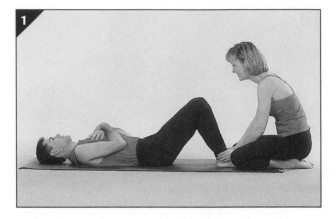

1. Lie flat on a surface. Bend your knees and tuck your feet under something that will help you keep them firmly down. Fold your hands across your chest and very gently tuck your chin in. This tucking action will lift the back of your head off the surface.

2. Translate the "tuck" into a continuous roll. Roll up slowly until your back is vertical and you are sitting up with your chest at your knees. Pause and then roll slowly back down, placing one vertebra at a time on the surface until your head is back down and you're relaxed. Prepare for the next rep. There is no need to rest between repetitions. Keep it going. Use a folded towel or a mat under your fanny if you're uncomfortable.

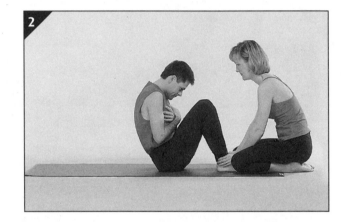

MODIFICATION

1. **Note:** If you're just beginning or are unable to do this exercise as we have described it, you can modify the move. If you are able, tuck your chin until your head leaves the surface and you feel your abdominals contract. Don't roll up. Just contract. Keep your back flat on the surface. Pause and then roll slowly back until your head is down and you're relaxed. Prepare for the next rep. There is no need to rest between repetitions. Keep it going.

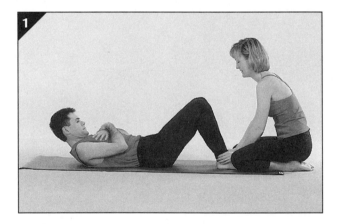

TRY PREHAB, NOT REHAB

36. OBLIQUE ABDOMINALS

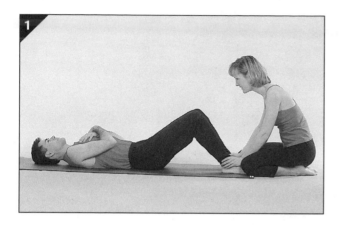

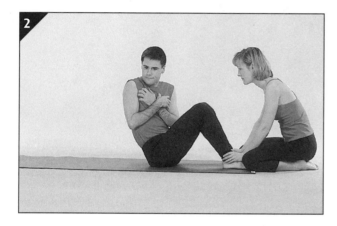

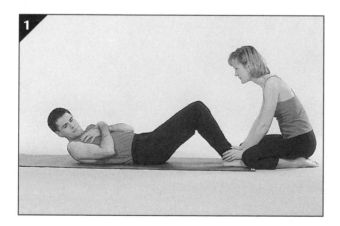

Muscles You Strengthen: Muscles on the sides of your abdomen

The Basic Lift: Flex your trunk with bent knees and rotate your torso

Pace of Lifting: Up slowly, pause, down slowly

Equipment: Heavy furniture or a companion to hold your feet down. When you are advanced, you can hold an ankle weight in your hands against your chest to add more resistance.

Reps: 10

1. Lie flat on a surface. Bend your knees and tuck your feet under something that will help you keep them firmly down. Fold your hands over your chest. Tuck your chin toward your chest. Rotate your torso to one side.

2. Roll up slowly until you're upright and can go no farther. When you can go no farther, pause and then, still in rotation, roll slowly back down, placing one vertebra at a time on the surface until your back is flat and your head is back down on the floor. Relax for a moment and then rotate again to the opposite side and begin an upward roll. There is no need to rest between reps. Keep it going. Use a folded towel or a mat under your fanny if you're uncomfortable.

MODIFICATION

1. **Note:** If you're just beginning or are unable to do this exercise as we have described it, you can modify the move. If you are able, rotate your torso and lift until your head leaves the surface and you feel your oblique abdominals engage. Don't roll up. Just contract. Keep your back flat on the surface. Pause and then, keeping your torso in rotation, roll slowly back down until the side of your back is flat, your head is back down, and you're relaxed. Prepare for the next rep on the opposite side. There is no need to rest between repetitions. Keep it going.

37. LOWER ABDOMINALS

Muscles You Strengthen: Muscles in your lower abdomen

The Basic Lift: Curl up, leading with your pelvis

Pace of Lifting: Up slowly, pause, down slowly

Equipment: Heavy furniture or a companion to support your weight. When you are advanced, you can strap an ankle weight to both ankles to add more resistance.

Reps: 10

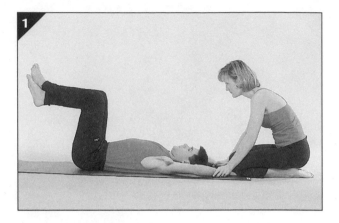

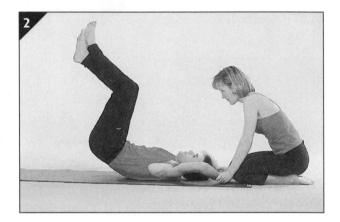

1. Lie flat on your back on a level surface. Bend your knees to get the tension off your back. Cross your feet at the ankles to focus your center of gravity, stabilize your torso, and help you isolate muscles. Reach back over your head and slip your hands under something heavy that will lock you down and resist your weight as you lift. Bring your knees up until your upper legs are perpendicular to the surface with which your lower legs are parallel. Your knees will be at 90-degree angles.

2. Pause for a second to make sure you're balanced and stable, and then thrust your lower body straight up toward the ceiling. Your buttocks will follow your knees and feet, and you'll feel your lower abdominals engage. When you're up as far as you can go and you're up on your shoulders, roll forward slightly. Pause and then return slowly to the starting position. Remember to keep your knees bent and resist the temptation to arch your back. There is no need to rest between repetitions. Keep it going. Use a folded towel or a mat under your fanny if you're uncomfortable.

Note: If you're just beginning or are unable to do this exercise as we have described it, you can modify the move. Lie flat on a surface. For a little more resistance, you can place your ankle weight on your abdomen right below your belly button. Bend your knees and place your feet flat. Keep your back on the surface, contract your lower abdominals, tilt your pelvis slightly, and lift your buttocks 2 to 3 inches. Pause. Slowly return to the starting position.

38. TRUNK EXTENSORS AND ROTATORS

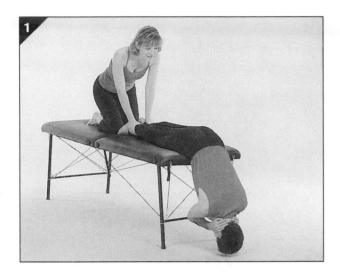

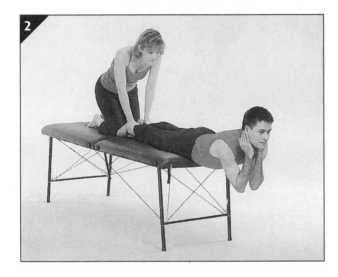

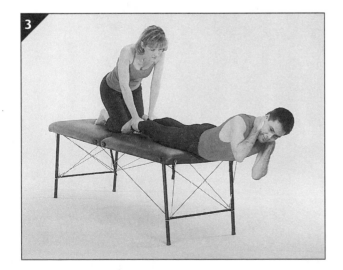

Muscles You Strengthen: All the muscles of your back

The Basic Lift: Roll your shoulder blades up toward the ceiling, like flying

Pace of Lifting: Up slowly, pause, down slowly

Equipment: You need a helper with this one.

Reps: 10 of each position—straight, right, left

1. You need help with this one! Lie flat on your stomach on a bed or a table and hang over the edge from your waist up. (In other words, your legs and pelvis are on the surface and your upper body is draped over the edge, head toward the floor.) You need a helper to hold your lower legs or ankles so that you won't slide onto the floor and to give you leverage so that you can lift your own weight without flipping off. Place your hands on your cheeks and tuck your elbows in tight. (Tucking your elbows in immobilizes traps and rhomboids—two muscle groups that rush to assist a lazy and ever-weakening mid- and lower back.) Relax and tuck your head down.

2. Lift your upper body up from your waist until you're cantilevered straight out. Hold your position. Lift your head. Pause. Slowly lower yourself back to the starting position.

3. Rotate your upper torso to one side as far as you can and lift your upper body while still in rotation. Pause. Return to starting position slowly. Rotate to opposite side and repeat.

Note: If your back is weak, or you don't have a partner to help you, you can modify this exercise. Lie flat on your stomach with your arms at your sides. Relax everything below your waist. Lift your head and chest off the surface and roll your shoulders back as far as you're able without discomfort. Your back will be arched. Hold for a moment and then slowly lower yourself back to the starting position.

39. TRUNK LATERAL FLEXORS

Muscles You Strengthen: Sides of your back

The Basic Lift: Lifting your trunk up from the side

Pace of Lifting: Up slowly, pause, down slowly

Equipment: You need a helper with this one.

Reps: 10 right, 10 left

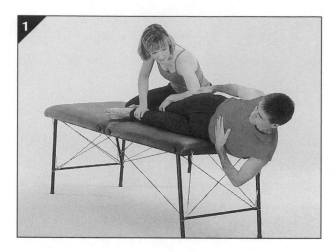

1. Lie on your side on a bed or a table. With a partner holding your lower calves and ankles, scoot over the edge until you are cantilevered straight off the surface from your waist. Keep your top arm and hand straight and on your side. Tuck your lower arm out of the way by putting your hand on your chest.

2. Bend and lower your torso, leading with your head, toward the floor. Remember to keep your body relaxed and in alignment. Go down as far as possible. You'll feel a stretch along your side. Slowly lift your upper torso back up until your body is back in a straight line. Lift your head and rotate to the side at the end of the movement. Pause. Repeat by lowering your torso slowly.

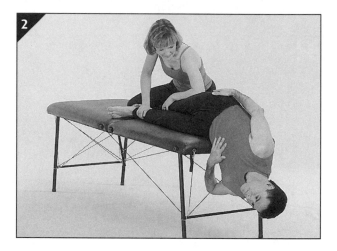

40. DELTOIDS

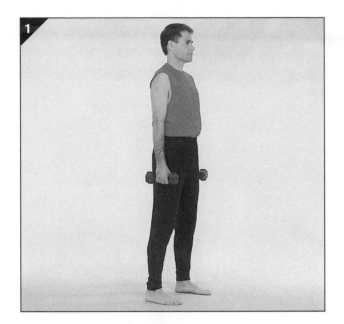

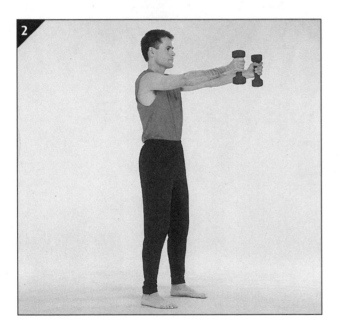

Muscles You Strengthen: Fronts of your shoulders, your upper back and middle shoulders, and backs of your shoulders and upper arms

The Basic Lift: Lifting your arms in sequence: up and forward, up and sideways, and up and backward

Pace of Lifting: Up slowly, pause, down slowly

Equipment: Handheld weights or ankle weights held in your hands

Reps: 10 of each of the three parts in the sequence

This exercise is done in three steps. Do 10 of each lift in sequence: forward, sideways, backward. When you have completed 10 of each of the three parts in sequence, this constitutes one set. There is no need to rest between sets unless you feel fatigued.

1. **Shoulder front:** Sit or stand. If you choose to stand, slightly bend your knees and tighten your abdominals to stabilize your back. Get a good grip on your weights, with your palms facing the midline of your body. Lift with both shoulders at the same time.

2. With your arms straight at your sides, slowly swing the weights straight up from your shoulders in arcs in front of you until they're level with your shoulders. Pause and then slowly return to the starting position. Hold your form and control the weights on the way back down.

(continued)

3. Upper back and middle shoulder: Stay in position. With your arms hanging straight down, the palms of your hands facing toward the midline of your body, and your elbows locked, slowly bring the weights out to the side and up to shoulder level. Pause and then slowly return to the starting position. Hold your form and control the weights on the way back down.

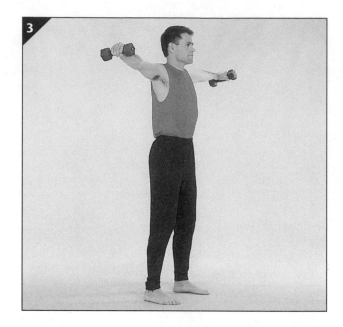

4. Backs of the shoulders and upper arms: Stay in position. With your back straight and relaxed, bend slightly forward at the waist. Dangle your arms straight down with the palms of your hands facing toward the midline of your body and your elbows locked.

Slowly arc your arms behind you and up, as shown, lifting the weights back as far as possible—maybe even beyond shoulder level. Pause and then slowly return to the starting position. Hold your form and control the weights on the way back down.

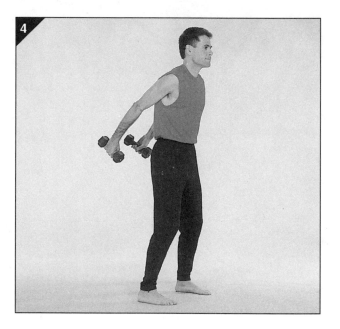

TRY PREHAB, NOT REHAB

41. PECTORALIS MAJORS

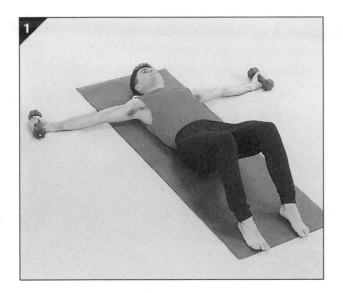

Muscles You Strengthen: Front of your chest

The Basic Lift: Lifting your arms straight up from a supine position

Pace of Lifting: Up slowly, pause, down slowly

Equipment: Rolled towel or small pillow, hand-held weights or ankle weights held in your hands

Reps: 10, right and left simultaneously

1. Lie face up on a surface with your knees bent and re-laxed and your feet flat. Tuck a rolled towel or small pillow under your neck and head. With weights in each hand, extend your arms straight out to your sides with your elbows locked and your palms up.

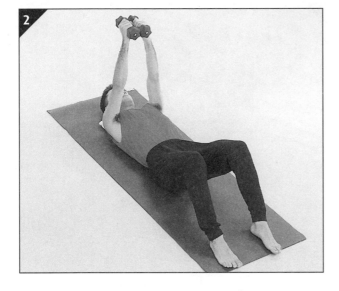

2. Lift from both sides at the same time and with equal weights. Bring your hands straight up toward the ceiling to meet above your face. Pause and then slowly return to the starting position. Hold your form and control the weights on the way back down.

42. TRICEPS—SUPINE POSITION

Muscles You Strengthen: Muscles in the backs of your upper arms

The Basic Lift: From supine position, extending your arms from bent elbow

Pace of Lifting: Down slowly, pause, up slowly

Equipment: Rolled towel or small pillow, hand-held weights or ankle weights held in your hands

Reps: 10, right and left simultaneously

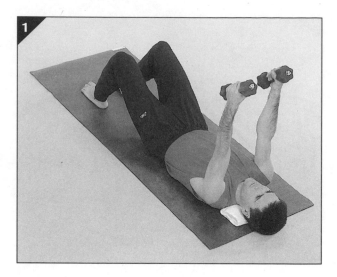

1. Lie face up on a surface with your knees bent and re-laxed, and your feet flat. Tuck a rolled towel or small pillow under your neck and head. Hold the weights up over your shoulders, perpendicular to the surface, with your palms facing to the midline of your body. Lock your elbows. Work both sides at the same time and with equal weights.

2. Bring the weights down by keeping your upper arm straight up and flexing your elbows until the weights are near the surface at your ears. Pause and then slowly return to the starting position. Hold your form and control the weights on the way back up. Be *very* careful when you are holding weight above your face. One false move will ruin your day.

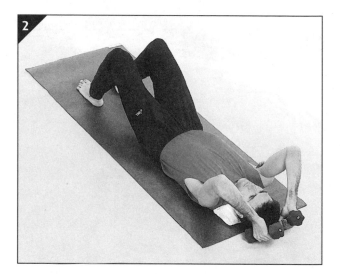

43. SHOULDER EXTERNAL ROTATORS

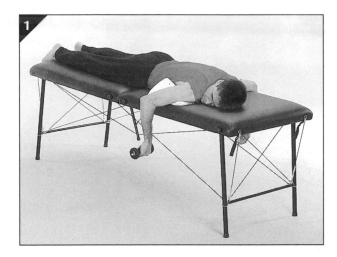

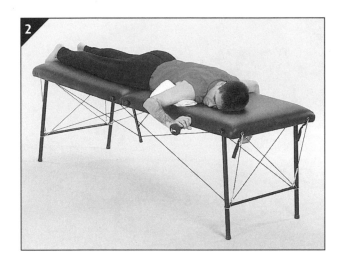

Muscles You Strengthen: Deep shoulder or rotator cuff

The Basic Lift: Externally rotate your shoulders

Pace of Lifting: Up slowly, pause, down slowly

Equipment: Handheld weights or ankle weights held in your hands, one or two rolled towels or small pillows

Reps: 10 right, 10 left (We assume that you will work one shoulder at a time. You can work out both sides simultaneously if your surface is very narrow and your weights are equal.)

1. Lie on your abdomen on a bed or a table. Place a rolled towel under your shoulder to take the strain off. Turn your head to one side and relax your neck. Extend your upper arm straight out from your shoulder over the edge and dangle your lower arm, hand holding a weight, toward the floor. Your elbow should be at 90 degrees with your knuckles facing forward.

2. Rotating from the shoulder, arc the weight straight up until it's level with your head. (Be *very* careful when you are swinging weight up toward your nose. Nothing ruins a perfectly good workout like a fracture.) Pause and then slowly return to the starting position. Hold your form and control the weight on the way back down.

44. SHOULDER INTERNAL ROTATORS

Muscles You Strengthen: Deep shoulder or rotator cuff, and sides of your chest

The Basic Lift: Internally rotate your shoulders

Pace of Lifting: Up slowly, pause, down slowly

Equipment: Handheld weights or ankle weights held in your hands, one or two rolled towels or small pillows

Reps: 10 right, 10 left (We assume that you will work one shoulder at a time. You can work out both sides simultaneously if your surface is very narrow and your weights are equal.)

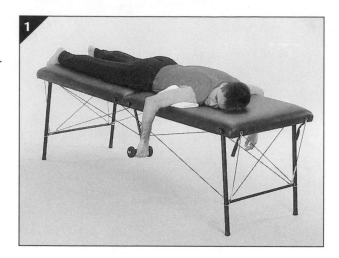

1. Lie on your abdomen on a bed or a table. Place a rolled towel under your shoulder to take the strain off. Turn your head to one side and relax your neck. Extend your upper arm straight out from your shoulder over the edge and dangle your lower arm, hand holding a weight, toward the floor. Your elbow should be at 90 degrees with your knuckles facing forward.

2. Lock your wrist and bring your hand straight back, leading with your palm as far back and up as you can go. (Resist recruiting back muscles to help lift this load. Beware the moment when your shoulder blade, your scapula, jacks up and your elbow moves skyward.) Pause and then slowly return to the starting position. Hold your form and control the weight on the way back down.

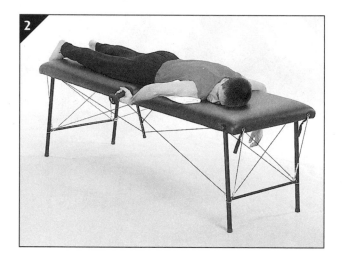

45. TRICEPS—PRONE POSITION

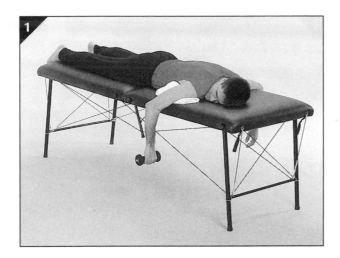

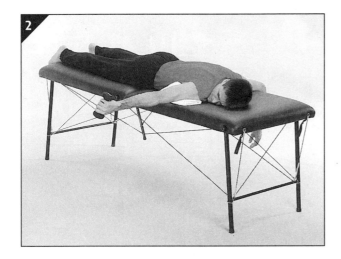

Muscles You Strengthen: Muscles in the backs of your upper arms

The Basic Lift: From face down, extending your elbows

Pace of Lifting: Up slowly, pause, down slowly

Equipment: Handheld weights or ankle weights held in your hands, one or two rolled towels or small pillows

Reps: 10 right, 10 left (We assume that you will work one shoulder at a time. You can work out both sides simultaneously if your surface is very narrow and your weights are equal.)

1. Lie on your abdomen on a bed or a table. Place a rolled towel under your shoulder to take the strain off. Turn your head to one side and relax your neck. Extend your upper arm straight out from your shoulder over the edge and dangle your lower arm, hand holding a weight, toward the floor. Your elbow should be at 90 degrees with your knuckles facing forward.

2. Lock your wrist, straighten out your elbow, and bring your hand straight out and up until your elbow is locked. Pause and then slowly return to the starting position. Hold your form and control the weight on the way back down.

46. TRAPEZIUS

Muscles You Strengthen: Outer group of muscles that stabilize and control your upper back, and the connection of your shoulder

The Basic Lift: From face down, lifting up and out from your shoulders

Pace of Lifting: Up slowly, pause, down slowly

Equipment: Handheld weights or ankle weights held in your hands

Reps: 10, right and left simultaneously

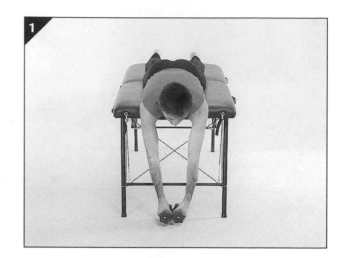

1. Lie on your abdomen on a bed or a table, and scoot your face and shoulders over the edge until you are suspended out as far as your armpits. You need to work both arms simultaneously. Make sure the weights in each hand are equal. Dangle your arms straight down from your shoulders. Keep your head and neck aligned straight with your body, and stay relaxed. Start with the weights directly below your nose. Keep your arms straight, your elbows locked, and your knuckles facing out.

2. Leading with your knuckles and rotating from your shoulders, arc the weights out to your sides and up as far as you can go. Pause and then slowly return to the starting position. Hold your form and control the weights on the way back down.

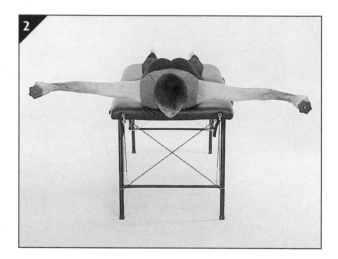

47. RHOMBOIDS

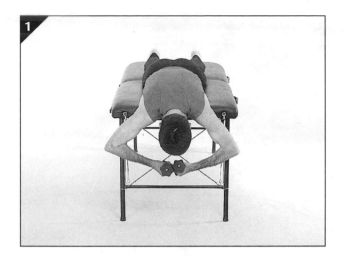

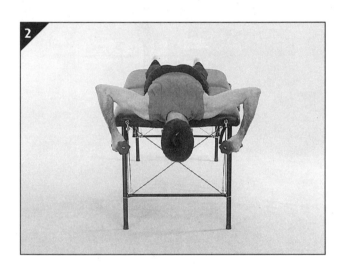

Muscles You Strengthen: Inner group of muscles that stabilize and control your upper back, and the connection of your shoulder

The Basic Lift: From face down and with elbows bent, lifting up and out from your shoulders

Pace of Lifting: Up slowly, pause, down slowly

Equipment: Handheld weights or ankle weights held in your hands

Reps: 10, right and left simultaneously

1. Lie on your abdomen on a bed or a table, and hang over the edge until you are suspended out as far as your armpits. You are going to work both arms simultaneously. Dangle your arms down over the edge. Relax your neck so that your head nods forward. Hold equal weight in each hand. Your knuckles should face each other, palms should face up, and your thumbs should point forward. Lock your elbows at 90-degree angles and bring the weights together until they touch.

2. Arc your locked elbows straight up toward the ceiling as far as you can go, separating the weights. Pause and then slowly return to the starting position. Hold your form and control the weights on the way back down.

48. BICEPS

Muscles You Strengthen: Fronts of your upper arms

The Basic Lift: Flex your elbow

Pace of Lifting: Up slowly, pause, down slowly

Equipment: Handheld weights or ankle weights held in your hands

Reps: 10, right and left simultaneously (As you progress to lifting heavier weight, you might prefer sitting to standing. You can work both arms at once with equal weights, or one at a time.)

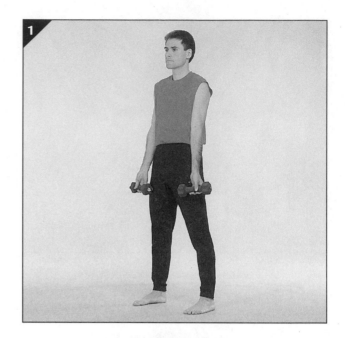

1. Stand on a flat surface with your feet apart and your knees relaxed. Start by holding the weights in your hands down at your sides with your elbows straight and your wrists locked. Your palms should be forward with your thumbs to the outside. To stabilize the lift, lock yourself into position by snugging your elbows tightly against your torso between your hipbones and waist.

2. Contract your biceps and slowly bend your elbows to bring the weights straight up in front of you to your shoulders. Keep your elbows and upper arms tightly against your body. Pause and then slowly return to the starting position. Hold your form and control the weights on the way back down.

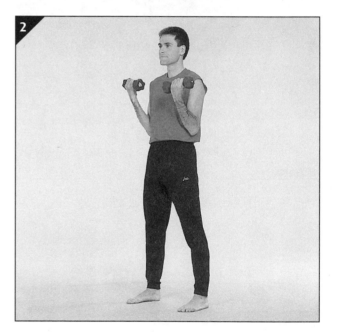

TRY PREHAB, NOT REHAB

49. SHOULDERS (THE ROLL)

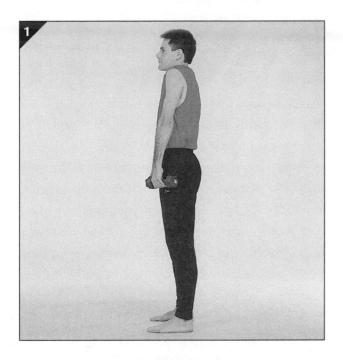

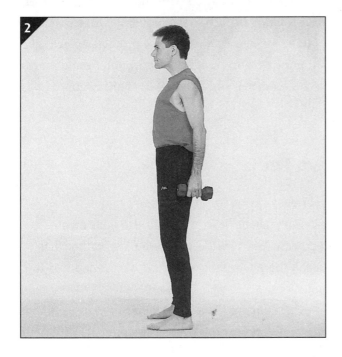

Muscles You Strengthen: Inner group of muscles that stabilize and control your upper back, and the connection of your shoulder

The Basic Lift: Rotate your shoulder joint

Pace of Lifting: This is a continuous roll.

Equipment: Handheld weights or ankle weights held in your hands

Reps: 10

1. Work both shoulders at the same time. Stand with your back straight and relaxed, feet slightly apart and knees slightly bent. Contract your abdominals for stability. Take a weight in each hand with your palms facing in and your thumbs facing forward. Hold your arms down at your sides. Straighten your elbows.

2. In a continuous, slow, and controlled motion, roll your shoulders forward, up, over, back, under, and down. You'll feel the pull in your shoulders and back through the resistance of the weights in your hands.

   The sequence of action will be: 1. Roll forward (lateral abduction); 2. Lift (elevation); 3. Roll backward (medial adduction); and 4. Lower or let down (inferior depression). For releasing tension, the most significant of the actions is rolling backward—when you adduct your shoulder blades (scapula). Be sure not to lose your focus through that one. Roll slowly and control the entire sequence. Pause between sequences and rest if you feel fatigued.

YOUR CARDIO PROGRAM

While there are nearly endless possibilities for boosting your heart rate for a good cardio workout, we've selected the most basic: walking. Despite being so basic that it's elemental to human activity, walking is a guaranteed butter-burning, blood-pumping, heart-pounding, energy-lifting, muscle-building, fat-melting, joint-pampering, metabolism-raising, mood-elevating workout. Unparalleled, in fact.

Dress so that you'll be comfortable and can move easily. When the weather is cool, you might start out dressed warmly and peel the layers down. You can tie your jacket or sweatshirt around your waist when it's too warm to wear.

Although you can walk barefoot—and many people do on the beach—most of us prefer shoes that are specifically designed for walking. If you don't have walking shoes, you can walk in *any* shoe that is comfortable and provides support. (See "Your Own Two Feet" below, for more suggestions on footwear.)

When enjoying your status as an "advanced" Active-Isolated-method athlete, try to remember a few of these suggestions.

Keep it simple. Walk as you normally do. Stride evenly and smoothly. Start off slowly, and gradually build to the pace at which you intend to walk. We suggest a good clip at a conversational pace, meaning that you can walk and still speak in full sentences without gasping between words.

When you're experienced, you can push this pace slightly so that conversation is a little more difficult, but still not impossible. Keep your torso upright, with your shoulders relaxed and back and your head up, so that you can get good deep breaths. Relax your hands and swing your arms rhythmically. As you speed up the pace, your arms will come up and "pump" energy into your stride. This means you're working. Good.

Be alert to your environment. Keep an eye on your walking surface so that you don't hit a rock or a pothole. Also, unless you're in a protected place (like an indoor track), remain alert to potential dangers such as cars that come too close, snarling guard dogs

---

Your Own Two Feet

When you shop for walking shoes, take along a pair of socks like the ones you intend to wear when you walk. Experts suggest that you try the shoes on at same time of day that you intend to do your walking workout, because the size of your foot may vary as much as half a size during the course of your day. When you find a pair of shoes you like, try on both shoes. Lace them all the way up, and walk around the sales floor. Put the shoes through their paces—slow, fast, left turn, right turn, pivot, and about-face. Don't be swayed by what they look like; evaluate shoes with

your eyes closed for at least a full minute. You care only about how they *feel.* Use your own judgment and buy the shoes you like, rather than taking the advice of a salesclerk whose job it is to sell shoes.

The right sock is a good investment in comfort and performance. You want a smooth, snug fit that's free from raised seams. Purchase socks that are designed to wick sweat away from your foot. This will prevent blistering, skin irritations, and odor. A clean pair of socks with every workout is a must.

who don't like your looks, and ill-intentioned strangers. If you walk a path and are nervous about people coming up behind you, walk the path in the opposite direction. You'll see everyone before they see you.

Carry identification. Carry a laminated I.D. card in your pocket, fanny pack, or shoe pocket. Or wear an I.D. tag around your neck. Include name, address, phone number, blood type, insurance information, and next of kin's name, address, and phone number. We're not trying to be alarmists, but in case of an accident, you'll want emergency personnel to know who you are, instead of referring to you as "that stranger in nylon shorts and a T-shirt."

Consider "filing a flight plan." Let someone know where you're going and when you'll be back. If you don't show up when you're supposed to, someone will know and be able to send out scouts.

Entertain yourself. If walking isn't stimulating enough for you and listening to books or music is fun, try a tape player or a CD player designed for working out. Look for a CD player with a no-skip feature so that the sound won't chatter as you jostle it. Leave one earpiece off so that you can stay attuned and alert to your surroundings.

If you are listening to music, make sure it has a beat that's in sync with your pace. It's nearly impossible to clip along when you're listening to Zen chants or to keep a slow pace when you're listening to salsa. Just make sure that you're matched in rhythms. As far as recorded books, select anything you're interested in, and enjoy.

Observe track etiquette. If you walk on a track, remember that walkers are "low men on the totem pole" among athletes who use the track. Be courteous and safe, and walk in a counterclockwise direction in the far outside lane, leaving the inside lanes for the runners. If you hear someone coming up behind you yelling, "Track!" you are being told that someone is trying to pass you, and you are being asked to get out of the way.

Drink water. Be sure to hydrate before, during, and after your walk.

Leave your weights at home. Do not carry hand weights. They don't add any benefit to walking and, in fact, may even be harmful during the unpredictable ups and downs of a cardio workout.

Bring a pal. Take your dog. Invite friends and family. Turn these brief moments of invigorating exercise into a mobile social club. Walking is wonderful fun to share.

YOUR COMPLETE PROGRAM

You now have all the facets to your complete program. We've assembled an at-a-glance chart so that you can see your workouts for each phase of our plan. (See pages 98 to 105 for details of each workout.) Phase 1, the beginning 6 weeks, emphasizes Active-Isolated Stretching. Phase 2, the intermediate 6 weeks, increases the number of Active-Isolated Strengthening workouts. Phase 3, the advanced 6 weeks, completes the program by adding cardio for total-body conditioning. There you have it—flexibility, strength, and cardiovascular endurance—your complete fitness program for a healthy back.

Phase 1: Beginning 6 Weeks

	Sunday	Monday	Tuesday	Wednesday	Thursday	Friday	Saturday
1	Rest	Stretch 1 & 2	Stretch 1 & 2	Stretch 1 & 2	Stretch 1 & 2	Stretch 1 & 2	Stretch 1 & 2
Notes:							
2	Rest	Stretch 1 & 2	Stretch 1 & 2	Stretch 1 & 2	Stretch 1 & 2	Stretch 1 & 2	Stretch 1 & 2
Notes:							
3	Rest	Stretch 1 & 2	Stretch 1 & 2	Stretch 1 & 2	Stretch 1 & 2	Stretch 1 & 2	Stretch 1 & 2
Notes:							
4	Rest	Stretch 1 / Strength 1	Stretch 1 / Strength 2	Stretch 1 / Strength 3	Stretch 1 / Strength 1	Stretch 1 / Strength 2	Stretch 1 / Strength 3
Notes: Now that your joints are opened up to a greater range of motion, add strengthening to the workouts this week.							
5	Rest	Stretch 1 / Strength 1	Stretch 1 / Strength 2	Stretch 1 / Strength 3	Stretch 1 / Strength 1	Stretch 1 / Strength 2	Stretch 1 / Strength 3
Notes:							
6	Rest	Stretch 1 / Strength 1	Stretch 1 / Strength 2	Stretch 1 / Strength 3	Stretch 1 / Strength 1	Stretch 1 / Strength 2	Stretch 1 / Strength 3
Notes:							

Phase 2: Intermediate 6 Weeks

	Sunday	Monday	Tuesday	Wednesday	Thursday	Friday	Saturday
7	Rest	Stretch 1 Strength 1	Stretch 1 Strength 2	Stretch 1 Strength 3	Stretch 1 Strength 1	Stretch 1 Strength 2	Stretch 1 Strength 3
Notes:							
8	Rest	Stretch 1 Strength 1	Stretch 1 Strength 2	Stretch 1 Strength 3	Stretch 1 Strength 1	Stretch 1 Strength 2	Stretch 1 Strength 3
Notes:							
9	Rest	Stretch 1 Strength 1	Stretch 1 Strength 2	Stretch 1 Strength 3	Stretch 1 Strength 1	Stretch 1 Strength 2	Stretch 1 Strength 3
Notes:							
10	Rest	Stretch 1 Strength 1	Stretch 1 & 2 (no strengthening)	Stretch 1 Strength 2	Stretch 1 & 2 (no strengthening)	Stretch 1 Strength 3	Stretch 1 & 2 (no strengthening)
Notes:							
11	Rest	Stretch 1 Strength 1	Stretch 1 Strength 2	Stretch 1 Strength 3	Stretch 1 Strength 1	Stretch 1 Strength 2	Stretch 1 Strength 3
Notes:							
12	Rest	Stretch 1 Strength 1	Stretch 1 Strength 2	Stretch 1 Strength 3	Stretch 1 Strength 1	Stretch 1 Strength 2	Stretch 1 Strength 3
Notes:							

Phase 3: Advanced 6 Weeks

	Sunday	Monday	Tuesday	Wednesday	Thursday	Friday	Saturday
13	Rest	Stretch 1 Strength 1 Cardio (20 minutes)	Stretch 1 & 2 Strength 2	Stretch 1 Strength 3 Cardio (20 minutes)	Stretch 1 & 2 Strength 1	Stretch 1 Strength 2 Cardio (20 minutes)	Stretch 1 & 2 Strength 3

Notes: Add cardio 20 minutes a day, 3 days a week.

	Sunday	Monday	Tuesday	Wednesday	Thursday	Friday	Saturday
14	Rest	Stretch 1 Strength 1 Cardio (25 minutes)	Stretch 1 & 2 Strength 2	Stretch 1 Strength 3 Cardio (25 minutes)	Stretch 1 & 2 Strength 1	Stretch 1 Strength 2 Cardio (25 minutes)	Stretch 1 & 2 Strength 3

Notes: Add cardio 25 minutes a day, 3 days a week.

	Sunday	Monday	Tuesday	Wednesday	Thursday	Friday	Saturday
15	Rest	Stretch 1 Strength 1 Cardio (30 minutes)	Stretch 1 & 2 Strength 2	Stretch 1 Strength 3 Cardio (30 minutes)	Stretch 1 & 2 Strength 1	Stretch 1 Strength 2 Cardio (30 minutes)	Stretch 1 & 2 Strength 3

Notes: Add cardio 30 minutes a day, 3 days a week.

	Sunday	Monday	Tuesday	Wednesday	Thursday	Friday	Saturday
16	Rest	Stretch 1 Strength 1	Stretch 1 & 2 Cardio (30 minutes)	Stretch 1 Strength 2	Stretch 1 & 2 Cardio (30 minutes)	Stretch 1 Strength 3	Stretch 1 & 2 Cardio (30 minutes)

Notes: Do strengthening three times this week. Add cardio 30 minutes a day, 3 days a week.

	Sunday	Monday	Tuesday	Wednesday	Thursday	Friday	Saturday
17	Rest	Stretch 1 Strength 1 Cardio (30 minutes)	Stretch 1 & 2 Strength 2	Stretch 1 Strength 3 Cardio (30 minutes)	Stretch 1 & 2 Strength 1	Stretch 1 Strength 2 Cardio (30 minutes)	Stretch 1 & 2 Strength 3

Notes:

	Sunday	Monday	Tuesday	Wednesday	Thursday	Friday	Saturday
18	Rest	Stretch 1 Strength 1 Cardio (30 minutes)	Stretch 1 & 2 Strength 2	Stretch 1 Strength 3 Cardio (30 minutes)	Stretch 1 & 2 Strength 1	Stretch 1 Strength 2 Cardio (30 minutes)	Stretch 1 & 2 Strength 3

Notes:

Training Log

(Photocopy for your use)

Dates_____ Week number_____

	Sunday	Monday	Tuesday	Wednesday	Thursday	Friday	Saturday
Stretch 1							
Stretch 2							

	Sunday		Monday		Tuesday		Wednesday		Thursday		Friday		Saturday	
		weight		weight		weight		weight		weight		weight		weight
Strength 1														
Strength 2														
Strength 3														

	Sunday	Monday	Tuesday	Wednesday	Thursday	Friday	Saturday
Cardio Training							
Time							
Route and Remarks							

	Sunday	Monday	Tuesday	Wednesday	Thursday	Friday	Saturday
Drank My Water							

Progress Update and Notes

_____

_____

_____

_____

_____

_____

Instructions

1. Stretching. Check the box when you have done the work.

2. Strengthening. Check the box and record the pounds of weight you used when you have done the work.

3. Cardio training. Check the box when you have done the work, record the amount of time you walked, and make notes about your route, the weather, and how you felt.

4. Water. Check the box to note that you drank eight full glasses of water.

STRETCH 1: Active-Isolated Stretching (Hip and Trunk)

This workout is the foundation of the Active-Isolated Stretching method and is featured in each week of the plan. Follow each exercise in the order specified here. (See pages 39 to 51 for detailed instructions.)

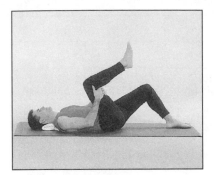

1. SINGLE-LEG PELVIC TILTS

Hold Each Stretch: 2 seconds

Reps: 10 right, 10 left

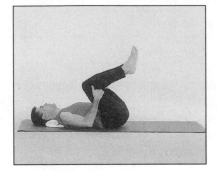

2. DOUBLE-LEG PELVIC TILTS

Hold Each Stretch: 2 seconds

Reps: 10

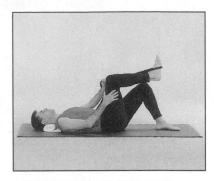

3. BENT-LEG HAMSTRINGS

Hold Each Stretch: 2 seconds

Reps: 10 right, 10 left

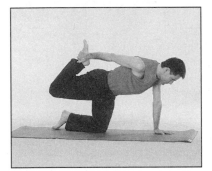

7. PSOAS

Hold Each Stretch: 2 seconds

Reps: 10 right, 10 left

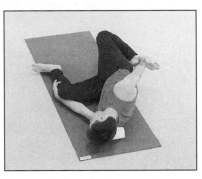

8. QUADRICEPS

Hold Each Stretch: 2 seconds

Reps: 10 right, 10 left

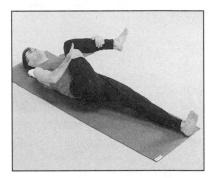

9. GLUTEALS

Hold Each Stretch: 2 seconds

Reps: 10 right, 10 left

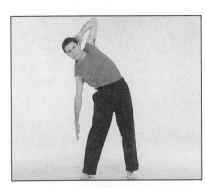

13. TRUNK L ATERAL FLEXORS

Hold Each Stretch: 2 seconds

Reps: 10 right, 10 left

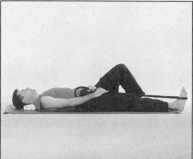

4. STRAIGHT-LEG HAMSTRINGS

Hold Each Stretch: 2 seconds

Reps: 10 right, 10 left

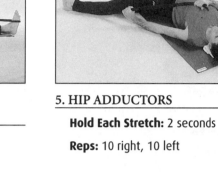

5. HIP ADDUCTORS

Hold Each Stretch: 2 seconds

Reps: 10 right, 10 left

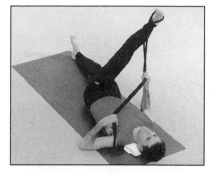

6. HIP ABDUCTORS

Hold Each Stretch: 2 seconds

Reps: 10 right, 10 left

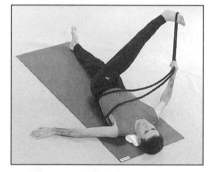

10. PIRIFORMIS

Hold Each Stretch: 2 seconds

Reps: 10 right, 10 left

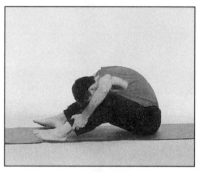

11. TRUNK EXTENSORS

Hold Each Stretch: 2 seconds

Reps: 10

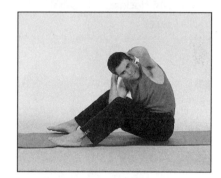

12. THORACIC-LUMBAR ROTATORS

Hold Each Stretch: 2 seconds

Reps: 10 right, 10 left

STRETCH 2: Active-Isolated Stretching (Shoulders and Neck)

The plans on pages 94 to 96 will tell you when to do this workout, which is essential for keeping your upper body limber. Follow the exercises in the order specified here. (See pages 52 to 62 for detailed instructions.)

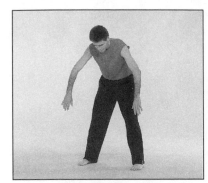

14. SHOULDER CIRCUMDUCTION

Hold Each Stretch: Technically, there is no stretch here.

Reps: 10 clockwise, 10 counter-clockwise

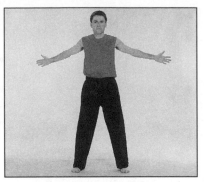

15. PECTORALIS MAJORS

Hold Each Stretch: 2 seconds

Reps: 10

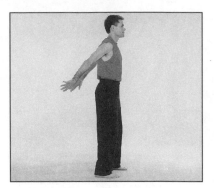

16. ANTERIOR DELTOIDS

Hold Each Stretch: 2 seconds

Reps: 10

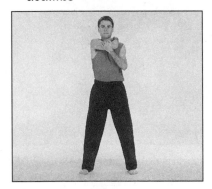

20. ROTATOR CUFF 2 (TRAPEZIUS)

Hold Each Stretch: 2 seconds

Reps: 10 right, 10 left

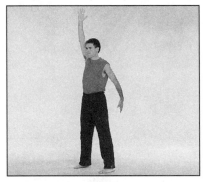

21. FORWARD ELEVATORS OF THE SHOULDER

Hold Each Stretch: 2 seconds

Reps: 10 right, 10 left (in opposition)

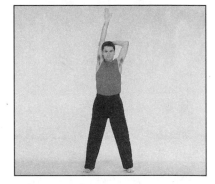

22. SIDE ELEVATORS OF THE SHOULDER

Hold Each Stretch: 2 seconds

Reps: 10 right, 10 left

TRY PREHAB, NOT REHAB

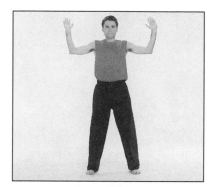

17. SHOULDER INTERNAL ROTATORS

Hold Each Stretch: 2 seconds

Reps: 10

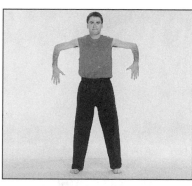

18. SHOULDER EXTERNAL ROTATORS

Hold Each Stretch: 2 seconds

Reps: 10

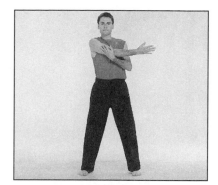

19. ROTATOR CUFF 1 (RHOMBOIDS)

Hold Each Stretch: 2 seconds

Reps: 10 right, 10 left

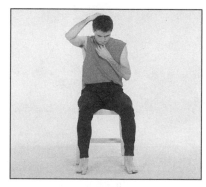

23. NECK EXTENSORS

Hold Each Stretch: 2 seconds

Reps: 10

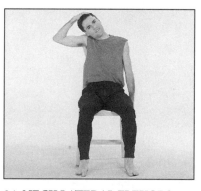

24. NECK LATERAL FLEXORS

Hold Each Stretch: 2 seconds

Reps: 10 right, 10 left

STRENGTH 1: Active-Isolated Strengthening (Muscles below the Belt Line)

You'll start this workout during the fourth week and continue through all three phases of your plan, as prescribed on pages 94 to 96. Perform the exercises in the order specified here. (See pages 64 to 73 for detailed instructions.)

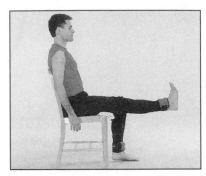

25. QUADRICEPS—KNEE EXTENSORS

Reps: 10 right, 10 left

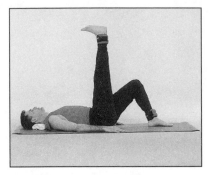

26. QUADRICEPS—HIP FLEXORS

Reps: 12 right, 12 left
(Remember: three positions!)

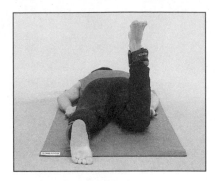

27. HAMSTRINGS

Reps: 12 right, 12 left
(Remember: three positions!)

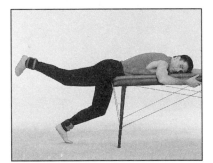

28. HIP EXTENSORS AND HAMSTRINGS

Reps: 10 right, 10 left

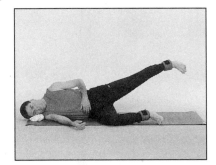

29. HIP ABDUCTORS

Reps: 10 right, 10 left

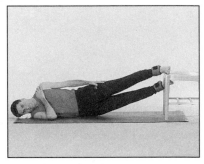

30. HIP ADDUCTORS

Reps: 10 right, 10 left

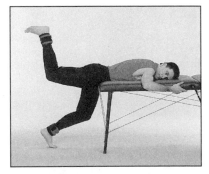

31. GLUTEALS

Reps: 10 right, 10 left

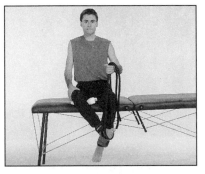

32. HIP EXTERNAL ROTATORS

Reps: 10 right, 10 left

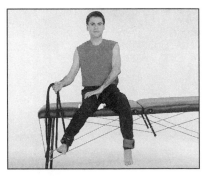

33. HIP INTERNAL ROTATORS

Reps: 10 right, 10 left

STRENGTH 2: Active-Isolated Strengthening (Muscles in the Pelvic Core)

You'll start this workout during the fourth week and continue through all three phases of your plan, as prescribed on pages 94 to 96. Follow the exercises in the order specified here. (See pages 74 to 80 for detailed instructions.)

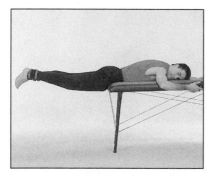

34. SACROSPINALIS

Reps: 10, right and left simultaneously

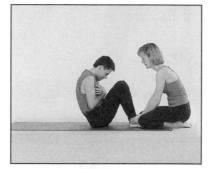

35. UPPER ABDOMINALS

Reps: 10

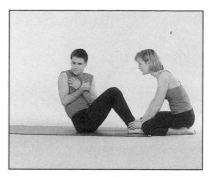

36. OBLIQUE ABDOMINALS

Reps: 10

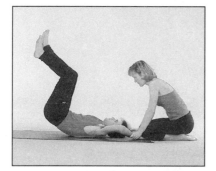

37. LOWER ABDOMINALS

Reps: 10

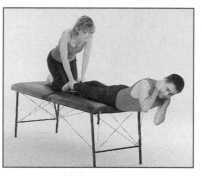

38. TRUNK EXTENSORS AND ROTATORS

Reps: 10 of each position—straight, right, left

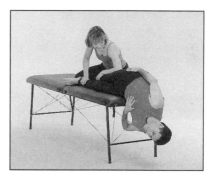

39. TRUNK LATERAL FLEXORS

Reps: 10 right, 10 left

STRENGTH 3: Active-Isolated Strengthening (Muscles in Upper Trunk and Shoulders)

You'll start this workout during the fourth week and continue through all three phases of your plan, as prescribed on pages 94 to 96. Perform the exercises in the order specified here. (See pages 81 to 91 for detailed instructions.)

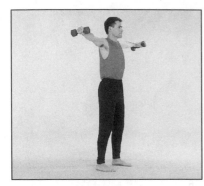

40. DELTOIDS

Reps: 10 of each of the three parts in the sequence

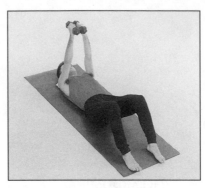

41. PECTORALIS MAJORS

Reps: 10, right and left simultaneously

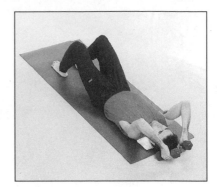

42. TRICEPS—SUPINE POSITION

Reps: 10, right and left simultaneously

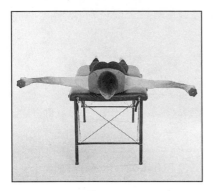

46. TRAPEZIUS

Reps: 10, right and left simultaneously

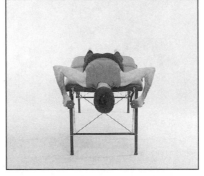

47. RHOMBOIDS

Reps: 10, right and left simultaneously

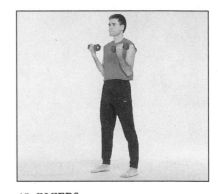

48. BICEPS

Reps: 10, right and left simultaneously

TRY PREHAB, NOT REHAB

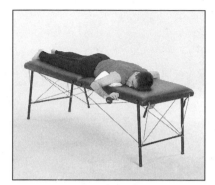 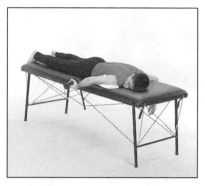 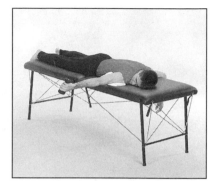

43. SHOULDER EXTERNAL ROTATORS

Reps: 10 right, 10 left; or 10 both sides simultaneously

44. SHOULDER INTERNAL ROTATORS

Reps: 10 right, 10 left; or 10 both sides simultaneously

45. TRICEPS—PRONE POSITION

Reps: 10 right, 10 left; or 10 both sides simultaneously

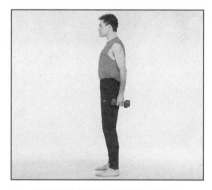

49. SHOULDERS (THE ROLL)

Reps: 10

Part 3

Stopping the Pain

Chapter 5

NAMING—AND TAMING— YOUR MOST COMMON ACHES

Pain is Mother Nature's loud, clear signal that your body is being damaged. In fact, your brain is programmed to instantaneously react to wrench you away from pain stimulus. In sports training and rehabilitation, pain is used as a diagnostic tool for pinpointing injury, getting an initial measure of its severity, and following up with subsequent readings on the progress of healing to see how things are going. Pain can be a very good and necessary thing.

About two-thirds of us will experience lower-back pain within our lifetimes. One in four of us admit to having chronic pain—that is, pain that will last a long time. In the United States alone, the cost of care for those with back problems is estimated to be in the billions every year. Physicians are inundated, and insurance companies are frustrated. They know, as we do, that most back problems can be mitigated or prevented altogether if people are lean, fit, flexible, and healthy.

THE NATURE OF PAIN

Thomas C. Chelimsky, M.D., is the director of the Pain Center at the University Hospitals Health Systems in Cleveland. Board-certified in Internal Medicine, Psychiatry, and Neurology, he has a triple perspective on pain.

Dr. Chelimsky makes a clear distinction between pain and the injury. A person experiencing pain focuses only on the pain. But pain isn't the problem—it's merely a signal sent from the site of injury to the brain through a pathway of nerves. The *injury* is the problem.

Let's say that you reach down to tie your shoe and have a sudden, sharp pain in your lower back. You will not intellectualize it by analyzing anatomy and physiology and the forces of physics and all the things that might have just gone wrong. No. You react only to the pain. Primally. Instinctively. In the first few minutes, you give little thought to the injury.

As for the concept of a "pain threshold"—the relative ability to feel pain—it doesn't exist, says Dr. Chelimsky. Studies show that the point at which all humans register pain is identical. The differences between the perception of high and low threshold are in how the pain is interpreted and how the person handles it, based on experience and attitude.

These differences can be radical. In fact, there can even be radical differences within the same person, who will change perception of the same pain from hour to hour. We've heard, "It feels better around midday" or "By 3:00, I was in so much pain, I couldn't stand it." Same injury. Same message to the brain. Different perception of the pain.

Because pain is a neurological signal interpreted differently by everyone, it is not used by physicians as a reliable diagnostic tool. Pain is, however, useful for leading the physician to the site of the injury, and it can be used to give clues for treatment. For example, determining if the injury feels better or worse when it is treated is very valuable information.

If that sounds cold and calculating, think again. Physicians take pain very seriously. In fact, pain has been designated as the fifth vital sign by physicians, along with temperature, pulse, respiration, and blood pressure. When you see your physician about back pain, you can expect full attention.

ACUTE PAIN VERSUS CHRONIC PAIN

Acute pain is a warning, an attention-getting mechanism that the mind and body use to sound the alarm that something is terribly wrong. The person in pain responds by jerking away from the source of the pain and "doing something" about it, such as yelling for help or running the injury under cold water. The medical response to acute pain is to quickly relieve it. From both the patient's point of view and the physician's point of view, acute pain is useful.

But when pain is chronic—it goes on for more than 3 months—it outlives its usefulness. There's no need for nerves to sound an alarm to the brain to alert it to an injury that can't be healed or pain that can't be relieved by immediate response. What then?

Centers like Dr. Chelimsky's are called pain-*management* centers rather than pain-elimination centers, with good reason. Although health-care professionals take pain very seriously and will do extraordinary things to relieve it, sometimes nothing works, and a patient has to just live with pain.

Chronic pain can set off a cascade of problems like depression, sleep disturbance, and anxiety. If chronic pain disrupts a person's ability to function at home or at work, feelings of worthlessness and hopelessness can set in. Even with professional help, it's not easy to learn to live with pain, because pain grabs all the attention. When a person is in pain, very little else comes into focus.

Pain management does everything medically possible to relieve pain and depression, redirecting attention, reframing the problem, and rehabilitating the patient so that he can return to as much function as possible. Counseling and fitness training are key components in the program. Let's look

Speak Up When You're in Pain

When you're in pain, even speaking hurts. Even the most articulate person can be so stressed from pain and fear that the ability to find the right words is impaired. Babbling is not uncommon. Neither is stoic denial, especially among athletes who view the inability to deal with pain as a character flaw.

We know one Broadway dancer who ignored a muscle strain in his lower back. Because he was so powerful, his body found a thousand ways to work around a muscle in rebellion. Each compensation caused another imbalance and problem. His situation reached a dramatic conclusion the night his back went into spasm on stage. He dropped his partner during a simple lift and injured them both. His explanation for not seeking a solution sooner? "My partner is a tank. Lifting is supposed to hurt. I took aspirin." Although whiners who obsess over every ache and pain can be frustrating, we are more concerned about stoics who ignore loud, clear signals that something's wrong or try to keep it secret.

Your physician can discern pain, even if you never say a word. Trained professionals are wizards at deciphering the clues. Even if you're unconscious, diagnostic tests will uncover problems. But let's hope your back problem doesn't come to this.

STOPPING THE PAIN

at some suggestions for what you can do when you've just begun to experience back pain.

Check your life for stress. Pain can be very real, but there could be reasons for it that are not physical. We seldom see back spasms in happy, relaxed people. Stress and tension head straight for the back.

Check for things that are bothering you or causing you anxiety. See if you can "fix" some of these, and you might be surprised that your pain will decrease or disappear altogether. (And, by the way, pain that is not physical in origin *can* be treated by a physician. Don't hesitate to seek help if you need it.)

Get exercise that includes stretching and light lifting. A fit, healthy, flexible, strong person doesn't have back pain very often. The program in this book is guaranteed to put you in that category. If you ever suffer a backache again in your life, chances are that the cause won't be that you're out of shape and vulnerable to injury.

If you're under stress, get a little more aerobic exercise, during which the body is likely to release endorphins, hormones that are nature's tranquilizers and painkillers. Your sense of well-being will be enhanced, and you'll work off some pent-up tension.

If you're depressed or anxious, get medical treatment. Depression and anxiety are both a cause and an effect of back problems. One of the first things a physician will ask a back patient is to clarify his state of mind. It's not unusual for a back patient to walk out of a physician's office with prescriptions for pain—as well as for depression and anxiety. If you think you might be depressed or if you feel anxious all the time, seek professional treatment before these problems affect your back.

Consult your physician to ensure that pain does not equal damage. No matter what the diagnosis or treatment, a person must not leave a physician's office until he is absolutely clear about what activities are allowed or advisable. When activity will cause more harm, lay off. If the activity will cause pain but no additional damage, the physician will allow the patient to "push through" the pain.

Get enough—or even more—sleep. Muscles get stronger by working hard to the point of breaking down then recovering through rest. During the period of rest and inactivity, the muscle fibers reorganize, regenerate, and get stronger. When the muscles are tested again, they can take a heavier load. When stressed harder, they break down again. In recovery, they come back even stronger.

This principle translates from the individual muscle to life itself. We work hard, we exhaust, we rest for a day, and we come back stronger. With a back injury, however, it's nearly impossible to have a hard day followed by an easy day. Every day is hard, so nothing ever regenerates and recovers fully to come back stronger. You must give your back the opportunity for that necessary time to repair.

Sleep is when the body repairs. Hard hours during the day should be followed by easy hours in sleep. Make sure you get plenty of sleep if you're recovering from an injury. In fact, try to get extra.

Pace yourself. Sometimes people just overdo it. They're having fun and get carried away. Or they overestimate their ability and make a mistake. When this happens, they pay the price. Often it's a back spasm. There's nothing wrong in pushing your own physical limits, but be smart about it.

Shed the extra pounds. One of the best ways to cure a bad back is to lose weight. Every extra pound of fat fatigues and strains the back even more. Physicians often send their back patients to consulting dietitians, who can develop diet plans for them. If your back is getting strained from excess pounds, consider losing weight by adjusting your diet and revving up your metabolism with exercise.

TAMING BACK SPASMS ON YOUR OWN

Of course, you're intending to become so fit, flexible, lean, and healthy that you'll never experience back pain! But in the meantime, let's look at a scenario in which something has gone wrong and you're hurting. Most of the time, back pain is merely muscle spasm in response to an injury or an inflammation. A

Increase Your Vocabulary

An accurate description of how your back feels will be useful to your physician in making a diagnosis. Here are some descriptive words that are commonly used. Although pressing your face into your doctor's stethoscope and reciting the entire list at the top of your lungs will certainly make your point, it won't really be helpful. We suggest that you select one or two from the following and speak them softly.

aching	dull	irritated	racking	stabbing
annoying	electric	jolting	radiating	startling
beating	explosive	nagging	raw	stinging
binding	fiery	nauseating	red-hot	suffocating
biting	flaming	only when I . . .	ripping	taut
blinding	flashing	pang	rubbing	tearing
blistering	flickering	paralyzing	scalding	tender
burning	fluttering	penetrating	searing	throbbing
chafing	gnawing	piercing	sharp	tight
cold	grating	pinching	shocking	tingling
constricting	grinding	pins and needles	shooting	trembling
convulsive	gripping	pounding	sizzling	tugging
cramping	heavy	pressing	sore	uncomfortable
crawling	hot	prickling	spasming	vibrating
cutting	immobilizing	pulling	splitting	whipping
dizzying	intense	pulsing	spreading	white-hot
drilling	intermittent	quivering	squeezing	wrenching

spasm is the involuntary contraction of a muscle (like a clenched fist that you can't open) and is nature's way of immobilizing muscles to serve as a sort of "splint" around an injury. If a spasm occurs in your back, it's doing its job: to freeze your spine and protect you from further injury.

The reasons that spasms occur are as varied as the injuries. Some are caused by overuse (like swinging a golf club all day when you're out of condition), an imbalance, or a single traumatic incident (like falling or getting hit or suddenly changing direction). You can also suffer a spasm if muscles are fatigued from poor posture or from holding a position too long (like keyboarding all day). Spasms can generate from injury or inflammation of the vertebrae, muscles, ligaments, tendons, or the disks between the vertebrae.

Spasms can be severe when they're in neutral position and intense when they're strained by movement. Although they usually clamp down and stay that way, spasms can fool you by letting go. You think you're better, but, when you move, they grab you again.

Don't suffer endlessly—there's really no need to hurt if the pain can be relieved. We've seen a bizarre human tendency: the "I Can Take It" syndrome. What's the matter with us? We shouldn't view pain as a chance for us to prove how tough we are.

Wanting to get out of pain is not a character flaw—it's smart. When your back is in pain and in spasm, your whole body tenses. This tension causes imbalances that torture the other muscles recruited to help you move. Blood flow is impeded. Metabolic waste from cellular activity isn't properly flushed.

The area becomes irritated. Your adrenaline rises, your heart rate increases, your breathing becomes rapid, and you become exhausted.

Instead of toughing out the pain, deal with it. (If you're unsure about the severity of your injury, dial 911 or get to your physician immediately. Remember, your spine encases your spinal cord, which is the information and communication conduit between your brain and your entire body. If anything goes wrong, it could mean trouble, so take no chances.)

This is how we handle a back problem in our clinic, step by step.

1. Take over-the-counter pain medication. Aspirin and nonsteroidal anti-inflammatory drugs (NSAIDs) such as ibuprofen might be your first line of defense when your back is hurting. Taken properly, they can reduce pain and inflammation in the muscles that support your spine and the soft tissues that surround it, such as tendons and ligaments, by blocking the production of prostaglandins (chemicals that cause inflammation and trigger transmission of the pain signal to the brain).

When you are in pain, you tense up to protect the injury from further harm. As we said earlier, your whole body forms a "splint" of sorts. Protection takes enormous energy and causes imbalances and tension everywhere. Relieving the pain, even temporarily, can allow you to move or flex the injured muscle just a

---

When Words Fail You

Back pain can be described in terms of a scale from 1 to 10, with "1" meaning a little pain and "10" meaning excruciating pain. Your physician will say, "On a scale of 1 to 10, how do you rate your pain?" You can get the physician to clarify and give you examples. For example, a "3" might be described as "pretty bad" and a "7" might be described as "really hurts a lot."

PAIN NUMBER SCALE

0	1	2	3	4	5	6	7	8	9	10
No pain										Worst possible pain

If language is such an impediment that neither words nor numbers will do the trick, your physician can help you describe back pain with the Wong-Baker FACES Pain Rating Scale. It's a simple drawing of six faces. The first one is smiling and looks relaxed. Each successive face looks less happy. The sixth one looks very sad. You simply point to the one that best describes your pain or how you feel about your pain.

WONG-BAKER FACES PAIN RATING SCALE

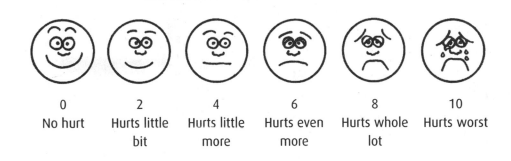

0	2	4	6	8	10
No hurt	Hurts little bit	Hurts little more	Hurts even more	Hurts whole lot	Hurts worst

From Wong, D.L.; Hockenberry-Eaton, M.; Wilson, D.; Winkelstein, M.L.; Schwartz, P.: *Wong's Essentials of Pediatric Nursing,* 6th ed. (St. Louis: 2001), p. 1301. Copyrighted by Mosby, Inc. Reprinted by permission.

---

little, because you have less need to protect yourself. You'll increase your range of motion and pump blood to the injury to promote healing and restore function. You'll also be more relaxed, sleep better, and allow your body to rejuvenate more quickly.

A few of words of caution: Pain is your body's way of communicating clear messages to you about the status of an injury. Don't use painkillers to mask pain that you need to be evaluating and using for information. And if you have had to take painkillers for a long period of time in order to be comfortable, there's something wrong and you need to take a different approach to deal with the pain.

NSAIDs have possible side effects of which you need to be aware: nausea, indigestion, diarrhea, and peptic ulcers. Aspirin could impede your blood's ability to clot and cause prolonged bleeding, colitis, gastrointestinal disorders, ringing in the ears, and aggravation of asthma, hives, and gout. Be careful.

2. Breathe and relax. Panic and tension amplify pain to an astonishing extent. As long as you're in overdrive, your adrenaline is pumping to rev you up for "fight or flight," but you're not battling or going anywhere. You have to consciously lower your heart rate and breathing to get control.

Stop making any voluntary sound that expresses pain. Relax your face completely and get rid of the grimace. Unclench your hands. Shake out your arms. Tell yourself that you can get this pain under control. Breathe deeply with your hand over your upper abdomen, just below your breastbone at your diaphragm. Exhale deeply so that your abdomen moves your hand in to the count of four. Push it out as you inhale to the count of four. Take 10 deep breaths. Relax your jaw by opening your mouth widely a couple of times to take the tension out of your temporomandibular joint, signaling your body to relax. This process, called "managing your state," will quiet the panic response that can aggravate pain.

3. Do a pain inventory. Move just a little by leaning forward a few inches, then back a few inches. Bend to the left side, to the right, then rotate from the waist just a little. What you feel will help you determine a course of action. If the pain is severe or if you experience any unusual symptoms other than pain, such as numbness or loss of function, stop immediately. You need professional attention. If you have full function and the pain is not severe, then proceed to step 4.

4. Get out the ice. We know it feels wonderful to sink an aching back into a hot bath, but that's the limit of the benefit. External heat can be comforting and relaxing, but when you're trying to throw the

Describing Pain with Drawing

Many people who can't speak English or who speak it well but can't find the right way to describe back pain find drawing useful, especially if they add colors. No artistic skill is necessary. Make a simple line drawing of your back and color the areas of intense pain in red, dull pain in blue. If you have no way to add color, just darken the area of pain with your pen, and draw arrows if you need to indicate that it radiates or travels.

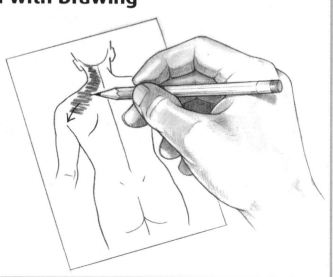

brakes on a spasm and facilitate muscle and tissue recovery, you need a little more.

Cold reduces swelling and initially restricts blood flow, providing a natural compress on the microscopic tears in the tissue that are leaking blood into the traumatized area and causing the spasm. Shortly, the body will recruit new blood to the cold area (notice how it turns a little red?) that flushes out metabolic wastes created by damaged cells.

If you have a localized "sore spot," you can treat it with a homemade ice pack. Fill a paper cup with water and keep it in the freezer. When you need it, simply peel down the rim to expose the surface of the ice. The paper cup, or what's left of it, serves as a little holder to keep your fingers warm and dry. Gently rub or swirl the ice surface on your injured or traumatized body part. Keep it moving and apply as much pressure as you can stand. In the first minute, it will feel uncomfortable, but this will ease. Treat yourself for 5 to 10 minutes. Watch your skin to make certain that it doesn't turn white, signaling frostbite.

When you are finished, return the cup to the freezer for next time. If the area you are treating is a little larger and harder to reach, a bag of frozen peas is a wonderfully pliable ice pack that can be refrozen frequently and reused for a long time. Lie down on top of it. Or press it between your back and the wall to hold it into place. If being cold is uncomfortable for you, wrap yourself in a blanket.

For a full-scale treatment (such as for postmarathon backache), you can fill a bathtub with cold water and add five to ten 5-pound bags of ice. Then grit your teeth and sink in for up to 10 minutes. The initial shock will wear off, and you'll soon be all right. This is very difficult, but it will put your recovery into warp drive. *Please note:* This is not for people with heart conditions or high blood pressure.

By the way, please do not rely on topical creams and ointments. They feel warm and tingly, but they are not going to help a back spasm. If anything, they will give you the misconception that you have done something good for yourself, resulting in a delay in

action that could actually be more helpful. The only exception might be a cream that contains capsaicin, the chemical "heat" extracted from hot peppers.

5. Stretch. Once you have quieted the inflammation and pain with ice, it's time to move, if only a little.

Remember the principles of Active-Isolated Stretching? Muscles work in pairs. When one contracts, the opposite muscle relaxes. When your back hurts, you want to relax it, which means you'll be firing muscles in your chest and abdomen to allow your back to let go. Go to the section of the workout program that outlines back stretches (pages 39 to 62), grab your stretch rope, and get to work.

Ideally, you'd be able to do the full stretch routine, because it unlocks joints and relaxes muscles in a sequence that would really help your spasm. But we're realistic. If you're desperate, go for the back stretches.

Now more than ever, it's important that you stretch correctly, allowing muscles in the front of your body to do all the work, while the muscles in your back enjoy gentle stretching. At first you might be able to move only an inch or so, but as the back relaxes, you'll see some progress. Do only a few repetitions in small, deliberate, careful movements. Remember to breathe. If for any reason stretching causes acute pain or any other new symptom, back off immediately and get yourself to your physician.

6. Ice again. When you've stretched your back for a few minutes, return to icing for 5 to 10 minutes.

7. Stretch again. Return to the back stretches and see if you can get a little farther on each stretch or do a few more of each one. Very likely, you'll be pleasantly surprised at your progress.

(If this icing and stretching seems redundant, we must tell you that we have been known to continue this routine for a full day with professional athletes who can't afford to be down for the count. Unless there is severe tearing or a fracture, we almost always succeed in restoring function and relieving pain with an aspirin, an ice cube, a stretch rope, and some patience.)

8. Drink plenty of water. Although you might be tempted to anesthetize yourself with a six-pack of beer (and who could really blame you?), alcohol will dehydrate you, and you need to hydrate. Consume at least a liter of water within the next 4 hours. Without adequate hydration, your body can't heal properly.

9. Have a light meal. Injury takes a tremendous amount of energy. If you're in pain, you're burning extra calories, even when you're standing still. You need fuel, but just a little. If you put too much food into your stomach, your body will divert blood away from your muscles and into all matters digestive. The idea is to keep your blood flowing easily, so it can bring in healing oxygen and take away all the metabolic waste that accumulates from injured and exhausted cells.

10. Get a good night's sleep. When your back is injured, you're mentally, physically, and emotionally exhausted by the effort to get out of pain. You need, and deserve, some rest.

You need rest, but your back also needs a break. Lie on your back; physiologists confirm that the forces on your spine are at a minimum when you're flat down. A small pillow is all right to use if it feels okay. If you flip over onto your side, you nearly double the forces. Do not sleep sitting in a chair. Forces are then nearly four times as great as when you're lying flat down.

Not only does sleep's relaxation of body and mind assist healing, a good night's rest will help you emotionally. Pain-management experts tell us that sleep deprivation or disruption is almost worse than the injury—it can unravel even the strongest person.

When you awaken, get up slowly. Roll over on your side, swing your legs over the side of the bed, and use your arms to push your torso vertically until you are seated. Do a quick inventory. If you feel all right, put your feet on the floor shoulder-width apart and lean forward very slightly. Keep your back straight and stand. Repeat the routines of aspirin or NSAIDs, ice, and stretch. If things aren't better, consider seeing your physician.

What Now?

How long your back spasm will last depends on the severity of your injury and how successfully your in-tervention has been. A mild injury can be gone in a day, but sometimes you could be sore for a couple of weeks.

Don't let that stop you from working out, however. You can, and should, continue to stretch, even from the moment of the onset of pain. You might even be able to walk. But save lifting, heavy work, and sports for when you're symptom-free.

If you experienced back spasm from anything other than an injury caused by trauma, you probably contributed to the problem. You need to be a lot stronger and more flexible than you are. Get out your stretch rope, ankle weights, and walking shoes, and get back in control.

"UH-OH! I WOKE UP WITH A CRICK IN MY NECK!"

We have yet to figure out the exact pathology of a crick, nor can we positively identify the muscles, tendons, and ligaments involved. We suspect the name comes from the scary sound you'd expect to hear when you attempt to turn your head the morning after a paralyzing night. Next to the common cold, the crick just might be the most common malady known to humanity. The good news is that it's easy to fix.

You know the scenario: Your back is fatigued from overuse or sitting in one position for too long, and the muscles tighten up so that you feel stiff or sore. No big deal. Then you climb into bed, and you sleep so soundly that, instead of redistributing weight and pressure on your body all through the night as you usually do, you don't change positions.

If you weren't contorted with your neck at an odd angle, held there by the weight of your head all night, this might not be a problem—but no such luck. You awaken with a crick. You can't move your neck. You're locked up. (We also see this commonly among people who sleep sitting up on airplanes or in the passenger seats of cars, where the neck relaxes and gravity causes the head to drop.)

Actually the crick is a simple, but painful spasm of neck muscles, easily stretched out into relaxation. All you need is some blood flow. Let's get started.

SEMI-CIRCUMDUCTION OF THE NECK

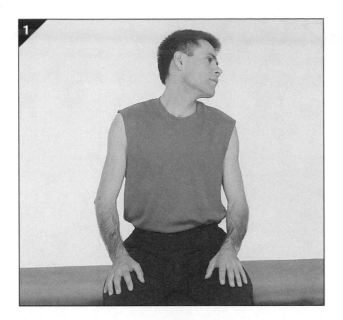

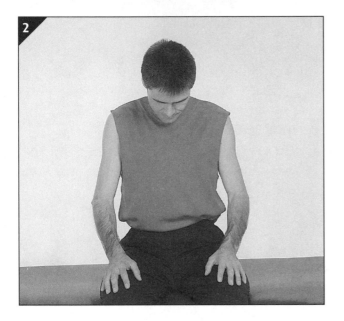

Active Muscles You Contract: None (This one's a warmup to increase the circulation of the neck.)

Isolated Muscles You Stretch: None (This is a warmup to increase the circulation of the neck.)

Hold Each Stretch: This is just a relaxed roll.

Reps: Back and forth 10 times

1. Sit on the edge of your bed with your hands on your knees. Face forward and then turn your head to the side until you're facing over one shoulder.

2. Relax your neck, allowing your head to roll gently toward the midline of your body until your chin is against your chest, as shown. Continue the gentle roll until your head is back up over the opposite shoulder and you are facing over that shoulder. Allow your head to fall forward again and roll back the other way.

(continued)

3. Face forward and then turn your head to the side, facing over one shoulder. Align your head directly over your body. Relax your neck. Allow your head to roll gently backward, as shown.

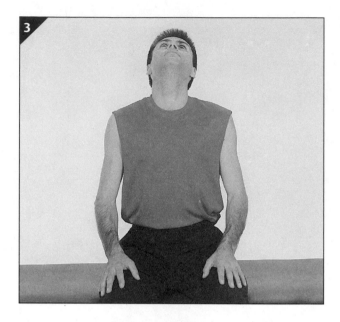

4. Continue to roll your head toward the opposite shoulder, extending your neck as much as you comfortably can. When you reach the opposite shoulder, roll back the other way. Do this a few times, gently.

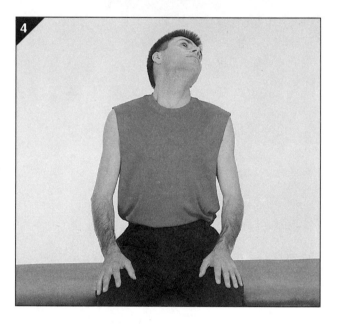

NECK EXTENSORS

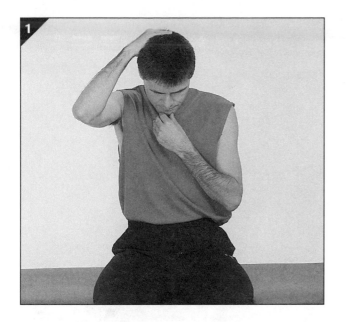

Active Muscles You Contract: Muscles in the front of your neck

Isolated Muscles You Stretch: Muscles in the back of your neck and the top of your back

Hold Each Stretch: 2 seconds

Reps: 10

1. Sit on the edge of your bed with your back straight and your feet flat on the floor. Place one hand on the back of your head and one hand on your chin to assist the stretch. Tuck your chin and roll your head forward until your chin meets your chest. You can gently assist the end of the movement with your hand at the back of your head. Keep your shoulders down.

NECK FLEXORS

Active Muscles You Contract: Muscles in the back of your neck and the top of your back between your shoulders

Isolated Muscles You Stretch: Muscles in the front of your neck

Hold Each Stretch: 2 seconds

Reps: 10

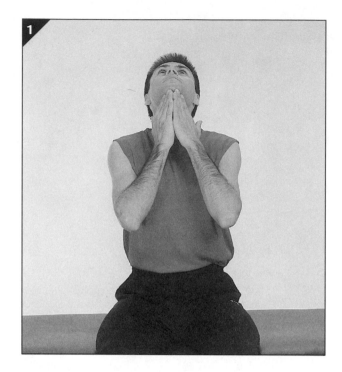

1. Sit on the edge of your bed with your back straight and your feet flat on the floor. Align your head over your body. Place your fingertips along your jawline just under your chin and roll your head backward very gently. You can gently assist the end of the movement with your fingertips. Keep your shoulders down.

STOPPING THE PAIN

NECK LATERAL FLEXORS

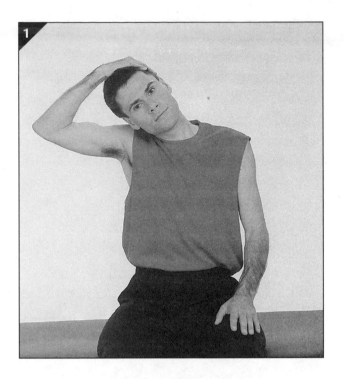

Active Muscles You Contract: Muscles in the side of your neck

Isolated Muscles You Stretch: Muscles in the opposite side of your neck

Hold Each Stretch: 2 seconds

Reps: 10 left, 10 right

1. Sit on the edge of your bed with your back straight and your feet flat on the floor. Look straight ahead. Cock your head to one side, lowering your ear straight down toward your shoulder. Reach up over the top of your head with the hand that is on the same side as the shoulder, gently place your fingertips on your temple, as shown, and press very gently down to assist the end of the movement. Keep your shoulders down and keep your body still.

NECK ROTATORS

Active Muscles You Contract: Muscles on the opposite side of your neck

Isolated Muscles You Stretch: Muscles in the side of your neck

Hold Each Stretch: 2 seconds

Reps: 10 right, 10 left

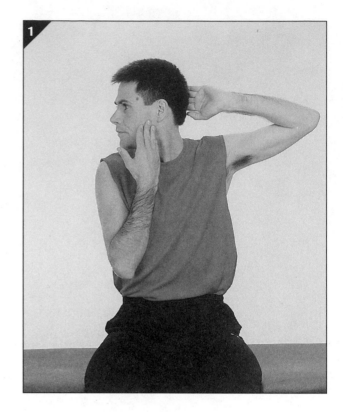

1. Sit on the edge of your bed with your back straight and your feet flat on the floor. Look straight ahead. Turn your head to one side, until your chin is over your shoulder. If you're turning to the right, reach up with your left hand and place it behind your head at the base of the skull. Apply gentle pressure to assist the end of the movement. Take your right hand and place your fingertips along your left jawline, as shown, and press very gently to guide. Be certain to keep your shoulders down and your body still. Stretch the other side.

NECK OBLIQUE EXTENSORS

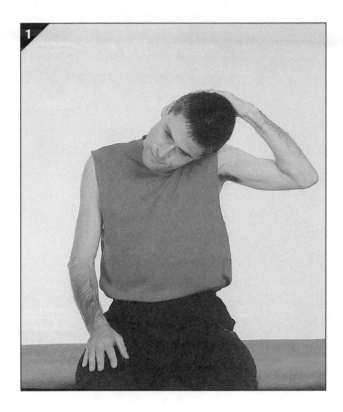

Active Muscles You Contract: Muscles in the front of your neck

Isolated Muscles You Stretch: Muscles in your upper shoulders to the side of the base of your neck

Hold Each Stretch: 2 seconds

Reps: 10 right, 10 left

1. Sit on the edge of your bed with your back straight and your feet flat on the floor. Turn your head right to a 45-degree angle. Maintaining the angle, drop your head forward with your ear toward your chest. Place your left hand on top of your head, as shown, and gently press down to assist the end of the movement. Be certain to keep your shoulders down and your body still.

NECK OBLIQUE FLEXORS

Active Muscles You Contract: Muscles in the base of your neck and upper back

Isolated Muscles You Stretch: Muscles in your neck and upper chest

Hold Each Stretch: 2 seconds

Reps: 10 right, 10 left

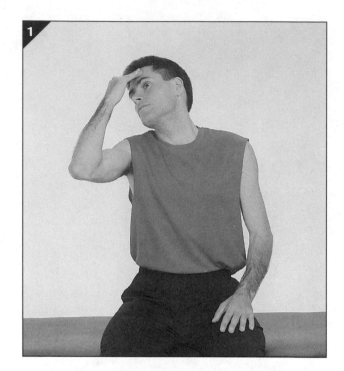

1. Sit on the edge of your bed with your back straight and your feet flat on the floor. Turn your head right to a 45-degree angle. Still at the angle, drop your head backward with your ear over your shoulder. Place your right hand on your forehead, as shown, and gently press back to assist the end of the movement. Be certain to keep your shoulders down and your body still.

WHAT YOUR DOCTOR CAN DO FOR PAIN

In the 18th century, Voltaire said, "The purpose of a doctor is to entertain the patient until the disease takes its course." Doctors today still sometimes "entertain" and wait, because about 85 percent of patients who suffer from lower-back pain can't be precisely diagnosed. The source of the pain remains vague until it eventually goes away. Some studies indicate that time heals as often as intervention. Unless something is horribly wrong, you'll probably be all right, in time.

That doesn't mean you should avoid the doctor and tough it out. In fact, we advise that when in doubt, seek help as quickly as possible. (See chapter 6 for advice on physicians.) Even if your doctor can't "fix" the injury, much can be done to keep you comfortable. Let's look at the different ways your doctor can help you manage the pain.

Prescription Medicines

Although over-the-counter medications can do a lot to ease an aching back, they have limitations. Your physician can widen the selection of medications with prescription drugs.

Nonsteroidal anti-inflammatory drugs. NSAIDs work to reduce inflammation and are often compared in results to aspirin. The difference is that NSAIDs have fewer side effects. They are most effective when taken continuously rather than taken only when the patient experiences pain. Many of these are available over the counter, but if you would like to try a new class of NSAIDs called COX-2 inhibitors, your physician will have to prescribe them. Sold under the names rofecoxib (Vioxx) and celecoxib (Celebrex), these medications selectively inhibit the chemical reaction that causes inflammation, but do a better job of protecting the stomach lining from ulcers.

Neuroleptic medications. These medications, such as gabapentin (Neurontin), stop or inhibit seizures. They're sometimes prescribed for patients with nerve pain or degeneration. Most often they're used for postsurgical leg pain, but they also may be used for back pain. They are not addictive and can be taken over a long period of time.

Antidepressants. Back pain is both a cause and an effect of depression. Recognizing this, physicians often prescribe both a pain medication and an antidepressant at the same time. Antidepressants that elevate mood and reduce anxiety, called tricyclics, are prescribed in low doses as sedatives to help a patient sleep, and, although no one is quite sure why, they diminish pain. They are not addictive. Examples are amitriptyline (Elavil), nortriptyline (Aventyl), and imipramine (Tofranil). Other drugs used to treat depression are selective serotonin reuptake inhibitors, or SSRIs. Serotonin is a neurotransmitter in the brain that governs mood. Enhancing levels seems to make a mood better. Among the most well-known of these are fluoxetine (Prozac), bupropion (Wellbutrin), and sertraline (Zoloft).

Nonnarcotic medications. These drugs, like tramadol (Ultram), act on the central nervous system to block pain, but have no value as an anti-inflammatory. They're stronger than aspirin but not as strong as narcotics. They're not usually addictive.

Steroids. With names such as methylprednisolone (Medrol), these are anti-inflammatory medications that can quiet a raging backache and reduce swelling. They are intended for use for only a short time. Also, once a patient starts, she must taper off rather than simply quit taking the pills. Side effects can be weight gain, excessive thirst, and ulcers.

Muscle relaxants. This group of drugs, which includes carisoprodol (Soma), cyclobenzaprine (Flexeril), and diazepam (Valium), sedates and relaxes the body. They act on the central nervous system, so they tend to quiet the entire body. Used in fighting spasm, they are generally prescribed for the short term.

Narcotics. When pain is severe, narcotics are used. They don't block pain, but work to disassociate the patient from it. As a tolerance is easy to develop, the medication becomes less effective during the course of treatment. They are usually prescribed for short periods of time to avoid addiction. Among the most well-known are oxycodone (Percocet, Oxy-Contin) and propoxyphene (Darvocet).

Stimulation

Your physician or therapist might be able to reduce pain and inflammation by introducing electric stimulation to the injury site. Additionally, steroids can be administered the same way. These treatments are done in the office.

TENS. This low-voltage electric stimulation is also known by its longer name: transcutaneous electrical nerve stimulation. The impulses from TENS interact with nerves to disrupt and override pain signals. The therapist holds the device in place, over the site of your injury.

It's also possible for your physician to surgically implant a peripheral nerve stimulator that works similarly to TENS for more consistent nerve disruption.

Ultrasound. This involves the use of deep heating generated by sound waves. The therapist glides the device over the site of your injury to penetrate into soft tissue, and, typically, you get a warm, tingling sensation. This treatment might relieve acute, spasmodic episodes and recruits healing blood flow to the area.

Iontophoresis. In this treatment, the therapist applies a steroid to the skin over the injury, then an electrical current is applied to send the steroid down through the skin to the injury. Steroids are anti-inflammatories that reduce swelling and pain.

Injections

Injections are used after a course of medications, physical therapy, or both have failed to solve the problem and before surgery is considered. Injections are more effective than oral medications, because they can zero in on the spot that is causing trouble and deliver pain relief directly and quickly. Injections are also sometimes useful as diagnostic tools. The physician can inject a numbing medication directly into an area suspected of being problematic. If the pain goes away, you've spotted the problem. If it doesn't, it lets the physician know that it's time to look elsewhere for the source of the pain.

Facet joint block. Each vertebra of the spine has facets, or flat surfaces, that make contact with each other where the vertebrae fit together. Facets are paired with cartilage between them, and these points of contact are called facet joints. Injuries from twisting or degeneration of cartilage can cause a facet joint to become irritated and inflamed. A steroid (anti-inflammatory) and lidocaine (painkiller) are injected directly into the joint to relieve the pain. The physician will use fluoroscopy, or a real-time x-ray, to make sure the injection is positioned in the right place.

Facet rhizotomy. If a few facet blocks are effective but can't sustain the relief, your physician may determine that the temporary results can be made permanent with a facet rhizotomy. A needle with a probe is inserted just outside the facet joint. The probe emits heat through radio waves to permanently disable the nerve. Once the nerve is deadened, it is unable to transmit pain messages to the brain.

Trigger point injections. A trigger point—a painful knot of muscle fibers in your back—is formed when small strains and microscopic tears in the muscle fibers fail to realign properly as they heal. They stick together in a wad called an adhesion, like scar tissue. (By the way, the back is not the only place knots form.) Medication can be injected directly into the knot to deaden the pain, so a patient can stretch the muscle and break up this adhesion.

Lumbar epidural injection. This is the most common of all spinal injections. Steroid is injected into the dura, the sac around nerve roots that contains cerebrospinal fluid in the lumbar spine, to relieve pain and reduce inflammation. The injection won't stop the pain, but it will relieve it enough to break the cycle for a time, so a patient can get moving again. Moving recruits blood supply, relaxes muscles, and reduces spasms.

The pain relief might take a day or two to kick in, and the injection works in only 50 percent of people who try it. The effects are temporary—from a week to a year. These injections are sometimes given in a series of three per year to keep a patient comfortable. Sometimes lumbar epidural injections are used to diagnose an injury by giving the physician a way to pinpoint the location. By injecting a specific dura, the physician can observe the effect of the medication. If you get relief, you're right on target. If you don't, it's time to look elsewhere for the culprit.

Selective nerve root block. When a nerve root is blocked, impinged, or inflamed, the pain can radiate through the back and legs. Your physician will try to determine which nerve root is in trouble with an imaging study, but sometimes they're hard to see. For this reason, a selective nerve root block can be useful as a diagnostic tool, helping to identify the source of your pain. A steroid and lidocaine are injected directly into the nerve where it exits the space between your vertebrae. The physician uses fluoroscopy to make sure he is on target. If your pain stops, bingo.

Sacroiliac joint block. The sacroiliac joint is the connection between the pelvis and the base of the spine called the sacrum. A steroid and lidocaine are injected directly into the joint. The physician uses fluoroscopy to make sure he is on target. Once the pain is deadened, the patient *must* get moving to improve range of motion. This block can be repeated three times a year.

Braces

When a lumbar spine has been fractured or fused, it's like any other broken bone: You need a period of time during which the bone can be immobilized so that it can remodel and knit back together. It also hurts, so keeping everything still can help a person feel better while the healing begins.

Rigid brace. This is a sort of removable body cast. Limiting spinal movement up to 50 percent, it's used when the physician wants a patient to keep still. Rigid braces are fitted to the individual torso and can be removed when the patient is lying down.

Corset. A corset is a fitted brace that keeps a patient from bending forward from the waist. They are used most often after lumbar fusion surgery, especially if the fusion was done without the use of appliances or stabilizing materials and the patient must rely on mending bones to heal. A corset can be removed when the patient is lying down.

Surgery

There are as many surgical procedures as there are injuries, conditions, and diseases. Your physician will know when and if it's time to consider this. See chapter 6 for a comprehensive look at selecting the right physician and getting the most out of your relationship.

WHEN IT'S TIME TO SEEK HELP:
A GUIDE TO BACK DOCTORS

When you have a back problem, getting well might begin when you put yourself in front of a health-care professional who specializes in diagnosing—figuring out what's wrong so that you'll be able to make the right decisions about treatment. Of course, it's human nature to try a few things on one's own first . . . and you will. But without an accurate diagnosis, at best you'll be taking a hit-or-miss approach to treatment and wasting valuable time. At worst you'll be putting yourself at risk of further injury in what can be a nightmarish cascade of other medical problems.

Promise us that you'll seek professional help—the best you can find. And promise us that you'll do it immediately, under the following circumstances.

- If the pain is severe and persists more than a day
- If the pain impedes your ability to move
- If you also have a fever and chills
- If the site of the pain feels hot or is swollen or reddened
- If the pain starts at your back but radiates down through your buttocks to your leg—especially below your knee
- If you can associate the pain with an injury such as a fall or a trauma

- If the pain is a result of a work injury, in which case you must see a physician in order to be in compliance with workers' compensation laws to receive assistance
- If one or both of your legs feels numb or weak
- If the pain is keeping you from enjoying your life or sleeping well
- If you have tried several remedies yourself without success
- If you have a history of cancer with sudden weight loss
- If you have sudden bowel and/or bladder incontinence

FIRST, LET'S FIND OUT WHAT'S GOING ON: DIAGNOSIS

In our practice, working with an injured athlete usually begins with a frantic phone call from a crazed coach who draws a deep breath; reels off a litany of symptoms; reviews in rapid succession the failed remedies they've tried; emphasizes the alarming ramifications of benching the athlete; gives us an unreasonable deadline to affect a complete healing, up to this time only possible at Lourdes; and then announces a flight number and an arrival time into LaGuardia. Then he draws his second breath.

Usually, as soon as we answer the phone and the coach knows that we're in our New York clinic, the athlete is dispatched to the airport. They must have worked out a hand signal. We pick up the ringing phone and say, "Hello?" Somewhere, out there in the world, a coach points to the door and an athlete hobbles toward a waiting cab while we get the details. And, thus, with the requisite pain, fear, and hope that are the signatures of sports medicine, another serious rehabilitation program begins.

Just as we have advised you to do, we start with a diagnosis. We have a cadre of physicians on speed dial and, like you, are faced with the challenge of choosing the right physician from the assortment. If we are certain about the type of injury, the choice is a specialist. But when the symptoms are unclear or confusing, we start with a generalist.

Our preference is to work with someone experienced with our athlete's particular problem. Each physician with whom we work was first highly recommended by other athletes or other physicians. We asked, so we knew.

PHYSICIANS WHO CAN GET YOU STARTED

When your back hurts, we suggest that you start with the basics. Although your instinct will be to run to the office of someone who you think can make the pain go away, you should try to stay focused on discovering *why* you're in pain.

Remember that back pain can generate from many sources, both subtle and surprising, so you need someone who can examine you from a broad, comprehensive perspective. We recommend that your first appointment be with a physician who has a general practice. Your selection should be based on the competence and experience of the practitioner, the ability of the practitioner to refer you to other qualified professionals, the facilities to which the practitioner has privileges and access, and, finally, your insurance company's willingness to re-imburse for services. Let's take a look at some of your options.

Primary-Care Physicians

Formerly called general practitioners, or GPs, these physicians are medical doctors (M.D.'s). They are the "gatekeepers" of your health care—men and women in various practices who have experience in a wide range of medical issues.

Even though they might refer you to more specialized practitioners, they're a good place to start. Moreover, they're a good place to finish. We make sure that all our medical records—no matter which practitioner generates them—are copied and sent back to our primary-care physician for safe keeping. Why? Medicine today is complicated. You might be consulting several physicians simultaneously, and it can be tricky for one physician who sees you infrequently to know what treatments you're receiving from everyone else. Medications prescribed from several sources might interact with each other, so it's advisable to have one person who has all your medical information at his fingertips.

Among the primary areas of practice are family-care doctors, internists, gynecologists, and pediatricians. They have 4 years of undergraduate college education, followed by 4 years of medical school, and at least 5 years of specialty training as medical residents and fellows.

Doctors of Osteopathy, or Osteopaths

In addition to medical doctors, doctors of osteopathy (D.O.'s) are recognized nationally as physicians with completed training. They are licensed in all 50 states to practice and have prescriptive privileges. (In fact, some M.D.'s are also D.O.'s.)

Most D.O.'s are in general practice with an emphasis on disease prevention through a healthy, balanced body, but some specialize in such disciplines as anesthesiology, physiatry, or orthopedics. All are graduates of a certified school of osteopathic medicine, with 1 year of supervised internship. Board-certified osteopaths who specialize must complete an additional 3- to 4-year residency.

HOW YOUR PRIMARY-CARE PHYSICIAN DECIDES A COURSE OF ACTION

When you arrive at the office, your doctor moves through a very systematic method of evaluating your back pain. She will:

1. Determine if the condition is urgent. Russell Hardy, M.D., from University Hospitals Health Systems in Cleveland has developed the Low Back Pain Management Algorithm that is widely used by primary physicians to evaluate patients and move them through diagnostics and treatment.

A patient is in an urgent situation in the following circumstances.

- Major trauma
- Minor trauma in a patient who may have osteoporosis
- Focal spine tenderness (meaning it hurts to the touch in a specific place)
- Fever
- Recent bacterial infection
- Immune system suppression
- IV drug use
- Severe pain at night
- History of cancer
- Very severe pain
- Numbing or paralysis
- New bladder dysfunction
- Severe lower-extremity deficits, such as numbness in the legs and feet
- Lax anal sphincter

If you go into the office with any of these conditions, your primary-care physician will refer you for immediate diagnostics and possible emergency referral to specialists who will get right into action. We'll talk about specialists in a minute.

2. Determine if it is garden-variety back pain. Physicians treat some back pain without extensive diagnostics or intervention by specialists. They include

sciatica (a pain that radiates from your butt down the back of your leg) and generalized lower-back pain (your grandmother used to call this lumbago).

If you have garden-variety back pain, the physician will likely educate you on what's happened and why and advise you on comfort measures that will likely help you feel better. She might administer epidural steroids for sciatica or prescribe oral steroids to reduce inflammation. You might be told to take nonsteroidal anti-inflammatory drugs (NSAIDs) such as ibuprofen. Bed rest might be suggested, but will be limited. You might be treated for depression and anxiety.

If you aren't getting better in a reasonable period of time, your physician might order more extensive diagnostics or refer you to an orthopedist, a neurosurgeon, or a chronic-pain-management expert who specializes in back problems.

3. Determine if you can be helped by a chiropractor. When your physician has ruled out serious neurologic and orthopedic problems and diseases, she may refer you to a chiropractor. (And good chiropractors will refer you right back to your primary-care physician if they take a look and decide that you have a problem beyond their scope of practice.)

You don't need a referral from a physician to see a chiropractor, so you can make your own appointment. In fact, many people bypass their primary-care physicians and go straight to chiropractors for initial diagnosis and treatment. If you are exhibiting *none* of the "red flag" symptoms and are very certain that your spine is merely out of alignment and balance, a chiropractor can be a pretty safe bet. (See "Chiropractors" on page 132.)

SURGICAL SPECIALISTS

Unlike any other mechanism in your body, your spine is a complex amalgamation of bone, spinal cord, soft tissues, connective tissues, and nerves. Diagnosis and treatment are matters of understanding *all* the systems involved. Only a few qualified specialists can help you, but don't get thrown by the word *surgeon.* A surgeon's toolbox is filled with a lot more

Board-Certified versus Board-Eligible

How do you know your physician is qualified? One way is to determine that she is board-certified.

When your physician is board-certified, this means that she has successfully completed an approved educational and training program and a rigorous evaluation process designed to assess the knowledge, skills, and experience necessary to provide quality patient care. Board certification is offered in 36 areas of medical practice.

After completing medical school and 3 to 7 years of specialty training (and sometimes a period of independent practice), the physician submits credentials to the governing board, which reviews them and determines whether or not the candidate is qualified to take the certification exam. If all goes well, the physician is board-certified.

The certifications are time limited, which means they expire every 6 to 10 years, requiring the physician to recertify several times in the course of a career. In addition, 88 subspecialties of medical practice exist in which a physician may be board-certified.

Some good physicians are not board-certified, but when you are working with board-certified physicians, you have some assurance that they meet the highest standards of their profession, must work continuously to keep education current, and "go the extra mile" in patient care. This designation doesn't automatically make her a good physician, but the chances are pretty good.

Please note: Beware the designation "board-eligible." The American Board of Medical Specialties has issued a statement declaring that "board-eligible" is an ambiguous term. It implies that the physician is in process and making progress toward becoming board-certified, but it has been used improperly by some physicians who claim "board-eligible" as a credential, rather than being board-certified. Even the requirements for entering the certification process change from time to time, making the term "board-eligible" less credible. Still, a young physician who claims to be board-eligible just might be, so be on the safe side—ask for clarification.

---

than scalpels. These doctors are adept at knowing when they need to step in with noninvasive therapies and when they need to operate.

The two surgeons who are uniquely qualified to handle back injury and disease are neurosurgeons and orthopedic surgeons. They overlap each other when back injuries are diagnosed and treated. Indeed, in choosing one, it's a hard call to make.

Each specialty suggests expertise in only one discipline. In fact, in the early days of spinal surgery, physicians from each of these two worked together in the operating room—one to handle the cord and nerves and the other to handle the bone. As medicine has become more specialized, a hybrid physician has emerged in each of the two professions: neurosurgeons who can handle the bone, and

orthopedic surgeons who can handle the cord and nerves. Make sure that the surgeon you're consulting is one of these physicians with expertise in spinal surgery—one with *both* sets of skills.

Neurosurgeons

While it's easy to think of neurosurgeons as "brain surgeons," many are expert in surgery of the spine, which includes bone. Just as orthopedic surgeons must be expert in the sensitive spinal cord and nerves, neurosurgeons who operate on spines must be expert in the mechanics of bone.

These physicians are either M.D.'s or D.O.'s trained in the diagnosis and treatment of disorders, injuries, and diseases of the brain and spine, and the nervous systems and blood supplies that serve and complement them. They have 4 years of undergraduate college education, followed by 4 years of medical school, and at least 5 or 6 years of specialty training as neurosurgical residents and fellows. In addition, this physician might extend training to include spine fellowship. To join this program, physicians must have completed 4 to 7 years of surgical residency and must be either board-certified or board-eligible in their specialties.

Orthopedic Surgeons (Orthopedists)

When your primary-care physician refers you to an orthopedic surgeon, she suspects that the source of your pain is in the bones of your spine.

These physicians are either M.D.'s or D.O.'s trained in the diagnosis and treatment of skeletal disorders, and injury and disease of bones. They have 4 years of undergraduate college education, 4 years of medical school, and at least 5 years of specialty training as orthopedic surgical residents and fellows. (If you're referred to an orthopedic surgeon, make absolutely certain that this physician has vast experience and plenty of success in working with spines.)

NONSURGICAL SPECIALISTS

While surgeons can provide skilled diagnostics that might or might not include surgery, other physicians can evaluate back problems and treat many of them without surgery. If your back problem does require surgical intervention, you'll be referred back to surgeons, but often, patients find successful treatment with nonsurgical specialists.

Chiropractors

These physicians are trained in the diagnosis and treatment of skeletal dysfunction, particularly that of the spine. As chiropractic medicine is often debated among people with back pain, we'll review their history.

Once viewed as alternative medicine, chiropractics have been recognized as "mainstream" since 1994 when the federal Agency for Health Care Policy and Research concluded that short-term spinal manipulation "appears to provide temporary relief of acute lower-back pain." Now, one out of three people with lower-back pain seeks the assistance of a chiropractor.

Practitioners are hands-on care providers who treat without surgery or drugs. Although they can recommend nutritional supplements, they cannot write prescriptions for medications, nor do they do surgery. Their practices are centered on diagnosis of imbalance and misalignment, noninvasive corrective procedures such as manipulation or adjustment, and therapies to promote healing such as ultrasound or massage. If you have bone disease, bone cancer, sciatica, rheumatoid arthritis, osteoporosis, or fractures, or if you are pregnant, consult your medical doctor before you undergo chiropractic treatment.

While many chiropractic colleges now require 4 years of general college credit with an emphasis on health sciences, many still admit students with only 2 years. The chiropractic curriculum is 4 years of academic training, followed by 1 year of supervised internship. Practitioners must successfully pass two or three levels of board certification, depending on the extent of their practices.

Chiropractors can also specialize. They are licensed in all 50 states and the District of Columbia, but requirements for licensure and laws governing scope of practice vary widely from state to state. The National Board of Chiropractic Examiners is the main testing agency for the profession, but all states maintain a registry and board of examiners. (Again, check credentials and interview other patients.)

Neurologists

These physicians are either M.D.'s or D.O.'s trained in the diagnosis and treatment of disorders, injuries, and diseases of the brain and spine, spinal cord, muscles, nerves, and all systems and functions involved. They do not do surgery.

Neurologists are brilliant at diagnosis of back problems, because their clinical knowledge is broad and their access to diagnostic procedures and equipment is vast. Some serve as consultants to other physicians and refer cases to them, but many maintain long-term management of patients with chronic disorders. They have 4 years of undergraduate college education, followed by 4 years of medical school, and at least 5 or 6 years of specialty training as neurology residents and fellows.

Rheumatologists

If the source of your back pain is a disease, you'll likely be referred to a rheumatologist. These physicians are either M.D.'s or D.O.'s trained in the diagnosis and treatment of arthritis and other chronic diseases of bone, connective tissue, and muscle such as osteoporosis and fibromyalgia. They do not do surgery.

Sometimes working with a rheumatologist will involve working with a team of health-care providers: medical consultants, rehabilitation therapists, psychologists, and pain-management experts. They have 4 years of undergraduate college education, followed by 4 years of medical school, and at least 5 or 6 years of specialty training as rheumatology residents and fellows.

Anesthesiologists (Pain-Management Physicians)

Anesthesiologists aren't just perched at the heads of tables in operating rooms to put patients to sleep and wake them up again. These physicians are either M.D.'s or D.O.'s and are also trained in pain management. For this reason, one might help you with your back problems. Many have emerged as pain-management physicians who work in pain-management clinics and multidisciplinary integrated-care centers. A pain-management physician can help mitigate chronic pain with medications and other interventional protocols. They have 4 years of undergraduate college education, followed by 4 years of medical school, and at least 5 or 6 years of specialty training as anesthesiology residents and fellows. In addition, they can spend an additional year in fellowship for a subspecialty.

Physiatrists (Physical Medicine and Rehabilitation Physicians)

These physicians are particular favorites among athletes because of their unique knowledge of biomechanics. If your back injury has been caused by an imbalance in your body or a dysfunction in the way you move, a physiatrist will spot it. They are either M.D.'s or D.O.'s trained in physical medicine and rehabilitation. Sometimes they are referred to as PM&R physicians. They diagnose and treat problems in muscle, bone, connective tissue, and nerve conduction. They do not do surgery.

Many are experts in pain management. Some-

Physicians Trained outside the U.S.: Okay?

Relax. The American Medical Association assures us that the Educational Commission for Foreign Medical Graduates evaluates and certifies physicians who were educated outside the United States and Canada. Termed International Medical Graduates (IMGs), these doctors may be citizens of the United States or Canada who chose to be educated elsewhere, or may be noncitizens who were admitted to the United States by U.S. immigration authorities.

The commission issues a certificate that is required before the IMG can enter an accredited training program. This certificate proves that the IMG has met the minimum standards, including proficiency in English, required to enter such programs. All IMGs must undertake residency training in the United States before they can obtain a license to practice medicine there, even if they were fully trained, licensed, and practicing in another country.

---

times working with a physiatrist will involve working with a team of health-care providers: medical consultants and rehabilitation experts. They have 4 years of undergraduate college education, followed by 4 years of medical school, and at least 4 years of specialized training as physiatry residents and fellows. It's not unusual for a physiatrist to have additional training in a subspecialty. You want a board-certified physiatrist. This means he has passed rigorous written and oral exams administered by his professional board. Additionally, physiatrists may have certifications in pediatrics, internal medicine, and neurology.

YOUR REHABILITATION TEAM

When the physician has made the diagnosis, treatment might include physical therapy—professional training to bring the body back into physical strength and balance. Often, not only can rehabilitation help heal, this training can teach you ways to move that will help you prevent injury in the future.

Physical Therapists

Rehabilitation of your back after an injury or surgery will likely include physical therapy. According to the American Physical Therapy Association, the physical therapist (P.T.) can help you prevent debilitating conditions or—once you've already experienced an injury, disease, or other precipitating event—can help you slow the progression of that condition. P.T.'s often help people with back and neck injuries, sprains, strains, fractures, arthritis, and many other conditions.

Basically, P.T.'s are experts in movement and function. They use exercise and training as their basic tools, but they also do hands-on assistance with joint range of motion, massage, heat and ice, ultrasound, and other advanced techniques to maximize function in your back. Most are covered by insurance. Your physician might refer you, or, if your state allows self-referral (and many do), you might be able to make an appointment on your own that might even be covered by insurance.

P.T.'s have a post-baccalaureate degree from an accredited education program and may also have a master's degree. In addition, a P.T. may earn a doctorate degree: doctor of physical therapy. P.T.'s are required to pass a national exam administered by each state. State regulations vary.

Occupational Therapists

Occupational therapists (O.T.'s) administer specialized assistance to people who have injuries or disabilities that make independent living difficult. This profession has been in the limelight for many years

---

How to Select a Physician

Picking the best physician for you involves more than just looking at credentials. When you set about finding a doctor to help you get or stay healthy, be sure you cover all these bases.

- Ask your primary-care physician to make recommendations.
- Ask family and friends.
- Call your insurance company and ask for a list of approved physicians.

- Call the physician's office and ask about experience with your specific problem.
- Determine whether or not the physician is board-certified.
- Check out the physician's access to diagnostic equipment and labs.
- Make sure the physician has privileges to practice in a hospital you like.
- Interview the physician and his staff to make sure you're comfortable.

as the "ergonomic experts"—the men and women who come into an office setting and redesign it from floor to ceiling to make it safe and comfortable for workers. But their skills extend far beyond the workspace. They can do the same job for your home.

Not only can they evaluate both the work environment and the home to spot problems and suggest specific adaptations, they can even follow you around for a while to assess your functional ability: how you move, how you handle tools and implements, how you sleep in bed, how you drive. After they have a checklist of possible problems and recommendations, occupational therapists can help you make adjustments and train you (and everyone in your environment) to be more effective.

Occupational therapists are credentialed at the professional level after completing a baccalaureate or an entry-level master's degree in occupational therapy. Occupational therapy assistants (O.T.A.'s) have a 2-year associate degree from one of more than 300 accredited programs at colleges and universities in the United States. Both the O.T. and O.T.A. must complete supervised fieldwork and pass a certification exam. The profession has established standards of practice and is regulated in all states.

STEPPING AWAY FROM CONVENTIONAL MEDICINE

When your back is in pain, you might be open to trying a few things aside from conventional medicine, sometimes even before you see your physician. We work all over the world, so we've seen medical practices that have run the gamut from dispensing teas made from blackened vegetation that looked as if it were raked out of the rain gutter to performing an animal sacrifice for transference of life force. Some were as ineffective as we thought they might be. Some worked like charms. All were well-intended. That experience pretty much sums up our opinion of complementary and alternative practices: Some of it is ineffective. Some of it works. And it's all well-intended when practiced by honorable people.

Four out of every 10 Americans have used some form of complementary and alternative medicine. They spend more than $30 billion a year on it, precious little of which is not covered by insurance. The American Medical Association has conceded that their patients are exploring options outside the clinical setting and has acknowledged that under some circumstances *both* traditional and nontraditional practices might work in concert for the benefit of the patient. A word to the wise: If you think that complementary and alternative medicine sure can't hurt and might even help, you would be only partially right. If you delay seeking medical attention because you're exploring alternatives, you could be wasting valuable time as your back problem deteriorates, making it more difficult to heal and putting you at risk for further injury. Use good judgment.

The National Center for Complementary and Alternative Medicine at the National Institutes of Health (NIH) suggests that you be an informed consumer. Do your homework regarding safety, effectiveness, risks, side effects, results you can expect, and length of treatment. On the Internet, go to the National Library of Medicine's PubMed system (www.ncbi.nlm.nih.gov/entrez) and Medline (www.nlm.nih.gov/medlineplus). Their databases can be searched using the keyword "CAM." If you don't have access to a computer, stop by your local library. If you can, ask your friends or other people with back symptoms like yours to tell you about the treatment they've undergone. Increasingly, you'll find physicians who can not only discuss protocols but also make recommendations and referrals. Keep asking questions.

We want you to know who you're dealing with, so check out the practitioner. Contact state and local agencies that regulate the practice you've selected. A few years ago, this would have been a long shot because there was little regulation, but, increasingly, complementary and alternative health-care practitioners are being called to task: regulated, certified, licensed, and accredited. Make sure that your caregiver is a professional practitioner with the required education and impeccable credentials to assure that you will receive the highest standard of responsible care and safety. Make sure that there have been no criminal charges or lawsuits filed or complaints registered. If you can, interview the practitioner in his own office. Get acquainted before you make an appointment. Know the costs before you allow yourself to be treated, and find out if any of them could be covered by your insurance.

Most important, remember the "complementary" aspect. The treatment you are considering probably shouldn't be the only thing you're doing to get well. Your personal physician should be involved and fully informed before and after you seek alternative medicine, so that there can be a seamless interface. And don't spend a lot of time exploring alternative medicine, especially if it delays a trip to your physician for accurate diagnosis and treatment.

We like to think that after you use the programs in this book, you will have no further need to seek alternative-healing protocols. You are holding the answer to your back problem in your hand. But just in case you're an adventurer, we are going to review some of the most common complementary and alternative medical practices used to treat back ailments.

Acupuncture

Channels of vital life energy, *qi,* or *chi,* (pronounced "chee"), run throughout your body. In order for a person to be healthy mentally, physically, emotionally, and spiritually, the channels must be clear and free flowing. When qi does not flow properly, it causes imbalance and disease. The purpose of acupuncture is to examine your channels, discover disruptions and impediments to the flow of qi, and clear the obstruction to restore free flow. It's done through the insertion of small needles or pressure. Sometimes the practitioner heats the needles or uses them to conduct small currents of electrical stimulation.

A skilled practitioner concerns himself with the total person and will also be trained in herbal medicine, Chinese psychology, and other disciplines of Chinese medicine. Among other things, acupuncturists treat back pain.

Although acupuncture might require multiple treatments to be effective, the NIH reports research that suggests acupuncture may be as effective for some conditions as the more widely accepted Western medical treatments, without as many side effects.

Practiced in China for thousands of years, acupuncture is now regarded as a credible medical discipline worldwide, including in the United States. Their regulatory board is the National Commission for the Certification of Acupuncture and Oriental Medicine (NCCAOM). In the United States, most states also regulate acupuncture practices with licensing, certification, or registration. These designations are: L.Ac. (licensed acupuncturist), R.Ac. (registered acupuncturist), and C.A. (certified acupuncturist).

Applied Kinesiology

When the musculature of your body and back is out of balance or badly toned, organs and glands do not function properly. These imbalances are caused by poor posture, allergies, stress, and injury. In order to make a diagnosis in applied kinesiology, the practitioner will apply force to a muscle, and the patient will resist. If the resistance is successful, the muscle is determined to be strong and balanced and the related organs and glands healthy. If, on the other hand, the patient can't resist the applied force, the muscle is determined to be weak and the related organs and glands unhealthy.

Allergies and food sensitivities are diagnosed similarly. The applied kinesiologist gives the patient a substance and tests specific muscular resistance. If the muscle is weak and the patient can't resist the applied force, the substance is suspect as being a source of sensitivity and allergy. By applying acupressure to reflex points on a muscle and chiropractic manipulation, the practitioner can balance the muscles and improve overall well-being. Long-term care can involve dietary changes and methods of stress reduction.

Practitioners are trained by the International

Building a Strong Relationship with Your Physician

Your physician is your partner in health care, so you want a good one. Ultimately, however, the responsibility for your body is *yours,* not anyone else's. You have to be a good partner, too. From your first appointment through your treatment and beyond, be efficient, honest, and conscientious. You expect a lot from your physician, and your physician expects a lot from you. In fact, the more you do to participate, the better your chances for a successful outcome.

To get your relationship off on a good foot, we recommend that you respect your doctor's time by being as prepared as possible. Hopefully, this preparation will buy you some extra attention and respect. Here are some tips for making sure that your first visit goes well.

1. Bring your medical records or have them transferred in advance of your visit.
2. Bring your insurance card and any other necessary documents.
3. Bring a notebook and pen.
4. Be considerate by making sure that your body and your clothes are clean when you know you'll be examined.
5. Write down your questions or list points you wish to discuss. Make sure that you cover them all during the appointment.
6. Write down your symptoms: what you feel like, when the symptoms started, what you think might be causing them, things that make them worse, things that make them better.
7. Prepare to discuss your medical history, your personal lifestyle, and medications you take—including vitamins, herbs, and over-the-counter remedies.
8. Be completely honest and forthcoming with information, knowing that the physician will protect your privacy.
9. Inform the physician of personal, cultural, and religious beliefs you hold that might influence treatment, such as being opposed to blood transfusion.
10. Come to an immediate understanding of financial arrangements and then honor them.
11. Be succinct in your conversation. Physicians are busy people who need to stay focused and on track.
12. Write down everything the physician tells you and make sure that you understand it completely before you leave the office. If you need to, bring another person who can help you take notes or remember what the physician has said.

College of Applied Kinesiology (a correspondence organization without an actual campus), where 100 hours of classroom work is required. The advanced level, diplomate, requires 300 hours of study, passing oral and written tests, and submitting two research papers. This industry is not regulated.

Ayurvedic Medicine

For more than 5,000 years, Ayurvedic medicine has been the cornerstone of patient care in India, made well-known in the United States by Deepak Chopra, M.D., medical director of the Chopra Center at La Costa and bestselling author of *Quantum Healing.* Healing is a matter of achieving health not by treating a single symptom, such as a pain in your back, but by treating you as a whole person in body, mind, and spirit. Ayurvedic practitioners do this by restoring and balancing three energies called doshas: Vata (space and air), Pitta (fire and water), and Kapha (water and earth). Disease is thought to be first a function of spiritual deprivation with consideration given to both internal and external influences.

Although the practitioner will treat you, this is a

participatory process. You will have to adjust your lifestyle and begin a slow healing process with personal responsibility. Treatment is as comprehensive as the word *Ayurveda* (meaning "knowledge of life") suggests. It includes massage, yoga, dietary counseling, herbal medicine, exercise, lifestyle counseling, meditation, aromatherapy, color therapy, chanting, cleansing, and other bodywork. Because of the extensive, comprehensive nature of diagnosis and treatment, Ayurvedic medicine is sometimes practiced in retreats or residential clinics, where a patient can expect to spend at least a few days.

At this time, Ayurvedic medicine is neither recognized nor regulated either nationally or by any state, although chiropractors, naturopaths, osteopaths, and medical doctors may have training. Ayurvedic practitioners have either been trained in India, have completed course work in the United States or through correspondence with an Ayurvedic center in India, or have apprenticed with an Ayurvedic practitioner.

Chinese Medicine

For thousands of years before the emergence of Western medicine, the Chinese have been practicing healing arts that are virtually unchanged from their origins. This is a broad classification of practice, but it generally centers on acupuncture, massage, qigong, and the use of herbs to regulate your vital life forces, the qi. Rather than treat symptoms of your back pain or dysfunction, the practitioner brings you into total balance so that pain or dysfunction simply cannot thrive.

Practitioners are called Oriental medicine doctors, or OMD's. This designation indicates that the practi-

---

Know Your Rights in the Doctor's Office

Entering the medical world with a back problem often requires that you deal with more than one professional diagnostician and caregiver. No matter how many people are involved, it's important to realize that you're in charge at all times—it's up to you to keep your recovery on track, so you have to be a good partner. Make sure that your physicians are accurately informed of your history, personal values, and health-care goals. In exchange for that, you will be treated respectfully and responsibly. Here are a few key things that you can expect from professional caregivers in the United States.

1. You have the right to obtain from physicians and other direct caregivers relevant, current, and understandable information concerning diagnosis, treatment, prognosis, and the immediate and long-term financial implications of your treatment. You can expect assistance in interpreting your bill and filing your insurance claims.
2. You have the right to know the identities of everyone involved in your care, including their names, titles, and job descriptions.
3. If you are medically able, you have the right to make decisions about the plan of care prior to and during the course of treatment.
4. If you must have surgery, and the risks might include death or permanent disability so that you might be no longer able to speak for yourself, you have the right to have an advance directive (such as a living will, health-care proxy, or durable power of attorney for health care).
5. You have the right to every consideration of privacy and confidentiality in every aspect of your care or interaction with medical and pharmaceutical personnel.
6. You have the right to review your medical records and to have the information explained or interpreted if you don't understand. Your medical records are yours. They will not be sent anywhere without your permission. You may have copies of everything.

STOPPING THE PAIN

tioner is trained in acupuncture, qigong, acupressure, herbal medicine, Chinese nutrition, and Chinese psychology, but does not indicate that the practitioner is licensed, registered, or certified by any governing board. Sometimes, however, an OMD will hold credentials as a medical doctor, a doctor of osteopathy, or an acupuncturist. As with acupuncture, regulations and scopes of practice by law vary from state to state.

Faith Healing

When your back is in pain, a faith healer may call upon a god or spirit to intervene and restore health. The healing can take place in a face-to-face meeting between you and the healer, or it can be invoked by thought, ritual, and prayer with you and the healer remote from one another. While the act of faith healing has not been validated by scientific study, prayer is supported and even encouraged by most physicians. There are studies that indicate that meditation or prayer lowers blood pressure, heart rate, respiration, and metabolism. The result is deep relaxation—good for a tight back. Additionally, belonging to a church or other spiritual organization appears to provide a strong support base for a patient. One small study in 1995 at Dartmouth Medical School evaluated older patients who had undergone open-heart surgery. Those who lacked spiritual support from a group or who had no spiritual belief in which to find comfort were three times more likely to die within half a year of their surgery than those who had spiritual support. (We're not saying you're going to die if you don't pray, but what does it hurt?)

Faith healers are not trained, regulated, or licensed. There are no requirements except intention and faith. Faith healers may be ministers, preachers, exorcists, spiritualists, lay clerics, priests, evangelists, shamans, or witch doctors affiliated with an organized faith.

Homeopathic Medicine

Homeopathic physicians evaluate you as an entire person, including the troubling symptoms in your back, and then select therapeutic substances that will match or simulate your symptoms to activate the body's own innate healing capacity, which is what finally triggers the cure. The principle is called "like cures like" or the "law of similars."

The more than 2,000 therapeutic homeopathic substances are classified as "drugs" by the FDA and administered as tiny sugared pellets soaked in a small amount of the selected substance. According to the principles of homeopathy, the smaller the amount of the remedy, the greater the effect. Homeopathic remedies are available in low dilutions over the counter for self-treatment. Some courses of homeopathic treatment work slowly, even over several months.

Homeopathic physicians are naturopathic physicians who have undergone formal training and have certification, but the availability of the substances and courses in homeopathy for laypeople make it easy for untrained enthusiasts to set up practice.

Hypnosis

In hypnosis, a trained therapist leads you into deep relaxation and concentration. In this focused state, you can be coached to modify behaviors and control pain, anxiety, and other chronic conditions that are exacerbated by tension in your back. Hypnotists don't diagnose or treat back injury or illness.

Although studies are limited and the medical community isn't quite ready to go out on a limb, hypnosis seems to be effective in pain management. In fact, it's used in some hospital settings.

Researchers have concluded that a person experiences pain in two ways: sensation and emotion. When something hurts, the anterior cingulate cortex is stimulated in the brain and influences how much pain is experienced and how much attention the patient will pay to it. This part of the brain can be quieted with hypnosis, blocking the sensation. (A word of caution: If you seek hypnosis to block back pain and you're very successful, you run the risk of further injury when you no longer sense or care about what is hurting. Clear this therapy with your physician.)

Hypnotists are trained in classes or in apprenticeships. As a profession, they are not regulated, but many are licensed counselors, psychologists, and therapists who practice hypnotherapy.

Massage

A good choice for a tired, aching back, massage is touch work, in which a trained therapist manipulates tissue. Nearly 150 recognized hands-on techniques are designed to improve health and well-being by loosening tightened and knotted muscles, relieving pain, easing tension, inducing relaxation, restoring movement, redirecting energy, and improving circulation. In addition, there seems to be an almost primal benefit to being touched and nurtured.

Most states require massage therapists to complete from 500 to 1,000 hours of academic instruction in a school accredited by the Commission on Massage Therapy Accreditation. Therapists are certified when they have completed their training and passed a written examination administered by the National Certification Board for Therapeutic Massage and Bodyworks. Advanced training and certification are available.

Therapists are licensed and regulated in most states, but even in states that do not, massage therapists are not authorized to diagnose or treat disease, order diagnostic tests, or engage in any activity that could be interpreted as the practice of medicine.

Naturopathic Medicine

Naturopathic medicine works on the assumption that your body contains a powerful, innate healing ability. Whenever possible, medical intervention should work in harmony with and support your body's natural ability. The practice centers on finding causes for problems rather than treating symptoms of your back pain: Eliminate the cause, and you will heal.

Naturopathic physicians are teachers, pointing you toward personal responsibility and attunement with your body's innate ability to heal. These physicians are trained to provide "natural medicine."

Depending on the regulations of the state in which they practice, naturopaths are qualified to use conventional diagnostics, natural therapeutics, dietary interventions, homeopathy, acupuncture, Oriental medicine, manipulation, physiotherapy, hydrotherapy, and counseling. The physicians train at recognized, accredited naturopathic colleges that offer 4 years of in-residence, post-baccalaureate naturopathic education. They are nationally licensed to practice.

Qigong

Qigong is an ancient Chinese practice of curing disease and promoting health. *Qi* (pronounced "chee") means energy or life force. *Gong* (pronounced "kuong") means practice. Qigong is the manipulation of energy by either meditation and visualization or physical movement.

Most visible among the qigong disciplines in the United States is tai chi, the slow dance of postures and positions that restore balance, build strength, remove disruptions in energy flow, and stimulate the flow of qi throughout the body. The back can be made stronger and more balanced along with the rest of the body. Men and women who practice the arts of qigong, including tai chi, report physical and spiritual benefits.

Practitioners are more teachers than clinicians. While many are trained by the Chi Kung School at the Body-Energy Center in Boulder, Colorado, most appear to be trained by apprenticeship with qigong instructors or within other disciplines: acupuncture, yoga, martial arts, and naturopathic medicine. They are not regulated.

Reiki

The practice of Reiki probably originated in Tibet, but it has been passed from master to master in a Japanese lineage that found its way to the Western world in 1937, when one of the masters from Japan, Hawayo Takata, moved to Hawaii. In Reiki, the practitioner acts as a passive conduit by drawing energy from the God-consciousness and the life force and then passing it through to your body, where it is drawn to areas of the body—specifically your painful back—where energy is blocked or disrupted. This influx of energy charges your own life forces and raises the vibration level in and around your physical body until the negative energies and disruptions are overcome and fall away.

The Reiki practitioner lays hands on you. Remember that scene in *Karate Kid* when Mr. Miyagi clapped his hands together and clamped them around Daniel-San's shoulder after an evil opponent had tried to rip his arm off at the tournament? Well, that was Reiki . . . sped up a bit by Hollywood. At more advanced levels, the Reiki practitioner is said to be able to send the energy from a remote location.

The techniques and philosophies of Reiki are taught by a master in a class. But those who practice Reiki believe that it's not a skill to be learned; rather, it's an attunement that is passed directly from the master to the student in a process that involves opening several chakras (energy centers in the body) and orchestrating a specific and ceremonial energy transference. Once the Reiki attunement has been given, it cannot be undone. It's with the student for life.

Reiki practitioners are not regulated, but they are credentialed by their profession, according to their advanced levels of training.

Rolfing

Muscles retain memories of specific incidents, both physical and emotional. A back problem might be the result of one such incident. Trained massage therapists can feel the tension through touch or observe it in your posture. A form of massage, Rolfing targets the muscle memory, releases it, restores energy, and returns you to mind-body integration and balance.

Rolfing has the reputation of being both physically and emotionally painful, but proponents swear by it. Therapists are generally licensed massage therapists with subspecialty training.

Yoga

Yoga classes might be useful for learning to relax your back and enhance your sense of well-being. Yoga is an ancient Hindu spiritual practice with healing and fitness benefits. A number of disciplines exist within yoga, with hybrid programs being developed every day. They all have three components in common: breathing, exercise, and meditation. Breathing increases oxygenation, helping you feel alert and focused. If your heart rate is also raised and combined with increased oxygenation, metabolic waste is removed from your body, promoting a feeling of well-being and healing. Yoga exercise is well-known for its postures through which the client develops balance, flexibility, and strength. And meditation, the last component of all the disciplines, slows down the pace of a busy person, lowering stress levels.

Instructors are neither licensed nor regulated, and therein lies our problem with a full-blown endorsement. We urge you to find a qualified instructor, attend a class before you sign a contract, and see if you like it before you make a commitment.

Chapter 7

AFTER THE DIAGNOSIS: GETTING OUT OF PAIN QUICKLY

Hopefully, your back will remain so healthy, strong, and flexible that you'll never have a problem requiring medical intervention. But if it happens, and your doctor takes you out of commission, we want to prepare you to be a good partner to your health-care team. Although medical people can do a tremendous amount to help you get well, the ultimate responsibility is yours. It's your back.

We have listed some of the most common diagnoses for back disorders and explained each one in simple terms. Of course, your physician will give you much more detail. Following the description of the diagnosis, we've made suggestions about getting into action, taking responsibility for getting out of pain, and restoring flexibility, strength, and balance to your body in general and your back specifically. If you were to come into our clinic with a particular malady, we would use the identical routines listed here to help ease your pain, quiet your inflammation, relax your raging muscles, restore your circulation, and increase your ability to move. You will feel progress from the first minute.

The stretches and strengthening exercises in this section are also in chapter 4. Please refer to the listings of individual exercises (page numbers are given below) for explicit instructions. We've included thumbnail photos for you here, as a quick, at-a-glance guide to the most critical poses for each condition.

Keep in mind that getting well is usually not a matter of performing miracles. (If it were this simple, we would just book you on the next flight to Lourdes.) Sometimes, recovery takes perseverance and patience and some time. We battle on. If we can make even a slight improvement, our client will feel better. We want full recovery for you. But if this can't happen, we want you to be able to recover as much comfort and function as you can.

Before you begin these or any exercises after a diagnosis of a back disorder, it is critically important that your physician knows in advance exactly what you would like to do and gives your plan his blessing. Take this book to your next appointment and study the suggestions together. Follow your physician's instructions to the letter. If you get the green light, begin immediately. If he wants you to modify a move, do it. If he denies you permission to work out, then take a break. When you're well and strong again, hopefully you'll be cleared to rejoin us. We'll wait for you.

Please note that we may repeat some general recommendations, with slight modifications for each condition. Often, you'll want to begin by drinking plenty of water, taking a mild nonsteroidal anti-inflammatory (unless otherwise directed by your doctor), and alternating stretching with icing the injury or condition. We'll modify this advice as necessary below.

In offering suggestions for short-term relief or for kick-starting recovery, we aren't implying that a full fitness program is no longer necessary. In fact, as soon as you are able, we urge you to return to the complete program for flexibility, strength, and cardio work. You need a well-rounded, lifelong workout plan of action to keep you fit and healthy and to make sure that back problems are things of the past.

DIAGNOSIS: ANKYLOSING SPONDYLITIS

Ankylosing spondylitis (AS) is a chronic, painful, rheumatic inflammatory disease that fuses the vertebrae in your spine from top to bottom. It can also appear in other joints, organs, connective tissues, and the chest wall. It's a form of inflammatory arthritis that's also called rheumatoid spondylitis or Marie-Strümpell disease. Ankylosing spondylitis usually presents itself in people between the ages of 20 and 40, attacking men over women three to one. No one knows the cause, but genetics appear to play an important role in predicting the likelihood of contracting the disease.

Because the joints between the vertebrae fuse, the patient will "lock up," frozen into position. The disease is painful and debilitating with flare-ups and progressive difficulties. Sometimes ankylosing spondylitis will trigger the vertebrae to generate bone spurs, protective coarsening of bone, like scarring. These spurs can compress and irritate the spinal cord and nerve roots, causing even more pain, numbness, weakness, and lack of coordination.

What You Can Do

While there is nothing you can do to stop an inflammatory disease, you can do a few things to relax and restore circulation to the muscles and soft tissues surrounding your spine and to take some of the compression off inflamed nerve roots. You also can slow down and possibly reverse this fusing phenomenon with stretching. You must get moving—the sooner the better.

Drink plenty of water to make sure you're always hydrated. Take a mild nonsteroidal anti-inflammatory (such as ibuprofen or naproxen) to get pain under control so that movement and subsequent relaxation are easier.

Stretch through the entire routine on pages 38 to 62. Do 10 repetitions of each. Move slowly and very gently and in the smallest ranges of motion. At no time should a movement hurt. Ice your back for 10 minutes to quiet down the area. Then stretch again. You can repeat the stretch-ice-stretch sequence several times, or until the pain lets up and you feel that you've restored range of motion to the smallest extent.

You must keep everything moving so that muscles are kept flexible and strong to support your back, circulation is restored and maintained, and the neurological connections and patterns between nerve roots and extremities remain sharp. And you have to fight the fusion of your vertebrae.

When you're ready, add the strengthening routines. Be patient, move slowly, and keep the weights light and the movements very small. At no time should a movement hurt.

The real problem in working out with ankylosing spondylitis are the bone spurs. Not only are they excruciatingly painful, they can impede movement. Frankly, they present a formidable impediment. Our only advice is to do the best you can. Work within the ranges of your own mobility and tolerance for discomfort, but don't push it.

DIAGNOSIS: BACK SPASM

Back spasm is a painful, involuntary seizure of the muscles in your back. It is literally a cramp. The spasm can last for a few minutes or a long time; it can even be intermittent (meaning it comes and goes). It might be caused by injury to or inflammation in muscles, the bones of your spine, the disks between vertebrae, ligaments, or tendons. The spasm is your body's way of immobilizing the area around the injury or inflammation. Locking up muscles creates a natural splint so that you can't move and cause more damage. The pain is a great gift, showing you where the problem is. Only your physician will be able to confirm the source of the spasm.

What You Can Do

Your mission is to relax the muscles to quiet the spasm. Drink plenty of water, so you'll stay hydrated. Relaxing a spasm is very tough when you're dehydrated, because the cells of your muscles are depleted. Take a mild nonsteroidal anti-inflammatory (such as ibuprofen or naproxen) to help with the pain so that movement and relaxation are easier.

If the spasm is in the lumbar region, or low in your back, immediately do the following two stretches. Do 10 repetitions of each. Ice the spasm for 10 minutes to quiet down the area. Then do the two stretches again. You can repeat the stretch-ice-stretch sequence several times, or until you feel the spasm relax and the pain lets up. When you're through stretching, lie flat on your back for a little while with a towel roll at the base of your neck and another at your lower back.

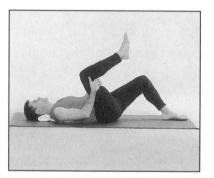

1. SINGLE-LEG PELVIC TILTS
See complete instructions on page 39.

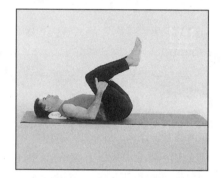

2. DOUBLE-LEG PELVIC TILTS
See complete instructions on page 40.

If the spasm is in the thoracic region, or the midsection, of your back, immediately do the following two stretches. Do 10 repetitions of each. Ice the spasm for 10 minutes to quiet down the area. Then do the two stretches again. You can repeat the stretch-ice-stretch sequence several times, or until you feel the spasm relax and the pain lets up. When you're through stretching, lie down flat on your back for a little while with a towel roll at the base of your neck and another at your lower back.

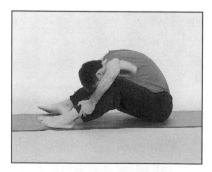

1. TRUNK EXTENSORS
See complete instructions on page 49.

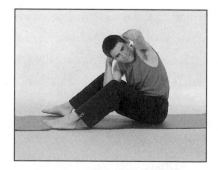

2. THORACIC-LUMBAR ROTATORS
See complete instructions on page 50.

STOPPING THE PAIN

If the spasm is in the upper thoracic region or the cervical region of your back—below your head and above your shoulder blades—immediately do the following two stretches. Do 10 repetitions of each. Ice the spasm for 10 minutes to quiet down the area. Then do the two stretches again. You can repeat the stretch-ice-stretch sequence several times, or until you feel the spasm relax and the pain lets up. When you're through stretching, lie down flat on your back for a little while with a towel roll at the base of your neck and another at your lower back.

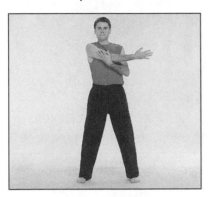

1. ROTATOR CUFF 1
See complete instructions on page 57.

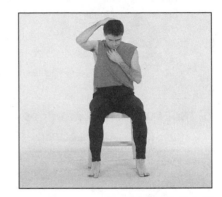

2. NECK EXTENSORS
See complete instructions on page 61.

DIAGNOSIS: BRUISE

Hardly an autumn weekend goes by without a news report of a football player removed from a game because of a deep-muscle bruise of the back or the thigh. The bruise is a well-known injury, but, fortunately, fairly uncommon among those of us who don't play contact sports.

The bruise is usually caused by a strain that rips tissue, a direct blow, or repeated blows to the body that crush the blood vessels, muscle fibers, and underlying connective tissue but don't break the skin. When blood vessels are damaged or broken, blood leaks out of the damaged vessel and into deep tissue, forming a raised, swollen bump that is bluish. This is called a hematoma. When the blood leaks out to the top layers of the skin, the bruise is a flat, purple mark called an ecchymosis.

The bruise is not an injury—it's only a leak. It's a sign the body uses to point the way to an injury. How easily a person bruises depends on many factors that have to do with the fragility of blood vessels and the clotting capacity of blood. When the back is bruised, the physician will be less interested in the bruise and more interested in the damage caused by the blow or rip.

What You Can Do

You need to relax and restore circulation to the muscles and soft tissues that surround the bruise.

Drink plenty of water. Take a mild nonsteroidal anti-inflammatory (such as ibuprofen or naproxen) for the pain. It will help make movement and relaxation more bearable. Until you can do a full stretch routine, choose from the four groups of stretches on pages 146 to 149. Do 10 repetitions of each, or as many as you can without discomfort. Bruises impede range of motion and make working out uncomfortable. Move slowly and gently and in the smallest ranges of motion. At no time should a movement hurt.

Ice your back for 10 minutes to quiet down the area. Then stretch again. You can repeat the stretch-ice-stretch sequence several times, or until the pain lets up and you feel that you've restored range of motion to the smallest extent. When you're through stretching, lie down flat on your back for a little while with a towel roll at the base of your neck, another at your lower back, one under the backs of your knees, and another under your heels. Try to position your legs a little higher than your head.

If the bruise is high on your back, restore circulation with these two stretches.

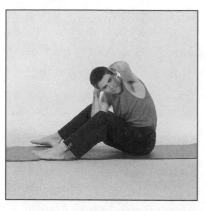

1. THORACIC-LUMBAR ROTATORS

See complete instructions on page 50.

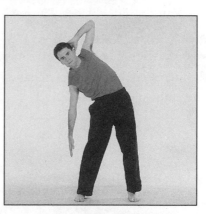

2. TRUNK LATERAL FLEXORS

See complete instructions on page 51.

If the bruise creates tension in the upper back, try these nine stretches.

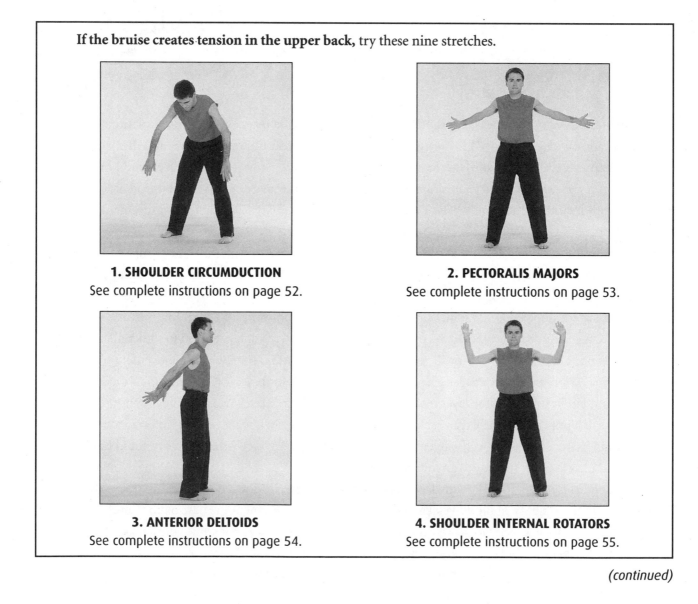

1. SHOULDER CIRCUMDUCTION

See complete instructions on page 52.

2. PECTORALIS MAJORS

See complete instructions on page 53.

3. ANTERIOR DELTOIDS

See complete instructions on page 54.

4. SHOULDER INTERNAL ROTATORS

See complete instructions on page 55.

(continued)

STOPPING THE PAIN

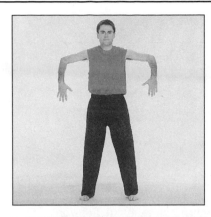

5. SHOULDER EXTERNAL ROTATORS
See complete instructions on page 56.

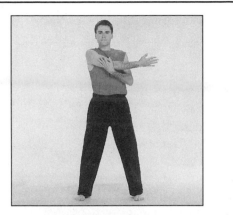

6. ROTATOR CUFF 1
See complete instructions on page 57.
Note: Rotator cuff 1 is the most important stretch in this routine for taking the tension caused by the bruising out of your upper back. Do it not only within this short routine but also frequently throughout the day.

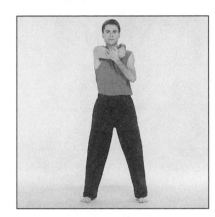

7. ROTATOR CUFF 2
See complete instructions on page 58.

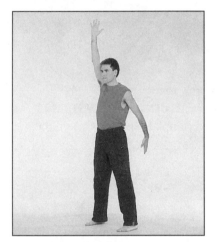

8. FORWARD ELEVATORS OF THE SHOULDER
See complete instructions on page 59.

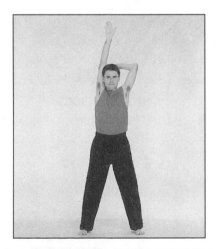

9. SIDE ELEVATORS OF THE SHOULDER
See complete instructions on page 60.

If the bruise is low on your back, restore circulation with these two stretches.

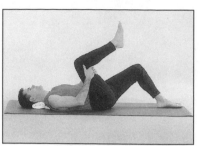

1. SINGLE-LEG PELVIC TILTS
See complete instructions on page 39.

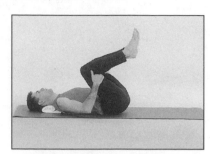

2. DOUBLE-LEG PELVIC TILTS
See complete instructions on page 40.

If the bruise creates tension in the lower back below your belt line, try these 10 stretches.

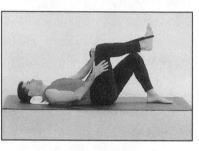

1. BENT-LEG HAMSTRINGS
See complete instructions on page 41.

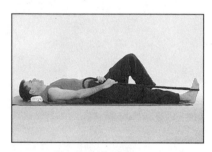

2. STRAIGHT-LEG HAMSTRINGS
See complete instructions on page 42.

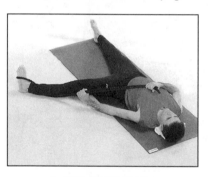

3. HIP ADDUCTORS
See complete instructions on page 43.

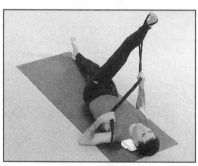

4. HIP ABDUCTORS
See complete instructions on page 44.

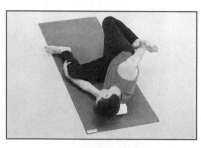

5. QUADRICEPS
See complete instructions on page 46.

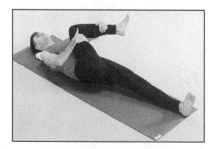

6. GLUTEALS
See complete instructions on page 47.

(continued)

STOPPING THE PAIN

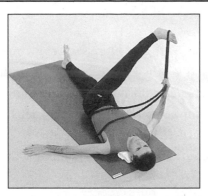

7. PIRIFORMIS
See complete instructions on page 48.

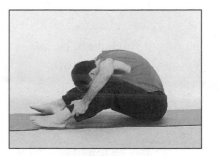

8. TRUNK EXTENSORS
See complete instructions on page 49.

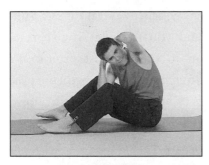

9. THORACIC-LUMBAR ROTATORS
See complete instructions on page 50.

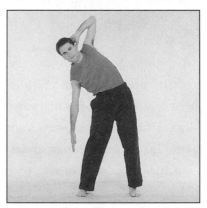

10. TRUNK LATERAL FLEXORS
See complete instructions on page 51.

DIAGNOSIS: CAUDA EQUINA SYNDROME

A small bundle of nerve roots at the base of the lower lumbar spine is called the cauda equina. These nerve roots are the transmitters of information from your brain through your spinal cord to your pelvic organs (including the bladder and bowel) and lower extremities, and back again the other way. When the cauda equina bundle is compressed or damaged, a lot can go wrong.

Cauda equina syndrome can cause permanent paralysis, dysfunction of the bladder and bowel, and pain and loss of sensation in one or both sides of your legs, buttocks, inner thighs, backs of legs, feet, or heels. The syndrome can be caused by herniated disk, tumor, infection, stenosis of the spinal canal, fracture, or trauma. If it's not corrected quickly, impairment can be permanent.

What You Can Do

How to treat cauda equina syndrome depends on the cause. This can be so serious that we urge you to rely on your physician and professional experience with this condition.

DIAGNOSIS: DEGENERATIVE DISK DISEASE

Degenerative disk disease is associated with the natural process of aging. Throughout life, vertebrae are cushioned from one another by soft, gel-like disks between them. The disks assist the flexion, extension, and rotation of the spine—just enough, but not too much. They help stabilize the spine, absorb shock, and distribute the ever-changing forces on your body.

When a disk is compromised by normal aging, injury from trauma, repetitive stress, instability, or inflammation, pain and weakness can step in. Interestingly, it's possible to have degenerative disk disease and have no symptoms at all. Still, it's good to know whether or not you have it, because a measure of caution can go a long way in protecting a fragile back from injury and insult. If you have degenerative disk disease and are bothered by it, your physician might suggest replacing the disk or fusing the spine to stabilize it. But he might also allow trying a few things first to strengthen the supporting muscles and connective tissues surrounding the disk.

What You Can Do

While there is nothing you can do to regenerate a disk, you can do a little to relax and restore circulation to the muscles and soft tissues that surround the degenerated disk. Drink plenty of water to make sure you're hydrated. Take a mild nonsteroidal anti-inflammatory (such as ibuprofen or naproxen) to get

pain under control so that movement and relaxation are easier.

Stretch with the exercises below, moving very slowly and gently. Do 10 repetitions of each. Small movements add up fast, so be patient. At no time should a movement hurt. When the stretching is completed, you need to strengthen the muscles that support your back to take the pressure off the disk. This workout routine has a little stretching and strengthening.

After completing one set of each exercise, ice your back for 10 minutes to quiet down the area. Then stretch again. You can repeat the stretch-ice-strengthen sequence several times or until the pain lets up and you feel that you've restored range of motion to the smallest extent. When you're through stretching and strengthening, lie down flat on your back for a little while with a towel roll at the base of your neck and another at your lower back.

If you've been diagnosed with degenerative disk disease, try these nine exercises.

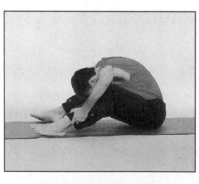

1. SINGLE-LEG PELVIC TILTS
See complete instructions on page 39.

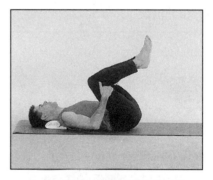

2. DOUBLE-LEG PELVIC TILTS
See complete instructions on page 40.

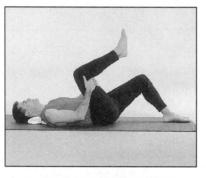

3. TRUNK EXTENSORS
See complete instructions on page 49.

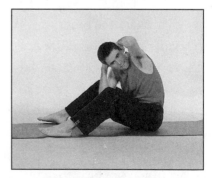

4. THORACIC-LUMBAR ROTATORS
See complete instructions on page 50.

(continued)

STOPPING THE PAIN

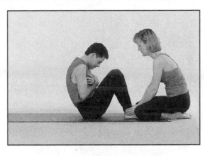

5. UPPER ABDOMINALS
See complete instructions on page 76.

Note: If you're just beginning or are unable to do this exercise as we have described it, you can modify the move. If you are able, tuck your chin until your head leaves the surface and you feel your abdominals contract. Don't roll up. Just contract. Keep your back flat on the surface. Pause and then slowly roll back until your head is down and you're relaxed. Prepare for the next rep. There is no need to rest between reps. Keep it going.

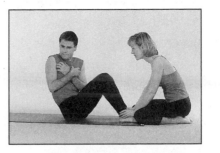

6. OBLIQUE ABDOMINALS
See complete instructions on page 77.

Note: If you're just beginning or are unable to do this exercise as we have described it, you can modify the move. If you are able, rotate your torso and lift until your head leaves the surface and you feel your oblique abdominals engage. Don't roll up. Just contract. Keep the side of your back flat on the surface. Pause and uncoil your rotation to roll slowly back down until your back is flat, your head is back down, and you're relaxed. Prepare for the next rep. There is no need to rest between reps. Keep it going.

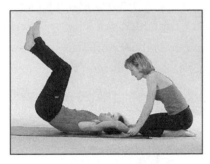

7. LOWER ABDOMINALS
See complete instructions on page 78.

Note: If you're just beginning or are unable to do this exercise as we have described it, you can modify the move. Lie flat on a surface. For a little more resistance, you can place your ankle weight on your abdomen below your belly button. Bend your knees and place your feet flat. Keep your back on the surface, contract your lower abdominals, tilt your pelvis slightly, and lift your buttocks 2 to 3 inches. Pause and then slowly return to the starting position.

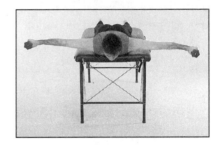

8. TRAPEZIUS
See complete instructions on page 88.

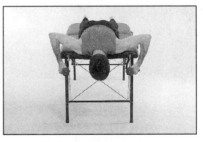

9. RHOMBOIDS
See complete instructions on page 89.

DIAGNOSIS: DISLOCATION

In everyday life, dislocations of the vertebrae are common reasons for visits to the chiropractor. They are actually *partial* dislocations, called subluxations, in which the vertebrae are no longer perfectly "stacked" and in alignment. The ligaments behind your spine keep everything together and stable, but the misalignment and strain cause pain and a possible degree of weakness and numbness in your arms and hands. Also, muscles surrounding the subluxation are pulled out of alignment when the vertebrae are torqued, and eventually those muscles fatigue in their efforts to keep the back in balance.

When the articulating joints between the vertebrae are no longer making any contact and the ligaments behind the spine are torn and can no longer support the spine, this is true dislocation. The vertebrae are out of whack, and it can be very painful.

What You Can Do

If ligaments are not torn, your strategy is to get strong and flexible to support your spine while it heals. You have to work to relax and restore circulation to the muscles and soft tissues that surround the dislocation. Tension in those muscles keeps the dislocation under pressure and will slow healing.

Drink plenty of water to make sure you're hydrated. Take a mild nonsteroidal anti-inflammatory (such as ibuprofen or naproxen) to help lessen the pain so that movement and subsequent relaxation are easier.

Doing a full stretch routine is best (see page 38). Go very slowly and work very gently. Nothing should ever hurt. If the smallest movement is all you can get, go for it. Small movements add up quickly.

If your diagnosis is dislocation *with* torn ligaments, you should do nothing except listen to your physician. You'll have to stabilize and immobilize the site of the tear so it can heal and your spine can stay aligned. You can resume working out later. Until then, keep the rest of your body moving—as long as you place no strain on the dislocation.

DIAGNOSIS:
EXERCISE-INDUCED MUSCLE SORENESS

Many people who are new to exercise experience discomfort as the body engages for the first time in a long time. And although we preach, "No pain," sometimes an athlete overdoes it and feels sore. There may be no injury, blood, or bone sticking through the skin, but the athlete still feels exercise-induced muscle soreness.

Sometimes the pain manifests itself immediately following the activity, as a function of simple fatigue. When the muscles are pushed, they can't flush the buildup of metabolic waste fast enough, so that accumulation of waste stays in the muscle, causing pain and weakness. Rest and a good stretch routine will flush the painful area, and the muscle will feel better.

Another, more confusing exercise-induced muscle soreness is delayed-onset muscle soreness (DOMS). DOMS doesn't show up immediately after the activity that caused it, but appears 24 to 48 hours later. Sometimes the delay is so lengthy and the pain is so severe that the person can't link the pain to the event and, in confusion, seeks medical attention. Muscles are stiff, sore, and weak. When a muscle is worked too hard, the muscle fibers tear very slightly as they strain. In addition to the tearing, the fibers swell, increasing pressure on surrounding tissue. For reasons not quite understood, DOMS is most common following activities where muscles contract while they are lengthening in braking actions, such as walking down stairs, running down hills, or lowering weights.

Although exercise-induced muscle soreness is usually not serious, only your physician can evaluate the magnitude of the damage that may accompany the pain and swelling.

What You Can Do

It's important that you relax and restore circulation to the muscles and soft tissues that surround the area of pain in your back.

Drink plenty of water to make sure you're always hydrated. Take a mild nonsteroidal anti-inflammatory (such as ibuprofen or naproxen) to keep pain in check so that movement and relaxation are bearable.

Start with the following stretches, and do 10 repetitions of each. Soreness, unfortunately, can be accompanied by slight swelling, which can impede range of motion and make working out uncomfortable. Move slowly and very gently and in the smallest ranges of motion. At no time should a movement hurt.

Ice your back for 10 minutes to quiet down the area. Then stretch again. You can repeat the stretch-ice-stretch sequence several times, or until the pain lets up and you feel that you've restored range of motion to the smallest extent. When you're through stretching, lie down flat on your back for a little while with a towel roll at the base of your neck, another at your lower back, one under the backs of your knees, and another under your heels. Try to position your legs a little higher than your head.

If the soreness is high on your back, restore circulation with these two stretches.

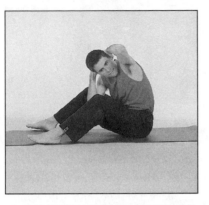

1. THORACIC-LUMBAR ROTATORS
See complete instructions on page 50.

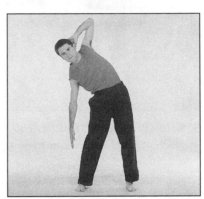

2. TRUNK LATERAL FLEXORS
See complete instructions on page 51.

If the soreness creates tension in the upper back, try these nine stretches.

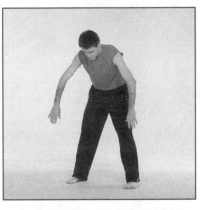

1. SHOULDER CIRCUMDUCTION
See complete instructions on page 52.

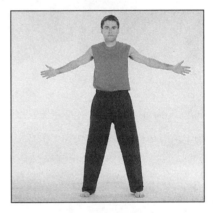

2. PECTORALIS MAJORS
See complete instructions on page 53.

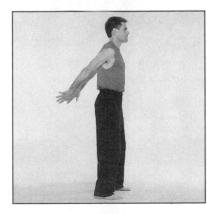

3. ANTERIOR DELTOIDS
See complete instructions on page 54.

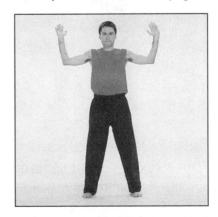

4. SHOULDER INTERNAL ROTATORS
See complete instructions on page 55.

(continued)

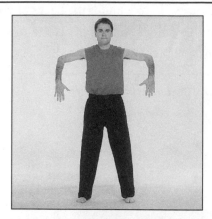

5. SHOULDER EXTERNAL ROTATORS
See complete instructions on page 56.

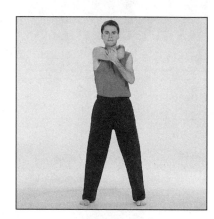

7. ROTATOR CUFF 2
See complete instructions on page 58.

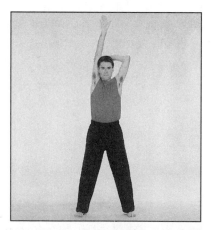

9. SIDE ELEVATORS OF THE SHOULDER
See complete instructions on page 60.

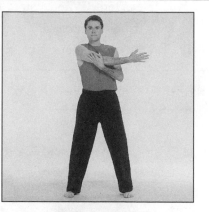

6. ROTATOR CUFF 1
See complete instructions on page 57.

Note: Rotator cuff 1 is the most important stretch in this routine for taking the tension caused by soreness out of your upper back. Do it not only within this short routine, but frequently throughout the day.

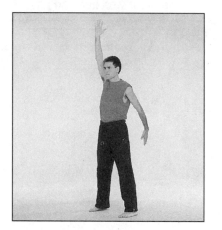

8. FORWARD ELEVATORS OF THE SHOULDER
See complete instructions on page 59.

STOPPING THE PAIN

If the soreness is low on your back, restore circulation with these 12 stretches.

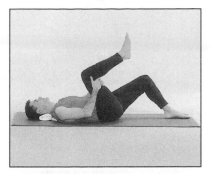

1. SINGLE-LEG PELVIC TILTS
See complete instructions on page 39.

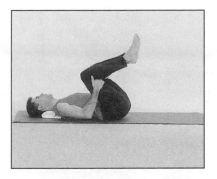

2. DOUBLE-LEG PELVIC TILTS
See complete instructions on page 40.

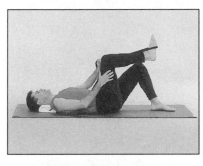

3. BENT-LEG HAMSTRINGS
See complete instructions on page 41.

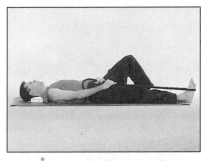

4. STRAIGHT-LEG HAMSTRINGS
See complete instructions on page 42.

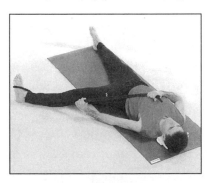

5. HIP ADDUCTORS
See complete instructions on page 43.

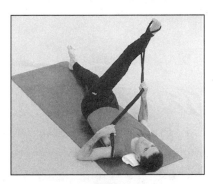

6. HIP ABDUCTORS
See complete instructions on page 44.

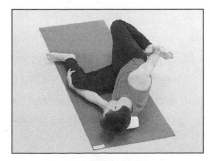

7. QUADRICEPS
See complete instructions on page 46.

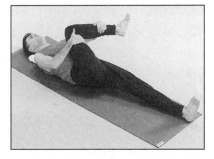

8. GLUTEALS
See complete instructions on page 47.

(continued)

AFTER THE DIAGNOSIS: GETTING OUT OF PAIN QUICKLY

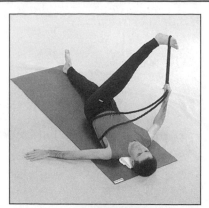

9. PIRIFORMIS
See complete instructions on page 48.

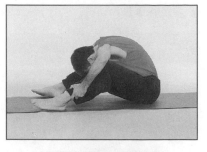

10. TRUNK EXTENSORS
See complete instructions on page 49.

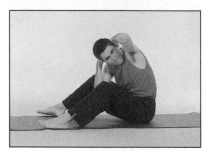

11. THORACIC-LUMBAR ROTATORS
See complete instructions on page 50.

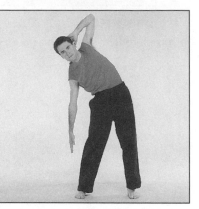

12. TRUNK LATERAL FLEXORS
See complete instructions on page 51.

DIAGNOSIS: FRACTURE

When vertebrae crack, it literally means that bones in your back have broken. Usually fractures occur with trauma, but when bones are weakened by disease, such as osteoporosis, they can also happen spontaneously.

In trauma, the type of fracture depends on the force of the blow, the location of the fracture in the spine, and the spatial orientation of the break. With a stable fracture, ligaments behind the vertebrae have not been disturbed, so the body still has a natural splint to support the spine. With an unstable fracture, the ligaments have been torn. The spine is without support, and the break is serious. In a simple compression fracture, the break appears to be minimal and is toward the midline of the vertebra. A vertical compression is like a simple compression, but the force of the break was more damaging. A comminuted cervical vertebral body fracture (a teardrop fracture) is caused by maximum force that causes explosive failure of the vertebral body—like a shatter.

When the vertebra shatters, the spinal cord can be in big trouble. Bone fragments can potentially penetrate or sever the cord, or the complete failure of the vertebra can cause serious compression of the cord.

Of all the bones in the body to be broken, a fractured vertebra has the most potential for disaster. No matter how large or small the fracture, an unstable vertebra can compress, damage, or sever a spinal cord. Unfortunately, with a vertebral fracture, it's impossible to isolate the broken bone and immobilize it in a cast. The entire area has to be immobilized to allow healing and, more important, protect the spinal cord from injury.

What You Can Do

If your diagnosis is fracture, you should do nothing except listen to your physician. You have to stabilize and immobilize the site of the break to allow the bones to knit back together. You can resume working out later. Until then, keep the rest of your body moving—as long as you place no strain on the break.

DIAGNOSIS: HERNIATED DISK

Also called a ruptured disk or a slipped disk, a herniated disk is sort of like the outcome of stomping on a jelly doughnut: the outer band of the disk bursts, allowing the soft, gel-like inner pulp to bulge out. The medical term for this is *herniated nucleus pulposus.*

The disks between each vertebra absorb shock and help hold the bones together in a stable, yet flexible way so that the back can move. When the outer band of a disk is herniated and the inner pulp bulges, that pulp can press against the spinal cord, causing extreme pain, nerve disruption, and coordination problems. In less severe cases, the escaped pulp can compress nerve roots, causing pain.

When the herniation or rupture is in the cervical spine, you can also feel pain and numbness in the neck, shoulders, arms, and hands. You can make the pain lesser or greater by positioning the neck to manipulate the bulge of pulp through the herniation. Wiggling around can take pressure off or put pressure on.

Interestingly, you can have a herniated disk without any symptoms at all. A herniation can take place quite suddenly or develop over a long period of time as the outer band deteriorates. Lack of regular exercise, poor nutrition, aging, normal wear and tear, dehydration, and bad posture can all contribute to the chance of developing a herniation.

What You Can Do

While there is nothing you can do to restore the integrity of a herniated, ruptured, or slipped disk, you can relax and restore circulation to the muscles and soft tissues that surround your spine, to take some of the compression off inflamed nerve roots.

Drink plenty of water to stay hydrated. Take a mild nonsteroidal anti-inflammatory (such as ibuprofen or naproxen) to control the pain. This will help make movement and subsequent relaxation easier.

Stretch through the entire routine on pages 38 to 62. Do 10 repetitions of each, moving slowly and very gently and in the smallest ranges of motion. At no time should a movement hurt.

Ice your back for 10 minutes to quiet down the area. Then stretch again. You can repeat the stretch-ice-stretch sequence several times, or until the pain lets up and you feel that you've restored range of motion to the smallest extent. When you're through stretching, lie down flat on your back for a little while with a towel roll at the base of your neck and another at your lower back.

You have to keep everything moving so that muscles are kept flexible and strong to support your back, circulation is restored and maintained, and the neurological connections and patterns between nerve roots and extremities are kept sharp.

When you're ready, add the strengthening routines. Be very careful, be patient, move slowly, keep the weights light, and keep the movements very small. It can't be repeated enough: At no time should a movement hurt.

DIAGNOSIS: JUVENILE RHEUMATOID ARTHRITIS

Juvenile rheumatoid arthritis (JRA) is an inflammatory arthritis that begins during childhood. The monoarticular form attacks only one joint, the polyarticular form attacks many joints, and the systemic form attacks several joints and organs of the body, causing not only arthritis symptoms but also high fevers and rashes.

The systemic and polyarticular forms commonly attack the cervical spine. At first, these forms of JRA cause pain and stiffness; later, they can interfere with the normal formation of the vertebrae and cause a fusion of the facet joints between the vertebrae.

In addition, ligaments that support the spine can be damaged by inflammation. When the ligaments are damaged and weakened, the vertebrae can't stay in alignment. When the vertebrae slip out of formation, the spinal cord and nerve roots are compressed, resulting in pain, weakness, numbness, and lack of coordination.

What You Can Do

Your mission is to get strong to support the spine so that no fusion can take place. Your first task is to relax, so you can restore circulation to the muscles and soft tissues that surround your spine and take some of the compression off inflamed nerve roots. At the same time, it's imperative that you strengthen muscles to support the spine.

Drink plenty of water to make sure you're hydrated. Take a mild nonsteroidal anti-inflammatory (such as ibuprofen or naproxen) to get pain under control so that movement and subsequent relaxation are tolerable.

We've designed a strengthening sequence to help with JRA symptoms. Do 10 repetitions of each exercise, moving slowly and very gently. Small movements add up fast. Be patient. At no time should a movement hurt. Ice your back for 10 minutes to quiet down the area after your workout.

If you're an adult dealing with juvenile rheumatoid arthritis, you may use light weights. If you're a young person, start with no weight at all and gradually progress to the lightest weights you can find. You'll discover that movement and the resistance of your own body weight are sufficient to make big changes in your fitness level. (And don't forget to make it fun! Crank up some tunes or recruit a workout partner.)

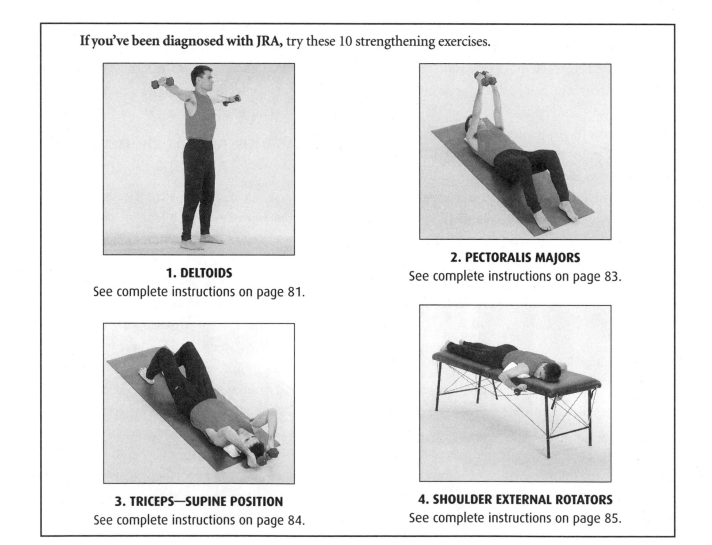

If you've been diagnosed with JRA, try these 10 strengthening exercises.

1. DELTOIDS
See complete instructions on page 81.

2. PECTORALIS MAJORS
See complete instructions on page 83.

3. TRICEPS—SUPINE POSITION
See complete instructions on page 84.

4. SHOULDER EXTERNAL ROTATORS
See complete instructions on page 85.

(continued)

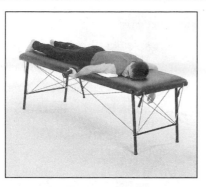

5. SHOULDER INTERNAL ROTATORS
See complete instructions on page 86.

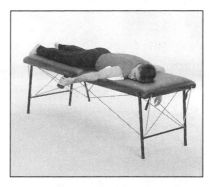

6. TRICEPS—PRONE POSITION
See complete instructions on page 87.

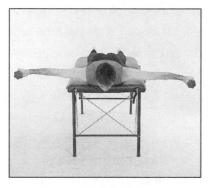

7. TRAPEZIUS
See complete instructions on page 88.

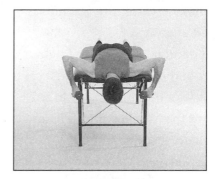

8. RHOMBOIDS
See complete instructions on page 89.

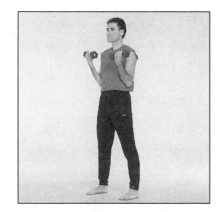

9. BICEPS
See complete instructions on page 90.

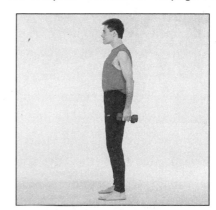

10. SHOULDERS (THE ROLL)
See complete instructions on page 91.

DIAGNOSIS: KYPHOSIS

Kyphosis, a term used to describe an abnormal hunching or curving of the thoracic or cervical spine, describes any spinal curve over 45 degrees. There are several types.

Postural kyphosis. Kyphosis is "hunchback." It's a rounded upper back that could be caused by something as simple as bad posture and slouching. When the abdominals are weak and a child slouches, this can stretch the ligaments in the spine—the connective tissue that connects bone to bone, in this case, vertebra to vertebra. That stretching can become significant and increase the natural curve of the spine.

(This is why parents are always yelling, "Stand up straight!")

Kyphosis usually shows up in teen years and is more common among females. Some young women might be sensitive to calling attention to developing breasts, so they slouch to allow clothing to hang loosely from their shoulders. Or, perhaps it is merely the increase in weight on the chest as breasts develop. The posture can become a permanent habit, and the curve can be forever. It is rarely painful, but like any curvature that is unnatural, it can become problematic as the child develops into adulthood. Most kids grow out of it and stand tall.

Weak abdominal muscles and tight hamstrings (the muscles in the back of the thighs) contribute to the slouch. When the child is able to strengthen the abs to support the back and get the hamstrings to let go and elongate, the situation improves immeasurably. By the way, weak abs and tight hamstrings are the signature problems of sitting too much. These problems are identical to those found in desk workers.

So what happens as a sloucher grows up? Because the natural curve of the thoracic spine is forward anyway, any weakness of the muscles or soft tissue in the back will draw it farther down. And an overdeveloped chest will do the same thing. A damaged or diseased vertebra will deteriorate and collapse its forward edge first (the edge toward the chest), so that will further pronounce the curve. (Hyperkyphosis is an exaggerated form of kyphosis characterized by rounded shoulders and a sunken chest.) But even if none of this happens, postural kyphosis in an adult can be painful and produce headaches, backaches, and joint pain.

Congenital kyphosis. In some infants, the spine never develops properly. The bones may not form correctly or a bone bar might develop between two vertebrae and cause a progressive hunch as the child grows up. If it's present from birth, it gets worse as the child matures. Children with such disorders as spina bifida can have severe kyphosis. The only treatment is a medical or surgical option. Intervention usually takes place by age 5.

Scheuermann's kyphosis. In this form of kyphosis, three or more vertebrae are irregular and wedged at 5 degrees each. Between them are small disks called Schmorl's nodes. Like postural kyphosis, it becomes obvious during teen years—however, it affects more males than females.

Scheuermann's kyphosis isn't usually painful, but it is an obvious cosmetic deformity that is disturbing to many people, and it can progress and become painful and cause neurologic symptoms. The only way to distinguish it for sure from postural kyphosis is with an x-ray. It can be treated with bracing that permits restricted remodeling of the bone in the vertebrae.

Kyphosis from compression fracture. The dowager's hump is a classic example of kyphosis that results from a compression fracture. It's caused when the vertebrae collapse because of osteoporosis (as is the case of dowager's hump), tumor, or infection. As with all fractures, and the accompanying soft-tissue damage and strain of deformity, this is painful. It can also lead to neurologic deficits. (Preventing osteoporosis *is* possible. See chapter 10 for more information.)

What You Can Do

For postural kyphosis, you can do a lot to correct the hunch. Remember that muscles work in pairs. So if the back is weak and extending into a slouch, then the chest is constricting and flexing to pull it forward.

Stability of the back is highly reliant on strong abdominals. When the abs are weak and the hamstrings are tight from sitting, then the back has no support. It tries to do all the work itself and shorts out. Over it goes.

For kyphosis from compression fracture stemming from osteoporosis, there's only so much one can do to relieve the imbalances. Fractures aren't so easy to fix. But osteoporosis can be prevented with calcium and load-bearing exercise, and if it's already set in, it can be slowed. Some medications on the market fortify bone so that it won't become porous and collapse. If the spine is already fractured, it might be able to be surgically stabilized, and the rest of the body can certainly be conditioned with strength and flexibility.

Until you're able to participate in a full workout, we suggest that you start with these four stretches. Work out on a soft surface such as your bed or a cushioned exercise mat.

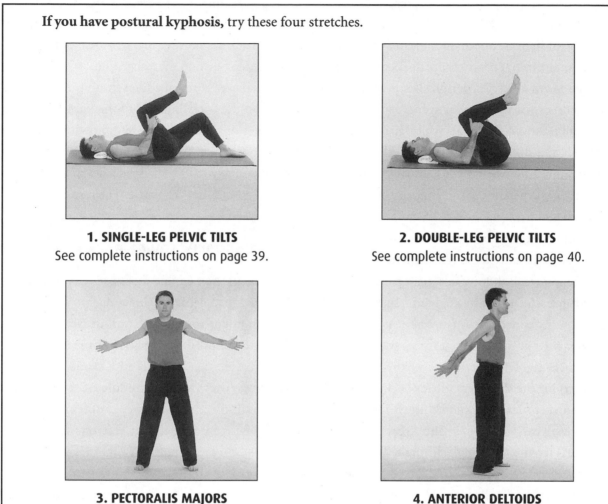

If you have postural kyphosis, try these four stretches.

1. SINGLE-LEG PELVIC TILTS
See complete instructions on page 39.

2. DOUBLE-LEG PELVIC TILTS
See complete instructions on page 40.

3. PECTORALIS MAJORS
See complete instructions on page 53.

4. ANTERIOR DELTOIDS
See complete instructions on page 54.

DIAGNOSIS: LORDOSIS

Lordosis (or swayback) refers to a severely arched back. The spine is naturally lordotic between the cervical and lumbar spine, but lordosis describes a curve that is excessive. As kyphosis describes a forward hunch, lordosis describes exactly the opposite—it's a swayback just above the buttocks, making the buttocks appear pronounced.

In fact, the prominence of the buttocks is the major clinical feature of lordosis. If you lay a child with lordosis on a flat surface, there will be visible air space between the lower back and the surface. If the child can flatten his back to the surface or if the lordotic curve is flexible and corrects when he bends forward, then lordosis is of little medical significance.

Lordosis can be a simple matter of poor posture. Or it can be present from birth or result from infection, injury, neurological and muscular problems, or back surgery. Symptoms vary, especially if there are accompanying defects such as muscular dystrophy. Sometimes lordosis is associated with bowel and bladder problems and pain in the back and down the legs. If it's anything other than postural lordosis, the only intervention should be medical and surgical options.

Hyperlordosis. Of particular interest to us are gymnasts and dancers, who assume a lordotic posture in many of their biomechanics. Studies suggest that although the initial postures are deliberate, they can become permanent. Hyperlordosis is an exaggerated curvature of the lumbar spine between L5 and S1 (lumbar 5 and sacral 1), which handles the greatest loads and stresses of the spine. It's also called hyperextension of the back. Although it produces a graceful line, it contributes to the majority of dance-related injuries.

Hyperlordosis can be both the cause and effect of a forward pelvic tilt caused by tight structures in the front of the hips, weak abdominals, tight psoas, weak inner thigh muscles that are unable to sustain the turnout, hyperextended knees (that appear to bend backward), a bow in the tibia that forces weight distribution back, tight hamstrings, weakness in the feet, and carrying the shoulders too far back, causing the upper torso to lean back and the chin to protrude. The result can lead to pain and stress fractures of the spine. If the dancer is male, lifting with hyperlordosis is dangerous for himself and the partner he'll drop when his spine collapses. The younger the dancer or gymnast who develops these bad habits, the greater the risk for injury.

Prenatal lordosis. As the weight of your unborn child puts pressure on your spine and unbalances your body, the natural tendency to arch your back for comfort takes over. Experts tell us that it will do no harm, nor will problems remain when returning to your former posture after your child is born and the weight is gone.

What You Can Do

Because lordosis is a swayback, we can assume that the abdominals are weak, the abductors are weak, the

hamstrings are tight, and the lumbar spine is compensating with contraction. Because these muscles work in pairs, straightening up the spine is a matter of tightening up the loose stuff and loosing up the tight stuff. As we said earlier, stability of the back is highly reliant on strong abdominals. When the abs are weak and the hamstrings are tight from sitting, then the back has no support. In the case of lordosis, it is pulled forward as the pelvis tilts.

The answer is simple: Loosen up the pelvis and strengthen the back. Loosen up the hamstrings and strengthen the abdominals. By following the complete program of Active-Isolated Stretching and Strengthening, you'll reverse the roles of the muscles in the pairs, and they'll balance. The result? The sway will go away.

DIAGNOSIS: LOWER-BACK PAIN

In light of all the possible diagnoses that might explain a back problem, hearing a diagnosis of lower-back pain might sound odd, but, in fact, it's a very real phenomenon. Lower-back pain is nonspecific discomfort in the lumbar and sacral regions—between the waist and the middle of the buttocks. This condition can become problematic when the pain is so intense that it restricts movement, disturbs sleep, or radiates through the buttocks to the legs.

Lower-back pain has many causes. Sometimes the source of the problem can be traced to muscle strain, overuse, ligament sprains, poor posture, spasm, injury, arthritis, weakness, or postural mistakes. Sometimes the source is more elusive and will require diagnostic imaging to rule out more serious conditions.

What You Can Do

You need to relax the muscles and restore circulation and movement. Drink plenty of water, so you'll stay hydrated. It's very tough to relax a muscle and restore circulation to an inflamed area when you're dehydrated, because the cells of your muscles are depleted. Take a mild nonsteroidal anti-inflammatory (such as ibuprofen or naproxen) to get pain under control so that movement and relaxation are easier.

When the pain gets especially acute, try the stretches below. Do 10 repetitions of each, but go very gently and settle for the smallest movements. Ice the site of pain for 10 minutes to quiet down the area. Then do the two stretches again.

You can repeat the stretch-ice-stretch sequence several times, or until the pain lets up. When you're through stretching, lie down flat on your back for a little while with a towel roll at the base of your neck and another at your lower back.

If the pain is in the lumbar region of your back or low in your back, immediately do these two stretches.

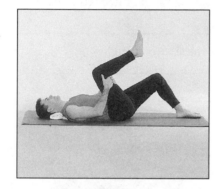

1. SINGLE-LEG PELVIC TILTS
See complete instructions on page 39.

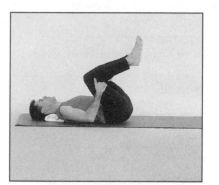

2. DOUBLE-LEG PELVIC TILTS
See complete instructions on page 40.

DIAGNOSIS: LUMBAR SPINAL STENOSIS

The word *stenosis* comes from the Greek word *stenos*, meaning "narrow." As we age, degenerative changes occur in our vertebrae, causing stenosis—a narrowing of the central spinal canal, through which the spinal cord runs. This narrowing can strangle nerve roots that run from the spinal cord through the vertebrae and branch out into the body. The net effect is pain, numbness, or weakness that can radiate down through the buttocks, thighs, and legs. Sometimes the pain can begin in lower legs and radiate up. The discomfort can sometimes abate with rest and flexibility that increases the area of the canal and decompresses the nerves.

The narrowing of the spinal canal is caused by a thickening and coarsening of the ligamentum flavum, a large connective band that runs along the inside of the spinal canal and holds everything together. In addition, extra bony, protective growths called osteo-

phytes form within the canal at sites of little traumas and irritations, narrowing the spinal canal.

Researchers are not sure why, but not everyone develops spinal stenosis as they age. They suggest that there might be a genetic predisposition to the condition.

What You Can Do

While there is nothing you can do to widen a narrowed spinal canal, you can relax and restore circulation to the muscles and soft tissues that surround your spine and take some of the compression off inflamed nerve roots. Drink plenty of water, so you'll stay hydrated. Take a mild nonsteroidal anti-inflammatory (such as ibuprofen or naproxen) to help with the pain so that movement and relaxation are easier.

Then stretch. Do 10 repetitions of each exercise on page 164, moving slowly and very gently. As you know, small movements add up fast, so be patient. At no time should a movement hurt.

Ice your back for 10 minutes to quiet down the area. Then stretch again. You can repeat the stretch-ice-stretch sequence several times, or until the pain lets up and you feel that you've restored range of motion to the smallest extent. When you're through stretching, lie down flat on your back for a little while with a towel roll at the base of your neck and another at your lower back.

These stretches will help your back, but stenosis is tricky because the pain radiates to and from sites that are not injured at all. It's very important that you work out your entire body—even those areas that hurt. One of the real dangers in dealing with stenosis is that an area of the body can be immobilized because of the perception of pain. Before you know it, a perfectly healthy set of muscles and connective tissues begins to deteriorate needlessly. You have to make sure that you're not pampering an area that needs no pampering. You can compound the damage of the stenosis and render your body more debilitated than it ever needed to be.

If you've been diagnosed with lumbar spinal stenosis, try these four stretches.

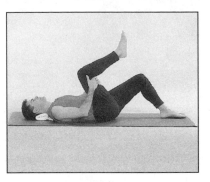

1. SINGLE-LEG PELVIC TILTS
See complete instructions on page 39.

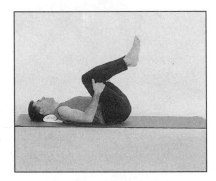

2. DOUBLE-LEG PELVIC TILTS
See complete instructions on page 40.

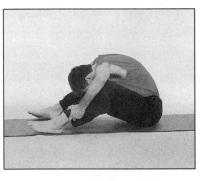

3. TRUNK EXTENSORS
See complete instructions on page 49.

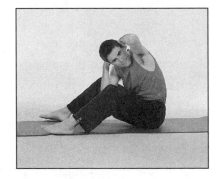

4. THORACIC-LUMBAR ROTATORS
See complete instructions on page 50.

DIAGNOSIS: MYELOPATHY

Whenever something goes wrong with the spinal cord, the condition is called myelopathy. This non-specific diagnosis merely describes difficulty rather than pinpoints cause. It's almost always accompanied by another diagnosis that is much more specific.

To say that you have myelopathy is to say that you have a specific disorder of bone, muscle, or connective tissue . . . and, oh yeah, the spinal cord is involved. Most commonly myelopathy presents itself in the elderly and is a result of other degenerative diseases of the cervical spine.

When degenerative diseases progress, they can

trigger bone spurs, in which the bone gets a protective coarsening similar to a scar. These spurs can press against the spinal cord or compress nerve roots, causing pain, numbness, and a lack of coordination.

The most common cause of myelopathy, however, is spinal stenosis, the narrowing of the spinal column (see the previous section for a full description). When the space through which the spinal cord travels is progressively constricted, function is disrupted. Not only is it painful, it could lead to problems with walking.

Myelopathy begins slowly and progresses gradually. The first symptoms are neck pain, difficulty with small motor skills, like buttoning a shirt, and difficulty in walking.

What You Can Do

How you deal with myelopathy will depend on your physician's diagnosis and advice. What we can say is that it's possible to get your back to relax to some extent and to restore circulation to the muscles and soft tissues that surround your spine and to take some of the compression off inflamed nerve roots that emanate from an irritated cord.

Drink plenty of water to make sure you're always hydrated. Take a mild nonsteroidal anti-inflammatory (such as ibuprofen or naproxen) to get pain under control. This will help make movement and subsequent relaxation more bearable.

Stretch through the entire stretch routine (starting on page 38). Do 10 repetitions of each. Move slowly and very gently and in the smallest ranges of motion. At no time should a movement hurt. Ice your back for 10 minutes to quiet down the area. Then stretch again. You can repeat the stretch-ice-stretch sequence several times, or until the pain lets up and you feel that you've restored range of motion to the smallest extent.

You have to keep everything moving so that muscles are kept flexible and strong to support your back, circulation is restored and maintained, and the neurological connections and patterns between nerve roots and extremities are kept sharp. Whatever you *can* move, move.

When you're ready, add the strengthening routine (starting on page 63). Be patient, move slowly, keep the weights light, and keep the movements very small. Remember, pain is a signal that you should stop.

Bone spurs can be a real problem when you work out with myelopathy. Not only are they excruciatingly painful, they can also impede movement. Actually, they present quite an obstacle. Our only advice is to do the best you can. Work within the ranges of your own mobility and tolerance for discomfort, but don't push it.

DIAGNOSIS: OSTEOARTHRITIS

Osteoarthritis is the most common of all joint diseases. It's an equal-opportunity disease, attacking men and women in equal proportion. In men, the onset is generally before age 45 and manifests most commonly in the hips, knees, and spine. In women, the onset is generally after age 55 and manifests most commonly in hands and knees. This disease attacks bone and cartilage, the specialized, dense connective tissue that forms parts of the skeleton and covers the ends of bone where they meet other bone.

Almost all people over age 65 have some of the bone and cartilage changes associated with osteoarthritis, but researchers tell us that it's not an inevitable part of aging. Many older people have the physical changes but no symptoms, such as pain or debilitation. The way people move and use their joints into their later years greatly affects the severity of symptoms.

Osteoarthritis is a low-grade inflammatory disease, like rheumatoid arthritis, that causes debilitating pits and cracks in cartilage. As the cartilage degrades, small bits may break and float into the liquid spaces that surround joints (the synovium), and bone is gradually exposed. Unprotected by cartilage, the action of bone on bone grates and irritates. Although the bone continually remodels to protect itself, the surface of the bone forms osteophytes, or bone spurs, "scars" that mark a site of injury or stress on the bone.

These uneven surfaces and spurs make joints less efficient and eventually cause deformities. Before long, the tissues surrounding the joint and connecting key parts struggle to compensate for biomechanical inefficiency. Inflammation engulfs the area and pain sets in.

At first, osteoarthritis is characterized by pain and stiffness when a person has "overdone it." As cartilage erodes, soft tissue surrounding the area inflames. The joint may eventually enlarge. When osteoarthritis strikes the lower spine, radiating pain to the buttocks and legs is often the result. When it sets into the hips, pain radiates to the buttocks, groin, inside the thigh, and knee. When it sets into the cervical spine, pain radiates to the shoulders and arms.

What You Can Do

While there is nothing you can do to restore the integrity of damaged cartilage and bone, you can relax and restore circulation to the muscles and soft tissues that surround your spine, to take some of the compression off inflamed nerve roots. Start with drinking more water to make sure you're always hydrated. Take a mild nonsteroidal anti-inflammatory (such as ibuprofen or naproxen) to help with the pain and make movement and subsequent relaxation easier. You have to keep everything moving so your muscles can remain flexible and strong to support your back, circulation can be restored and maintained, and the neurological connections and patterns between nerve roots and extremities are kept sharp.

Stretch through the entire routine (starting on page 38). Do 10 repetitions of each. Move slowly and very gently and in the smallest ranges of motion; at no time should a movement hurt. Ice your back for 10 minutes to quiet down the area, then stretch again. You can repeat the stretch-ice-stretch sequence several times, or until the pain lets up and you feel that you've restored range of motion to the smallest extent. When you're through stretching, lie down flat on your back with a towel roll at the base of your neck and another at your lower back, and rest for a little while.

When you're ready, add the strengthening routine (starting on page 63). Again, be patient: Move slowly, keep the weights light, and keep the movements very small. At no time should a movement hurt.

The real problem in working out with osteoarthritis is the bone spurs, which not only are excruciatingly painful but also can impede movement. Frankly, they can be a difficult hindrance. Our only advice is to do the best you can. Work within the ranges of your own mobility and tolerance for discomfort, but don't push it.

DIAGNOSIS: OSTEOPOROSIS

In some older people, bones become porous as a result of slowed bone remodeling and diminished calcium content. These fragile bones are more likely to fracture. In the spine, it's possible for a fracture or collapse of one or more vertebrae to occur without impact or apparent reason. Sometimes severe and disabling, this pain can affect not only the back but also the extremities when the nerve roots are involved. See chapter 10 for a more complete discussion of this disease.

DIAGNOSIS: PSYCHOSOMATIC BACK PAIN

Hearing someone proclaim your pain to be "all in your head" is perhaps an even greater hurt than the pain itself. But the truth is in the word *psychosomatic.*

Psycho means "mind." And *somatic* means "of the body." In other words, the mind and body are clearly linked. When you're under great stress, the back can undergo attack. Don't be embarrassed if your back pain appears to be without physical cause. The cause might not be physical, but the symptoms are.

Physicians treat psychosomatic back pain as *real* pain, because it is. Keep your body loose by regularly doing the stretch series, and refer to chapter 12 for a complete discussion of the role of tension on your back.

DIAGNOSIS: RADICULOPATHY

The word *radiculopathy* is used to describe pain, numbness, weakness, or tingling in arms and hands or legs and feet that is caused by an injury or disruption to nerve roots in your spine. A good way to remember the word is that it sounds like "radiating," referring to pain that radiates from your back to your extremities. But the word is really a derivative of the Latin words *radix* (roots of a tree) and *pathos* (disease).

The nerve roots are the communication conduits between your spinal cord and the rest of your body. When a nerve root is injured or disrupted, communications can become unclear and problems begin. The injury or disruption can be caused by compression or inflammation of the spinal cord and the nerve roots caused by a herniated disk or some other degenerative disease.

Sensory problems, such as pain, are more common than motor problems, such as weakness. In fact, if motor problems are present, it's a clue that the nerve root compression or inflammation might be more serious.

What You Can Do

Treatment depends on the cause of the radiculopathy. If your physician gives you the green light, get to work relaxing and restoring circulation to the muscles and soft tissues that surround your spine and taking some of the compression off inflamed nerve roots.

Drink plenty of water to make sure you're hydrated. Take a mild nonsteroidal anti-inflammatory (such as ibuprofen or naproxen) to control the pain so that movement will be easier.

Do 10 repetitions of each stretch below, moving slowly and very gently. Small movements add up fast. Be patient. At no time should a movement hurt. Ice your back for 10 minutes to quiet down the area. Then stretch again. You can repeat the stretch-ice-stretch sequence several times, or until the pain lets up and you feel that you've restored range of motion to the smallest extent. When you're through stretching, lie down flat on your back for a little while with a towel roll at the base of your neck and another at your lower back.

These stretches will help your back, but radiculopathy is tricky because the pain radiates to and from sites that are not injured at all. It's very important that you work out your entire body—even those areas that hurt. One of the real dangers in dealing with this condition is that an area of the body can be immobilized because of the perception of pain. Before you know it, a perfectly healthy set of muscles and connective tissues begins to deteriorate needlessly. You have to make sure that you're not pampering an area that needs no pampering. You can compound the damage of the original injury and render your body more debilitated than it ever needed to be.

If the pain is radiating to the arm, wrist, elbow, or hand, get fast relief with these two stretches.

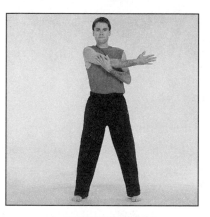

1. ROTATOR CUFF 1
See complete instructions on page 57.

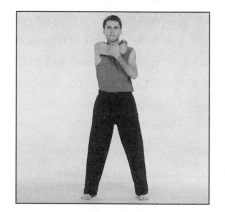

2. ROTATOR CUFF 2
See complete instructions on page 58.

If the pain is radiating to the buttocks and legs, get relief with the following stretches.

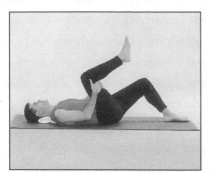

1. SINGLE-LEG PELVIC TILTS
See complete instructions on page 39.

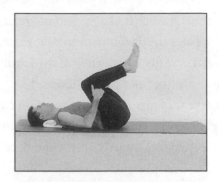

2. DOUBLE-LEG PELVIC TILTS
See complete instructions on page 40.

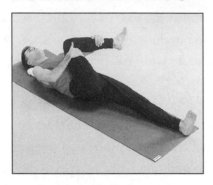

3. GLUTEALS
See complete instructions on page 47.

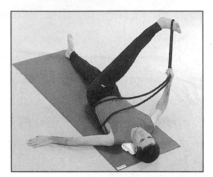

4. PIRIFORMIS
See complete instructions on page 48.

DIAGNOSIS: RHEUMATOID ARTHRITIS

Rheumatoid arthritis is an inflammatory, degenerative condition of the synovial membrane, the tissue that lines the joints. This condition usually presents itself between the ages of 20 and 50, and attacks women over men three to one.

Although the disease attacks the entire body, including hands and fingers, feet and toes, and hips, the back is in danger. The vertebrae in the neck just below the head—the atlas and the axis—are especially susceptible to damage, particularly in people who have had rheumatoid arthritis for more than 10 years.

When the atlas and axis are attacked and begin to degenerate, too much movement between the vertebrae makes the cervical spine unstable. As the disease progresses, the tip of the first bone might protrude up into the base of the skull, compressing the brain stem and causing difficulty in balance and coordination.

Finally, rheumatoid arthritis can cause the lower vertebrae in the cervical spine to slip forward, forcing a thrusting posture of the head and a hunch forward of the neck. If you have been diagnosed with rheumatoid arthritis, there is a 60 percent chance that it will progress into your spine. Being vigilant about monitoring and treating the condition is very important.

What You Can Do

The mission here is to get circulation back into inflamed, congested joints. You have to get blood flow to carry oxygen in and remove waste products to keep the bone remodeling and the tissues healthy. You also have to restore range of motion.

While there is nothing you can do to stop rheumatoid arthritis by yourself, you can do a few things to

STOPPING THE PAIN

restore circulation to the muscles and soft tissues that surround the attacked vertebrae. Drink plenty of water to stay hydrated. Take a mild nonsteroidal anti-inflammatory (such as ibuprofen or naproxen) to help with the pain—movement and subsequent relaxation will be more bearable.

Do 10 repetitions of each stretch below, moving slowly and very gently. Small movements add up fast. Be patient. At no time should a movement hurt. Ice your cervical spine for 10 minutes to quiet down the area. Then stretch again. You can repeat the stretch-ice-stretch sequence several times, or until the pain lets up and you feel that you've restored range of motion to the smallest extent.

If you feel your cervical spine tightening, do these two stretches frequently throughout the day.

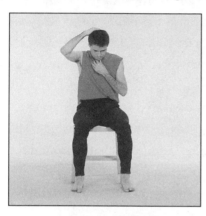

1. NECK EXTENSORS
See complete instructions on page 61.

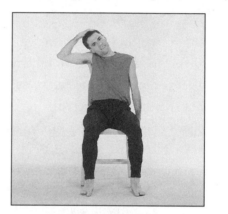

2. NECK LATERAL FLEXORS
See complete instructions on page 62.

DIAGNOSIS: SCIATICA (OR PIRIFORMIS SYNDROME)

The largest nerve in your body, the sciatic nerve is as wide as your thumb and runs from your lower back through your buttocks and into the backs of your thighs, all the way down to your feet. When that nerve is compressed or strained in your lower back in some way, the nerve becomes irritated. Instead of transmitting messages for movement from your spinal cord to your legs, it transmits messages of pain. This condition is called sciatica.

Many things can cause the compression: arthritis, a tumor, a herniated disk, an infection in the spine, or an injury. The pain is generally on one side only and most often starts in the buttocks. Occasionally, it manifests as numbness or weakness in the leg and foot, which makes walking difficult. Patients generally complain of a deep pain in the buttocks that becomes ex-

cruciating when sitting, climbing stairs, or squatting. Studies in Finland reveal that the predisposition to back problems in general, and sciatica in particular, is mainly genetic. Researchers have identified a genetic mutation that damages the protein charged with helping the body maintain the integrity of cartilage between the disks. If your parents suffered from sciatica, research suggests that you have to be extra vigilant.

One of the most common causes of sciatic pain is piriformis syndrome. The piriformis muscle is the external rotator muscle in the center of your pelvis that shoots right through the buttock over to the greater trochanter of the femur—the large, protruding bump on the outside top of the thigh. The sciatic nerve passes underneath the piriformis.

In about 15 percent of the population, however, that nerve runs right through the fibers of the piriformis muscle. When the muscle is contracted and compresses the sciatic nerve, the piriformis strangles it, causing irritation and all the symptoms of sciatica listed above.

Intense repetitive activity that hammers the lower back, buttocks, and hip can cause this muscle to swell. Sitting on something that puts pressure directly on the muscle will do it—like sitting on a wallet. Being out of shape can do it, too. Weakness in the hip muscles and gluteals in your buttocks will tighten up the piriformis and strangle the sciatic nerve.

What You Can Do

It's important to relax and restore circulation to the muscles and soft tissues that surround your lower back and to get the piriformis to relax and let loose its stranglehold on the sciatic nerve.

Drink plenty of water to make sure you're always hydrated. Take a mild nonsteroidal anti-inflammatory (such as ibuprofen or naproxen) to control pain so that movement and subsequent relaxation are easier.

Start with stretching, doing the exercises below. Do 10 repetitions of each. Soreness can be accompanied by slight swelling that can impede range of motion and make working out uncomfortable. Move slowly and very gently and in the smallest ranges of motion. At no time should a movement hurt. Ice your back for 10 minutes to quiet down the area. Then stretch again. You can repeat the stretch-ice-stretch sequence several times, or until the pain lets up and you feel that you've restored range of motion to the smallest extent.

Take a look at your lifestyle and see what you're doing to cause this impingement. Are you overweight? Do you wear your wallet in your back pocket? Do you do one activity repeatedly, without giving your body a rest? Pay attention to this signal, and think of a way to give your overtaxed sciatic nerve a break.

This stretching sequence is designed in a specific order to relax muscles that surround the piriformis and then sneak up on it. One day of work will not alleviate the problem, but patience will prevail. Stop all stretches short of pain.

If you have sciatica, try the 10 stretches in this sequence.

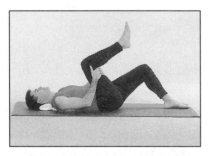

1. SINGLE-LEG PELVIC TILTS
See complete instructions on page 39.

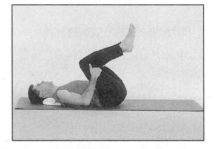

2. DOUBLE-LEG PELVIC TILTS
See complete instructions on page 40.

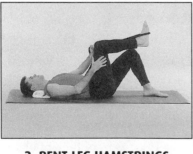

3. BENT-LEG HAMSTRINGS
See complete instructions on page 41.

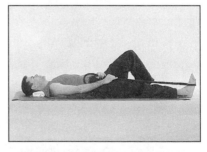

4. STRAIGHT-LEG HAMSTRINGS
See complete instructions on page 42.

(continued)

STOPPING THE PAIN

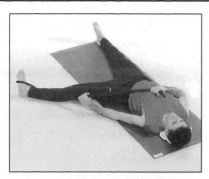

5. HIP ADDUCTORS
See complete instructions on page 43.

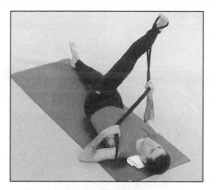

6. HIP ABDUCTORS
See complete instructions on page 44.

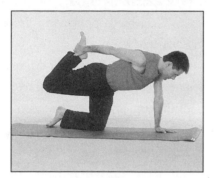

7. PSOAS
See complete instructions on page 45.

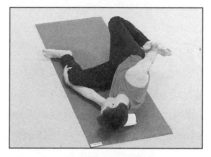

8. QUADRICEPS
See complete instructions on page 46.

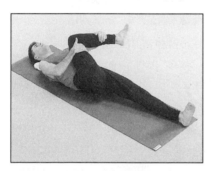

9. GLUTEALS
See complete instructions on page 47.

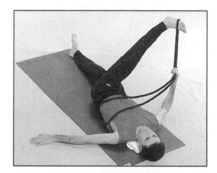

10. PIRIFORMIS
See complete instructions on page 48.

DIAGNOSIS: SCOLIOSIS

If you take an x-ray of a healthy spine from the back, it appears to be a straight line up and down. But if that line looks more like the sideways curve of the letter C, or worse, the letter S, then you're looking at scoliosis.

Pediatricians are always on the lookout for scoliosis, as are school nurses (remember those moments in the cold nurse's office, bending over so the nurse could feel your back?). Scoliosis can be caused by spinal deformities from birth, genetic disorders, neuromuscular disorders, leg-length discrepencies, spina bifida, cerebral palsy, atrophy of muscles surrounding the spine, and tumors, but more than 80 percent of scoliosis cases have no explanation or origin. This idiopathic scoliosis "just happens." Most of the time, it presents itself in childhood between ages 10 and 15, but it can develop as we grow older. Or it can go undetected in childhood and then become obvious and problematic as we grow older.

Scoliosis runs in families, and it occurs equally in males and females. Nonetheless, females are seven to nine times more likely to have a severe curve that progresses more aggressively and that will require some sort of intervention. No one is really certain why this happens.

Several types of scoliosis can develop.

The C-shaped curves. Scoliosis, if serious and untreated, can pull the rib cage out of its normal position, compressing and crowding the ribs on the inside of the curve and pulling apart the ribs on the outside of the curve. If the C-shaped right thoracic curve shifts the ribs on the right side, it can constrict the heart and lungs. Breathing is difficult. Or the if the C-shape is lower—in the lumbar region—it can distort the hips. Extreme curves can certainly make some activities difficult and most others painful.

The S-shaped curves. The most common S-shaped curve is a double curve—a combination of major curves. One will distort the thoracic spine and the chest, and the other, going the other way, will distort the lumbar spine and hips. Although this sounds horrendous, and it can be, generally, the two curves in opposition sort of balance each other out and cause less deformity.

The rotation phenomenon. Another problem with serious, uncorrected scoliosis is that as the spine grows and develops, the forces of the scoliosis cause it to rotate on its own axis. This rotation pulls the rib cage around so that one side of the rib cage appears higher than the other in the back. While that's going on, the ribs on the inward side of the rotation are bunched together and the ribs on the outward side are spread. This can contribute to respiratory difficulty and cardiac problems later in life.

Neuromuscular scoliosis. When scoliosis is present in children with other neuromuscular disorders (spina bifida, muscular dystrophies, spinal cord injuries), the scoliosis is called neuromuscular scoliosis. As these children grow and their trunks grow weaker, the scoliosis worsens from progressive deformity and collapse of the spine. Neuromuscular

scoliosis requires medical and surgical intervention.

Congenital scoliosis. If scoliosis is congenital—that is, if the child is born with it—the culprit is a malformation of the vertebrae. This form of scoliosis is frequently accompanied by other physical abnormalities in systems that develop in the fetus at about the same time the spinal column is forming, such as urinary anamolies. It's also possible that a birth defect may cause an imbalance in the way the spine grows, causing it to become crooked as the child matures.

Under these circumstances, scoliosis can be a serious matter. Treatment options in these cases are strictly medical and surgical.

In most cases of scoliosis, the curve is minimal and causes no real problems, and rarely is it painful. But the condition should be handled when your child is young, because the curve can become more pronounced in adulthood and cause problems. (If you notice any pain or loss of function, the condition warrants serious and immediate attention.)

Once the scoliosis is confirmed by x-ray, it's often appropriate to take a "wait and see" approach, especially if the angle of the curve is not severe (less than 20 degrees). Some curves never progress beyond a few degrees, while others increase rapidly. Researchers have not been able to determine why these differences exist.

Whether or not your child's physician will advise treatment will also depend on the child's developmental stage of growth. An 18-year-old girl whose physician discovers scoliosis during a physical is already mature skeletally. Major changes in the curve are not likely to happen. If she has been symptom-free, the physician will probably not recommend intervention. On the other hand, a 5-year-old girl who has not yet reached peak maturity might be a candidate for intervention.

What You Can Do

We have a soft spot in our hearts for people who experience curvature of the spine. You may recall Phil's story from chapter 1: During an intense training period at college, Phil was nearly incapacitated by pain in his back. No rest, massage, Rolfing, chiropractors, or medication could touch the pain—he was in agony. When a doctor suggested implanting rods in his spine and forbade him from continuing to run, we were desperate to find another, nonsurgical solution. That's what brought us to Aaron Mattes and the Active-Isolated method—and the rest is, thankfully, vital, energetic history!

As a parent, few things are scarier than suspecting your child has scoliosis. Before you panic, first go through this checklist of early-warning signs of the condition.

■ Shoulders are of different heights.
■ One shoulder blade appears more prominent than the other.
■ Hipbones are uneven.
■ Waistline is uneven.
■ Bottoms of each sides of the rib cage don't line up.
■ Body leans to one side.
■ Head appears to be off center with the pelvis.
■ One arm appears longer than the other.
■ Hemlines of skirts and pants are uneven.
■ When the child bends over, ribs form a hump on one side.
■ Head appears to be tilted.

Another option is to do a home version of the nurse's office test, officially called "Adam's Forward-Bend Test." Have your child wear a tight T-shirt or no shirt at all, and stand directly behind him. Have him put his feet together, and with his back straight, have him bend from the waist 90 degrees. His torso will be parallel with the floor. Look straight over his back, and you will be able to see if it's even and symmetrical. If it's not, then you might suspect scoliosis.

In our clinic, we've frequently found scoliosis to be nothing more than the result of a compensation by the body to bring itself back into balance when one side of the back is weaker than the other. When the physician has ruled out neuromuscular scoliosis or congenital scoliosis, we take over. As long as most physicians take a "wait and see" attitude with scoliosis, why not try a few things?

When the body is out of balance, one side is weak,

and the other side is constricted from trying to bring the body into alignment and balance. Muscles work in pairs. When one flexes, the other elongates. Scoliosis can be a battle of muscle pairs. By strengthening weak muscles and relaxing and elongating constricted ones, we are frequently able to correct scoliosis.

By the time scoliosis has set in, the child may have a lot of muscular and connective tissue imbalances and weaknesses, so correction is not instantaneous. Old habits are hard to break—even at the cellular level. Use the complete Active-Isolated program to restore structural integrity, and build new neural patterns so that the body will know how it's supposed to align. Then make sure everything is strong and flexible enough to sustain the new positions. Small results are nearly immediate, but full correction does take time. It can be done, however! Phil is living proof.

DIAGNOSIS: SPONDYLOLISTHESIS

In some people, the architecture of the individual vertebra is defective. When the bone on the back of a vertebra is deformed, it's possible for the vertebra to move forward out of alignment. This migrating vertebra may tease the vertebrae above it out of alignment as well, setting off a cascade of discomfort.

Spondylolisthesis can result in sciatica, lower-back pain that travels through the hips and buttocks to the thighs. Athletes who bear weight and torque in their backs—such as football players, weight lifters, and javelin throwers—appear to be prone to this condition. Degenerative spondylolisthesis is deformation of the architecture of the vertebrae due to wear and tear that erodes the facet joints between the bones. Of particular risk are people with diabetes, who are four times more likely to develop degenerative spondylolisthesis than the average person. Among our patients, it's not uncommon for a person to have spondylolisthesis and scoliosis (curvature of the spine) at the same time.

What You Can Do

Because spondylolisthesis deforms the spine and is sometimes accompanied by scoliosis, it's important for you to begin stretching out your body immediately. You need to relax and restore circulation to the muscles and soft tissues that surround your lower back, and generally to strengthen your body and bring it back into balance.

Drink plenty of water to make sure you're always hydrated. Take a mild nonsteroidal anti-inflammatory (such as ibuprofen or naproxen) to get the pain under control so that movement is tolerable.

Start with stretching. Do 10 repetitions of each described below. Soreness, unfortunately, can be accompanied by slight swelling that can impede range of motion and make working out uncomfortable. Move

slowly and very gently and in the smallest ranges of motion. At no time should a movement hurt. Ice your back for 10 minutes to quiet down the area. Then stretch again. You can repeat the stretch-ice-stretch sequence several times or until the pain lets up and you feel that you've restored range of motion to the smallest extent.

Also, take a moment to examine the repetitive movements you make, to see if they may be contributing to your problem. If diabetes is the root cause of your spondylolisthesis, we trust you have a lot of reasons to try to control your weight and the progression of this dangerous disease—consider the relief of your back pain to be another incentive.

If you've been diagnosed with spondylolisthesis, try this sequence of 10 stretches.

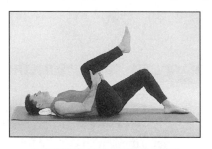

1. SINGLE-LEG PELVIC TILTS
See complete instructions on page 39.

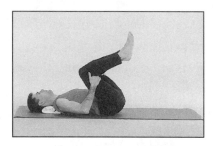

2. DOUBLE-LEG PELVIC TILTS
See complete instructions on page 40.

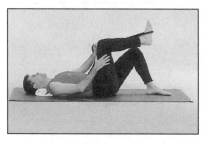

3. BENT-LEG HAMSTRINGS
See complete instructions on page 41.

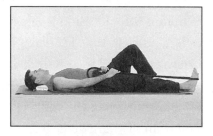

4. STRAIGHT-LEG HAMSTRINGS
See complete instructions on page 42.

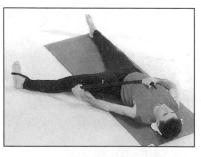

5. HIP ADDUCTORS
See complete instructions on page 43.

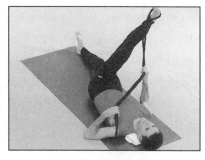

6. HIP ABDUCTORS
See complete instructions on page 44.

(continued)

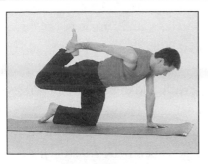

7. PSOAS
See complete instructions on page 45.

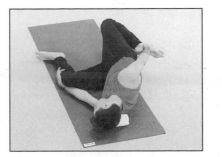

8. QUADRICEPS
See complete instructions on page 46.

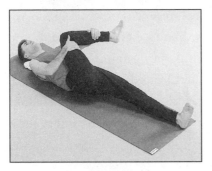

9. GLUTEALS
See complete instructions on page 47.

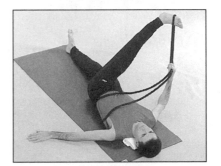

10. PIRIFORMIS
See complete instructions on page 48.

DIAGNOSIS: SPONDYLOSIS

Spondylosis is a common degenerative disease of the spine, most likely caused by age-related changes in intervertebral disks. Also called spinal osteoarthritis, the disease may attack the cervical, thoracic, or lumbar spine, or a combination of all three.

As we age, the structures of the disks change. The collagen content and water content of the anulus fibrosus (the bands of collagen that encase the gel-like interior of the disk) diminish. The disk actually decreases in height. Without the stability and spongy shock absorption of the anulus fibrosus, the vertebrae become less secure. Also, each vertebra has four facet joints, or hinges, that allow the spine to bend forward and backward, rotate, and do all of these in combination. Each of these facet joints is covered with cartilage that allows the bones to glide over each other without grating. Spondylosis causes degradation of cartilage where the vertebrae lay down osteophytes—extra mineralization in places they perceive to be injured.

These osteophytes, also called bone spurs, are nasty. Not only do they hurt, they can impede the blood supply to the vertebrae and irritate nerve roots from the spinal cord to the body. As if this isn't bad enough, the ligaments that hold the spine in position, and yet allow it to move, degenerate or thicken and weaken and are no longer able to hold the spine in alignment.

When spondylosis attacks the cervical spine, it's painful. Those pesky bone spurs can cause nerve root compression and consequent weakness from your shoulders down through your arms and hands (otherwise known as radiating pain and weakness). In extreme cases, bone spurs at the front of the cervical spine can even interfere with the neural signals that the brain sends to swallow. When spondylosis attacks the thoracic and lumbar spine, it causes pain when you move to bend forward or backward. Additionally, the stress and pressure of sitting can cause compression of the lumbar spine, no longer able to absorb and dissipate the forces of your body's weight.

What You Can Do

While you cannot stop the disease, you can do a lot to make yourself more comfortable. You should relax and restore circulation to the muscles and soft tissues that surround your spine and take some of the compression off inflamed nerve roots. It's especially hard to restore circulation to the ligaments, so you must concentrate on restoring circulation to everything that surrounds them. You have to restore balance to your muscles, but this is going to take time. You have to be diligent and patient.

Drink plenty of water to make sure you're always hydrated. Take a mild nonsteroidal anti-inflammatory (such as ibuprofen or naproxen) to dampen the pain and make movement and subsequent relaxation easier.

Start with the stretches below. Do 10 repetitions of each. Soreness, unfortunately, can be accompanied by slight swelling that can impede range of motion and make working out uncomfortable. Move slowly and very gently and in the smallest ranges of motion. At no time should a movement hurt. Ice your back for 10 minutes to quiet down the area. Then stretch again. You can repeat the stretch-ice-stretch sequence several times, or until the pain lets up and you feel that you've restored range of motion to the smallest extent.

The real problem in working out with spondylosis is the bone spurs. They are not only excruciatingly painful, they can impede movement. Actually, they can be a formidable impediment. Our only advice is to do the best you can. Work within the ranges of your own mobility and tolerance for discomfort, but don't push it.

If you have spondylosis, try this sequence of 10 stretches.

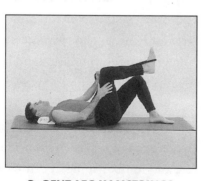

1. SINGLE-LEG PELVIC TILTS
See complete instructions on page 39.

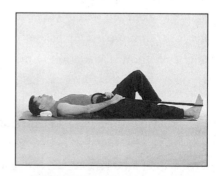

2. DOUBLE-LEG PELVIC TILTS
See complete instructions on page 40.

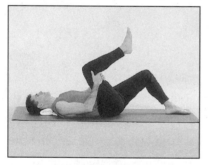

3. BENT-LEG HAMSTRINGS
See complete instructions on page 41.

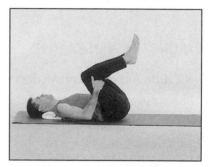

4. STRAIGHT-LEG HAMSTRINGS
See complete instructions on page 42.

(continued)

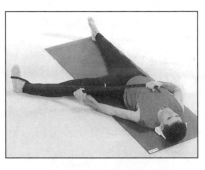

5. HIP ADDUCTORS
See complete instructions on page 43.

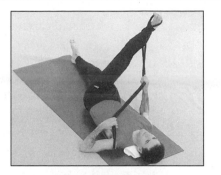

6. HIP ABDUCTORS
See complete instructions on page 44.

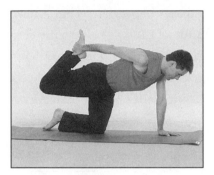

7. PSOAS
See complete instructions on page 45.

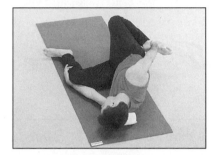

8. QUADRICEPS
See complete instructions on page 46.

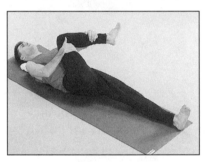

9. GLUTEALS
See complete instructions on page 47.

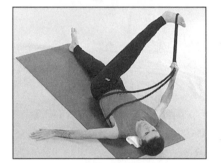

10. PIRIFORMIS
See complete instructions on page 48.

DIAGNOSIS: SPRAIN

Ligaments are cordlike bands in a fibrous sheath that connect bone to bone in your joints. They hold the skeleton together so that joints can move, but ligaments also restrict movement so that joints don't move too much and drop you into a heap on the ground like a rag doll.

When a ligament is injured, the joint it serves is also injured, and its structural integrity and function are compromised. This is called a sprain. The bad news is that if trauma is severe enough to damage a ligament, the chances are good that surrounding soft tissue is also damaged.

Sprains can be difficult to heal. Ligaments are connectors; they are fairly free of blood and therefore fairly isolated from the healing powers of circulating blood that brings in oxygen and carries away metabolic waste generated by the injury.

When your back is sprained, the ligaments that hold your vertebrae in alignment are damaged, and pain and dysfunction are the result. As in a strain, physicians view a sprain as possibly overlying more serious injuries, so it's always treated carefully.

What You Can Do

Relax and restore circulation to the muscles and soft tissues that surround your spine, and take some of the compression off inflamed nerve roots. It's hard to restore circulation to the ligaments, so you must concentrate on restoring circulation to everything that surrounds them. You have to be diligent and patient.

Drink plenty of water to make sure you're always hydrated. Take a mild nonsteroidal anti-inflammatory (such as ibuprofen or naproxen) to get pain under control so that movement and subsequent relaxation are easier.

We would like to direct you to the entire stretch routine (starting on page 38), but if you can't tackle the entire routine, start with the few stretches below to get things moving. Do 10 repetitions of each. Move slowly and very gently and in the smallest ranges of motion. At no time should a movement hurt. Ice your back for 10 minutes to quiet down the area, then stretch again. You can repeat the stretch-ice-stretch sequence several times, or until the pain lets up and you feel that you've restored range of motion to the smallest extent.

When you're through stretching, lie down flat on your back for a little while with a towel roll placed at the base of your neck, at your lower back, under the backs of your knees, and under your heels. Try to position your legs a little higher than your head.

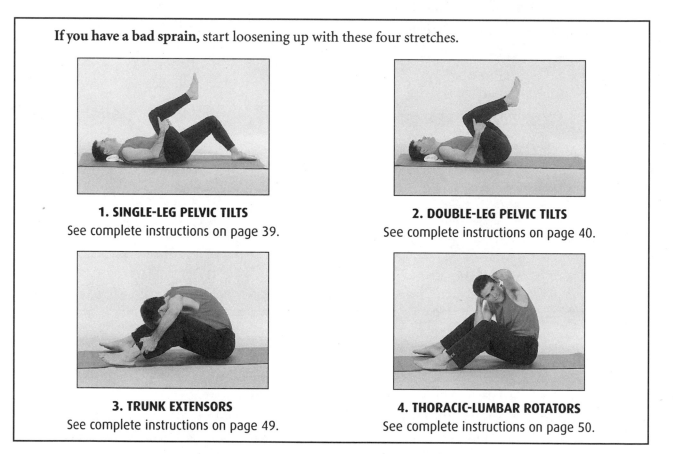

If you have a bad sprain, start loosening up with these four stretches.

1. SINGLE-LEG PELVIC TILTS
See complete instructions on page 39.

2. DOUBLE-LEG PELVIC TILTS
See complete instructions on page 40.

3. TRUNK EXTENSORS
See complete instructions on page 49.

4. THORACIC-LUMBAR ROTATORS
See complete instructions on page 50.

DIAGNOSIS: STRAIN

Strain usually occurs in the lower back in the lumbar region. A strain is an injury characterized by overstretching or tearing of the muscles, tendons, or liga-

ments. You can strain your back by overuse, such as when you rake leaves all day when you're out of shape, or by trauma, such as when you lift something too heavy.

Your back muscles are among the largest in the body, and the erector spinae muscle group runs from the bottom of your lower lumbar spine all the way to the base of your head. This muscle group works in perfect concert to keep you standing upright and allows you to bend forward and backward, rotate, and do all that together. To keep the erector spinae from fatiguing—because it's always on duty—the individual components of the group trade off functions, firing in sequence to keep you upright and moving seamlessly.

When the erector spinae is strained, the group can't function properly, and nearly every move can be painful. The erector spinae isn't the only vulnerable muscle group. Another is the psoas, which runs through the pelvis. If it's strained, its dysfunction places incredible exertion on the lumbar spine. Your physician knows that a strain sometimes overlies a more serious injury, such as a disk injury that's not yet evident, so caution is always advised.

What You Can Do

The good news is that there's a lot you can do. Most strains heal 100 percent. Focus on relaxing and restoring circulation to the muscles and soft tissues that surround your spine and taking some of the compression off inflamed nerve roots. Drink plenty of water to make sure you're hydrated. Take a mild nonsteroidal anti-inflammatory (such as ibuprofen or naproxen) to control the pain and make movement and relaxation easier.

Start with the stretches below. Do 10 repetitions of each. Move slowly and very gently and in the smallest ranges of motion. At no time should a movement hurt. Ice your back for 10 minutes to quiet down the area. Then stretch again. You can repeat the stretch-ice-stretch sequence several times, or until the pain lets up and you feel that you've restored range of motion to the smallest extent. When you're through stretching, lie down flat on your back for a little while with a towel roll placed at the base of your neck, at your lower back, under the backs of your knees, and under your heels. Try to position your legs a little higher than your head.

If you're trying to heal a strain, start with this sequence of four stretches.

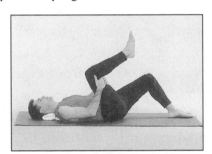

1. SINGLE-LEG PELVIC TILTS
See complete instructions on page 39.

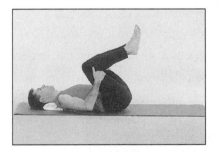

2. DOUBLE-LEG PELVIC TILTS
See complete instructions on page 40.

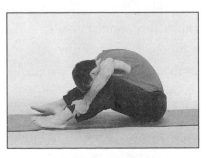

3. TRUNK EXTENSORS
See complete instructions on page 49.

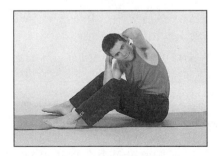

4. THORACIC-LUMBAR ROTATORS
See complete instructions on page 50.

AFTER THE DIAGNOSIS: GETTING OUT OF PAIN QUICKLY

DIAGNOSIS: STRESS FRACTURE

Normal bone is a dynamic organ that continuously remodels itself. As needed, it deposits minerals, called osteoblasts, and reabsorbs minerals, called osteoclasts. Bone reacts to stress by increasing density, or laying down osteoblasts to fortify the site of stress and make it stronger.

But there's a limit to how much deposit a bone can lay down. When stress—continued and repeated trauma to the same site on the bone—exceeds the bone's ability to regenerate, reabsorption occurs faster than the rebuilding. The results are microfractures of the trabecular layer of the bone, the inner layer. If the forces and stresses continue, eventually the fracture deepens to the cortical bone, the outside. When the cortical bone is cracked, it's called a stress fracture. If the stress continues, a full-blown fracture can occur.

Two types of stress fracture have been identified: fatigue fractures in which normal, healthy bone is exposed to continued stress (like distance running) until it cracks, and insufficiency fractures in which porous, unhealthy bone cracks under normal stress (like osteoporosis, bone cysts, osteoid osteoma, or malignancies such as osteosarcoma).

The pelvis and sacrum are vulnerable sites for fatigue fractures in distance runners. A stress fracture, however, can be a big warning sign, an intermediate step between bone bruising (made up of multiple microfractures of the outer layer of the bone) and a full fracture. For example, an insufficiency fracture in a person with osteoporosis could be the precursor to compression fractures of the vertebrae, femoral neck fractures, and fractures of the sacrum. Obviously, a stress fracture is a sign that your body is being taxed—be sure to get a bone scan to see where your particular problem may lie.

What You Can Do

A stress fracture is a break in the bone. It's important to let it heal with rest. Work around the injury site with stretching and strengthening, so that your body doesn't deteriorate and you have plenty of circulation, but stay away from the stress fracture.

If you want to speed up healing, start with drinking plenty of water to make sure you're hydrated. Take a mild nonsteroidal anti-inflammatory (such as ibuprofen or naproxen) to lessen the pain so that movement and subsequent relaxation are easier.

Check with your doctor before doing any exercise. Show him the photos of the specific exercises you intend to do. If you do stretch, do so slowly and very gently. Small movements add up fast. Be patient. At no time should a movement hurt. Ice your back for 10 minutes to quiet down the area. Then stretch again. You can repeat the stretch-ice-stretch sequence several times, or until the pain lets up and you feel that you've restored range of motion to the smallest extent.

Above all, stay off the stress fracture.

DIAGNOSIS: WHIPLASH

Whiplash is the injury made famous by car accidents. When a car is struck from behind, the passengers' heads in the front car are snapped forward and backward in an action very similar to that of a whip. Wearing seat belts make no difference. The term itself is more of a nickname coined by the legal community for a group of injuries, not a medical diagnosis.

The word *whiplash* describes a hyperextension-hyperflexion injury of the neck. When the head (which weighs about 8 pounds in an adult) is suddenly jerked forward and backward beyond the physiological limits of the neck's support, the neck muscles and connective tissues can be strained, sprained, or torn. In extreme cases, the disks between the vertebrae can suddenly herniate (also called slipped disk or bulging disk).

Herniation occurs when the neck is snapped so explosively that the outer band of the disk bursts, allowing the soft, gel-like, inner pulp to escape. That pulp can press against the spinal cord, causing extreme pain, nerve disruption, and coordination problems. In less severe cases, the escaped pulp can compress nerve roots, causing pain. When the herniation or rupture is in the cervical spine, you will feel pain and numbness in the neck, shoulders, arms, and hands.

You might appear to be fine and, in fact, have no serious injury, but muscles that have been traumatized can soon tighten up in response to small microtears. Or they can tighten in a defensive response designed by Mother Nature to form a natural splint to protect the neck from further snapping.

Either way, tightened muscles can cause huge problems, starting with headaches. Also common are back spasms of overtaxed muscles that are trying to compensate for imbalances and a neck that appears to be out of order. At its very worst, whiplash can cause a brain injury.

What You Can Do

While your physician will probably never say that you have whiplash (because it's not a legitimate diagnosis), he might compare a specific injury to whiplash to help you understand how the trauma happened.

When they're caused by whiplash, injuries of the neck can be tricky. The problem is that the jolt of impact shocks your entire body, and you have to relax it in sequence, working from the lower back up to the neck. If you unlock only your neck, the traumatized muscles and structures below will soon pull it back into misalignment. You need to relax and restore circulation to the muscles and soft tissues that surround your lower back and then work toward your neck.

Drink plenty of water to make sure you're always hydrated. Take a mild nonsteroidal anti-inflammatory (such as ibuprofen or naproxen) to get pain under control so that movement and subsequent relaxation are easier.

Stretch, using the sequence below. Do 10 repetitions of each. Move slowly and very gently and in the smallest ranges of motion. At no time should a movement hurt. Ice your back for 10 minutes to quiet down the area. Then stretch again. You can repeat the stretch-ice-stretch sequence several times, or until the pain lets up and you feel that you've restored range of motion to the smallest extent.

This stretching sequence is designed in a specific order to relax muscles in the lumbar region first and then work toward the neck. One day of work will not alleviate the problem, but patience will prevail. Stop all stretches short of pain.

If you have whiplash, first start working in the lumbar region, with these nine stretches.

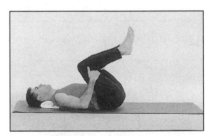

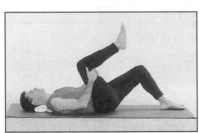

1. SINGLE-LEG PELVIC TILTS
See complete instructions on page 39.

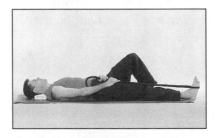

2. DOUBLE-LEG PELVIC TILTS
See complete instructions on page 40.

3. BENT-LEG HAMSTRINGS
See complete instructions on page 41.

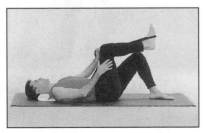

4. STRAIGHT-LEG HAMSTRINGS
See complete instructions on page 42.

(continued)

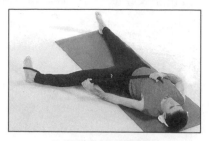

5. HIP ADDUCTORS
See complete instructions on page 43.

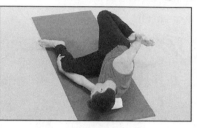

7. QUADRICEPS
See complete instructions on page 46.

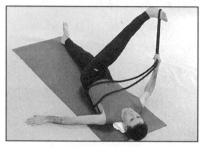

9. PIRIFORMIS
See complete instructions on page 48.

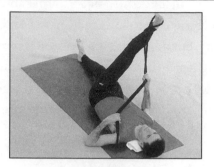

6. HIP ABDUCTORS
See complete instructions on page 44.

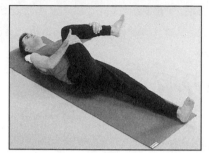

8. GLUTEALS
See complete instructions on page 47.

From the lumbar region, we now move up closer to the injury in the neck.

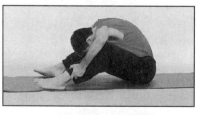

1. TRUNK EXTENSORS
See complete instructions on page 49.

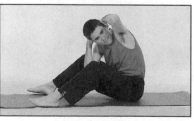

2. THORACIC-LUMBAR ROTATORS
See complete instructions on page 50.

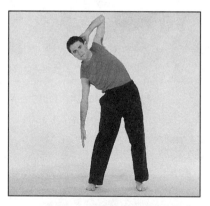

3. TRUNK LATERAL FLEXORS
See complete instructions on page 51.

Moving from the trunk and even closer to the neck, do these stretches.

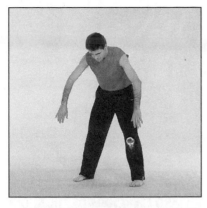

1. SHOULDER CIRCUMDUCTION
See complete instructions on page 52.

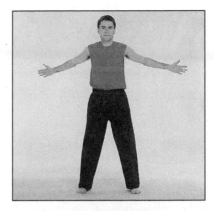

2. PECTORALIS MAJORS
See complete instructions on page 53.

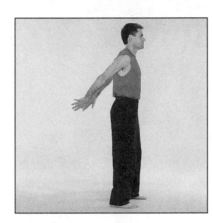

3. ANTERIOR DELTOIDS
See complete instructions on page 54.

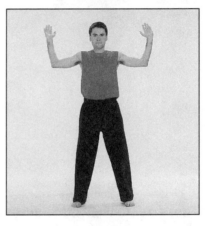

4. SHOULDER INTERNAL ROTATORS
See complete instructions on page 55.

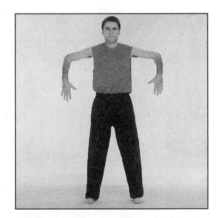

5. SHOULDER EXTERNAL ROTATORS
See complete instructions on page 56.

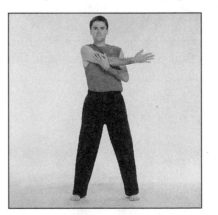

6. ROTATOR CUFF 1
See complete instructions on page 57.

(continued)

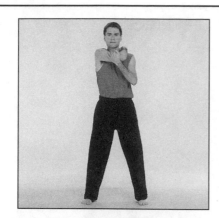

7. ROTATOR CUFF 2

See complete instructions on page 58.

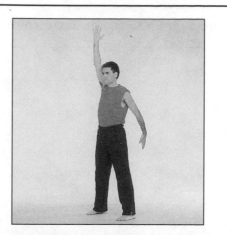

8. FORWARD ELEVATORS OF THE SHOULDER

See complete instructions on page 59.

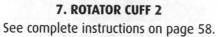

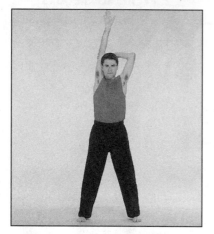

9. SIDE ELEVATORS OF THE SHOULDER

See complete instructions on page 60.

Now that you're warmed up and the back below your neck is relaxed, stretch the neck.

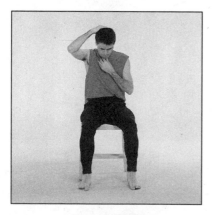

1. NECK EXTENSORS

See complete instructions on page 61.

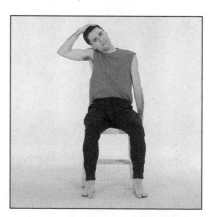

2. NECK LATERAL FLEXORS

See complete instructions on page 62.

STOPPING THE PAIN

Throughout the day, to keep everything unlocked and circulation flowing, do the following four stretches.

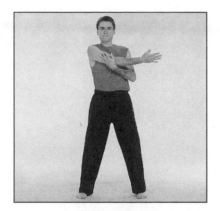

1. ROTATOR CUFF 1
See complete instructions on page 57.

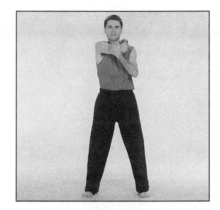

2. ROTATOR CUFF 2
See complete instructions on page 58.

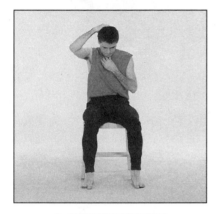

3. NECK EXTENSORS
See complete instructions on page 61.

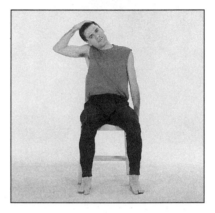

4. NECK LATERAL FLEXORS
See complete instructions on page 62.

Part 4

Protecting Your Back As Your Body Changes

Chapter 8

TAKING OFF THE POUNDS

Hank Biloxi is an award-winning Broadway producer who has enjoyed many hits. He's also one of our long-term clients.

When we met him, his back was in constant spasm. He was in so much pain that he tried to stay immobilized much of the time. Still, being a producer meant that Hank was constantly sitting through meetings, dashing in and out of cars, dining, socializing, and enduring grueling workdays in the office. When he wasn't on the go, he was on the floor in his apartment in agony.

Hank was miserable, and his world was winding down into a spiral of pain and exhaustion. On a weekly basis, he hobbled into our clinic, and we worked with him to unlock his back, relax his muscles, and get him out of pain.

For a little while, he felt great, but his body simply wasn't strong enough to sustain the results we could give him on the table. But exercising to get stronger was out of the question for Hank. He was too busy, and, even when he had time, his pain was an undeniable impediment to his motivation. His body felt too fragile to go through a vigorous workout.

Hank's weight had crept up over the years primarily because he was sedentary most of the time, and his muscles had lost a lot of their tone. We loved Hank, but we were used to getting results in our clinic, so seeing him hobble in week after week was

becoming disheartening. At one point, we had a meeting to determine if we were wasting our time and his money. We all decided to press on.

The one thing we had not tried was helping him knock off some pounds. After months of gentle nudging, he consulted our favorite dietitian, who put him on a healthy, low-fat diet. The results were immediate and astonishing. As each pound melted away from his body and lightened the load that his spine was carrying, Hank felt better and stronger. Today, when we put him through a stretch routine, it sticks.

EXTRA POUNDS ARE HARD ON YOUR BACK

In the past two decades, obesity in the United States has risen dramatically and has been conclusively identified as a strong risk factor for some well-known killers: cardiovascular disease, cancer, high blood pressure, stroke, and endocrine disorders. What has not been as well-publicized is the link between excess weight and back pain.

In 2002, results of a study conducted by Dartmouth Medical School in Hanover, New Hampshire, conclusively linked obesity to back problems. Nearly 16,000 patients with spine disease were evaluated to determine the association between obesity and their health status. One theory supposed that the weight and bulk of the obese body place abnormal mechanical loads on the spine. Another study looked at whether an initial injury to the spine leads to a sedentary lifestyle, which leads to obesity. The researchers concluded that while other factors may make spinal conditions worse, obesity is the only factor that can be changed relatively simply, either through diet, exercise, and behavior therapy, or, in more extreme cases, through surgery and medications. In fact, the Dartmouth researchers state, "it is conceivable that as a patient's obesity improved, functioning and symptoms would also improve."

In our experience, we can tell you that it is almost guaranteed.

Extra weight has to be supported by the spine. When you're too heavy, those pounds put extra compression on the disks in your spine. In addition, every time you bend or rotate, your spine has to help you support and balance against more weight than it was designed to handle. For example, if you have excess fat in your abdomen in the form of a potbelly, you're carrying too much weight forward, forcing your back to sway to counterbalance to keep you upright. The strain can be enormous and can lead to muscular dysfunction as your body compensates for the overload. Some muscles will overdevelop. Some will weaken. The net effect is a body that can't work properly, and things start to go wrong over time. This compression caused by excess weight also works from the bottom up.

Being too heavy affects the arches of your feet. They can no longer work as shock absorbers to put spring into your step. When your arches are flattened under crushing weight with each foot fall, your ankles roll to the inside, throwing off the alignment of your knees. Shortly, the insides of your knees strain and weaken, transmitting the misalignment to your hips. The hips transmit it directly to your back.

Fat gets in the way of range of motion. Heavy and encased in bulky padding, one can't move. We have heavy clients who can't touch their knees when they first come to us. It's not that they have no flexibility. That might well be the case, but we'll not know that for a while because they have so much body fat

that they can't reach around it. This immobilization that creeps in as weight creeps up is a nasty double whammy. The less you can move, the more sedentary you become. The more sedentary you are, the less able you are to burn calories—and the more easily you gain weight. Before you know it, you're in real trouble.

Being overweight puts your heart and lungs into constant overdrive. The additional pounds give your body extra tissue that still demands circulation and oxygen, which your heart and lungs must work extra hard to provide. One of the treadmill tests we use to determine cardiovascular fitness, the VO_2 max, is a sort of stress test to measure how much oxygen gets into the bloodstream. With heavy clients, we find that their VO_2 max is significantly lower than that of lean or fit people. Without sufficient oxygen making its way into tissues, and with a heart working far too hard to make up that deficit, the body tires easily. A tired body is a sedentary body. And once again, the more sedentary you are, the less able you are to burn calories and the more easily you gain weight. You're in a full-blown vicious cycle.

Results of a 20-year study at Purdue University in West Lafayette, Indiana, give us a disturbing glance into the future of an obese person, finding that risk of disability later in life is twice that of a lean person, even when weight alone is associated with the impairment. (The study defined disability as being unable to do simple things like walk ¼ mile, get in and out of a car, and do light chores.) And here's the really bad news. Even if the people managed to lose weight during the study, the elevated risk for disability persists, albeit to a lesser degree. The study builds a compelling case for getting weight under control as quickly as possible and keeping it there.

Being overweight can be very painful. When your body doesn't work properly, your back hurts. Joints are strained. Soft tissue is torn. Muscles are brutalized. Effort is agonizing. Systems break down. Healing is difficult. Medical treatment is difficult. Therapy is difficult. Surgery is difficult, even dangerous. But almost more than all that, being overweight—even moderately so—can also be emotionally painful.

So why go through all this risk and heartache for something that's preventable and probably completely unnecessary?

We want to help you get a handle on your love handles right now. The longer you wait, the harder it is to get control. Middle-age spread is one of the very real challenges of growing older. As we age, our metabolism—the rate at which our bodies burn calories—naturally slows. From the time you're 30, your metabolic rate starts to decrease by about 2 percent per decade. By age 80, you're burning 200 fewer calories every day than you did when you were 30.

One would think that we could compensate by cutting back on food intake in direct proportion to the slowdown, but nothing in life is that simple. As we grow older, most of us also tend to decrease our activity. Getting less activity causes muscle mass to decline. Muscles are the furnaces that burn calories, so when they get smaller, the body burns fewer calories. The net effect is weight gain—unless you maintain discipline and remain active throughout your lifetime.

EXERCISE IS THE ANSWER

"I've gained 10 pounds! I guess it's time to go on a diet."

If these words are familiar to you, you may be looking at both your best intentions and the primary reason for your downfall.

When you drop your calorie intake quickly or dramatically, your body is programmed to interpret your new diet as pending starvation and slows down to hang on to fat stores. The theory goes that each time you attempt a diet and drop your calorie count, your body gets even more efficient at triggering "conservation mode," resulting in an uphill battle against a slower metabolism. You might gain that pesky weight back quickly, and, even worse, gain back more than you lost.

So you try again. And again. It's this cycle of losing and gaining that we call yo-yo dieting.

We used to think that at some point, when the metabolism was lowered one time too many and one calorie too far, dieting to lose weight would be impossible. But according to the National Institutes of Health, most studies have shown that weight cycling does *not* affect your long-term metabolic rate. More important, the fact that you've been a yo-yo dieter will not adversely affect the success of your future diet attempts. No matter how many times you have failed in the past, a new attempt just might be the one that succeeds. And we have the secret that will help you succeed this time: exercise.

Diets fail because they are only one component of what should be a two-part system. Let's look at the statistics: While the average number of calories consumed by Americans each day fell from 1,826 calories in 1977 to 1,774 in 1991, the percentage of obese adults climbed from 14.5 percent to 22.5 percent. Most recently, that number is 31 percent. Many people try and fail to lose weight, or they lose and then put the weight back on. According to a study conducted by the National Weight Control Registry, the people who succeed at weight loss and sustain that loss for a period of time have one thing in common: Exercise is a key component to their plans.

HOW DOES EXERCISE CONTROL WEIGHT?

Don't just take our word for it. Here are 10 proven ways that exercise helps you shed pounds and keep them off, more healthfully and predictably than cutting calories.

1. Exercise burns the right kind of calories. These calories come from two different sources: glycogen, made from converted sugars and stored in the muscles and the liver; and fat, stored in the fat cells.

During high-intensity exercise, you burn mostly glycogen; during low-intensity exercise, such walking (suggested for the cardio portion of the Active-Isolated method), you burn mostly fat. A good rule of thumb is that if you can talk while you're exercising, you're burning more fat than glycogen. If you can't gasp out a word, you're burning more glycogen.

As you adapt to a training program and you get stronger and fitter, the effort you exert drops. In other words, a previously tough workout gradually becomes easier. And—voilà!—your body goes back to burning fat as its primary fuel source. The workout program that will work for you is in chapter 4.

2. Exercise builds muscle. Muscle cells are eight times more metabolically active than fat cells. The more lean muscle mass you have, the higher the demand for energy, the more efficiently you burn calories, and the faster you dip into and reduce fat stores. For every pound of muscle you add, you burn an average of 50 to 100 calories every day.

3. Exercise increases fat-burning enzymes. Muscles contain enzymes that burn only fat. Research has demonstrated that regular exercisers, as opposed to sedentary people, have developed muscles with more fat-burning enzymes. The more enzymes you have, the more fat you burn.

4. Exercise helps build and maintain healthy bones, muscles, and connective tissues. When your body feels stronger, your body movements will be more fluid and seem more natural. Feeling great in your own skin is the best incentive to exercise— and once you make that connection, you'll understandably become more active and burn more calories.

5. Exercise helps control blood pressure. When your blood pressure is lower, you'll feel better able to be more active. As your activity level increases, you'll burn more calories, and your weight will drop even faster.

6. Exercise helps regulate appetite. Even though one might assume that a good workout would work up an appetite, the opposite is true. Exercise helps keep cravings and overeating in check.

7. Exercise changes your body's fat-storing chemistry. When the body is sedentary, it lowers its metabolism to conserve energy. Unfortunately, stored energy is fat. When the body is active, hormones signal a release of energy, so working out can help boost your fat-burning potential by improving the profiles of many hormones related to fat storage, such as insulin, adrenaline, and cortisol.

8. Exercise is physically addictive. When exercise is intense, your body releases endorphins, chemicals that enhance a sense of well-being, and reduce stress.

9. Exercise helps you sleep better. When you're rested, you have more energy to be more active. When you're more active, you burn more calories.

10. Exercise increases your motivation to eat well. Once you've started to exercise and treat your body better, you'll be less likely to treat it poorly by polluting it with junk foods.

Getting active brings great joy to your life. Once you've had a little taste of the fun of fitness, you're less likely to backslide.

THE WHARTONS' "SHED FAT, SPARE YOUR BACK" PLAN

We've sold you, right? You're ready to take responsibility for your back pain and start putting your body's health first.

First, it's time to set some goals. Turn to "How Much Should I Weigh?" on page 194 to see your ultimate goal. Know that the most long-lasting, safest weight loss is an average of 1 to 2 pounds a week.

Then, work on getting your diet in line with your active lifestyle. Turn to page 194 and read "Eating to Maximize Your Exercise." You'll learn how many calories you should be eating, as well as a number of the strategies that have helped our clients shed hundreds of pounds. You're taking responsibility for your body, and you've earned the right to give it the highest quality fuel possible.

And finally, our favorite part. Exercise. You already have the best plan for all of your needs: Active-Isolated Stretching to get your back out of immediate pain and increase your flexibility, Active-Isolated Strengthening to rebuild your muscles and prevent pain in the future, and cardio training to rev up that fat-burning engine to banish those pounds forever. Turn to chapter 4 and get started today. (In order to get your calorie-burning activity ramped up right away, feel free to begin the cardio portion of the program at the same time you begin Phase 1. Simply add one 20-minute walk three times a week. By the time you get to the Advanced phase, you will be light years ahead of where you began, and you can step up your cardio training with confidence.) And, as always, check with your doctor before beginning any exercise program.

In the beginning, we realize that those extra pounds may be putting more strain on your lower back, hips, legs, and feet. In that case, you may need to start with baby steps.

If you need to start slowly, try out these exercises for 30 days, or until you feel comfortable beginning the full program.

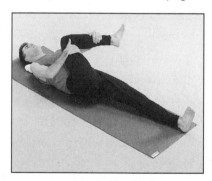

1. SINGLE-LEG PELVIC TILTS
See complete instructions on page 39.

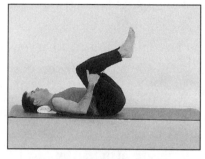

2. DOUBLE-LEG PELVIC TILTS
See complete instructions on page 40.

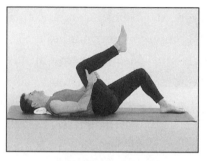

3. GLUTEALS
See complete instructions on page 47.

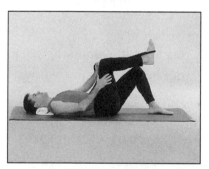

4. BENT-LEG HAMSTRINGS
See complete instructions on page 41.

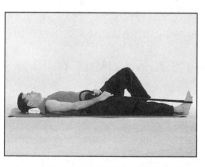

5. STRAIGHT-LEG HAMSTRINGS
See complete instructions on page 42.

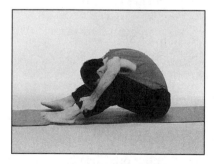

6. TRUNK EXTENSORS
See complete instructions on page 49.

HOW MUCH SHOULD I WEIGH?

We have a confession to make: What you weigh is unimportant. It's true. Keep your scale if you like, but pay very little attention to it on a daily basis.

The truth is that you need to be concerned with how much *fat* you're carrying in relation to your total weight. The number on the scale reflects that fat, to be sure, but it also registers the weight of tissue, organs, skeleton, water, and clothing. Total weight will vary from day to day, even from hour to hour. We've seen clients take off their shoes and rip off their clothes or go without water for hours before weighing in order to register a lower number, but the simple truth is that nothing you do right before you step on the scale will diminish your fat content. You are what you are.

Determining your exact body composition will take the assistance of a health-care professional using skin-fold calipers or one of the high-tech electronic measuring devices, but you can get a general idea about whether you are fat or lean by calculating your body mass index (BMI), a ratio between your height and weight, with a formula that correlates with body fat. Here's how.

1. Multiply your weight in pounds by 703.
2. Multiply your height in inches by your height in inches.
3. Divide the answer in Step 1 by the answer in Step 2 to get your BMI.
4. Round that number off.

Here's an example of how it would work for a person who is 5 feet 5 inches tall and weighs 140 pounds.

1. Multiply your weight in pounds by 703.
   $140 \times 703 = 98,420$
2. Multiply your height in inches by your height in inches. $65 \times 65 = 4,225$
3. Divide the answer in Step 1 by the answer in Step 2 to get your BMI. $98,420 \div 4,225 = 23.29$
4. Round that number off. The person's BMI is 23.3.

The higher the BMI, the greater your risk for cardiovascular disease, cancer, high blood pressure,

Health Risk Based on BMI

BMI	Risk
Below 25	Minimal
25–26.9	Low
27–29.9	Moderate
30–34.9	High
35–39.9	Very high
40 and above	Extremely high

stroke, endocrine disorders, and back pain. Having a low ratio is important for your health. The American College of Sports Medicine recommends that adults with a BMI over 25 get their fat under control. (To get a sense of what your calculated BMI means, see the table "Health Risk Based on BMI.")

Where you carry your weight is important, too. "Apple-shaped" people, who carry their weight around their waistlines, are at greater risk of weight-related disease than "pear-shaped" people, who carry their weight on their hips, buttocks, and thighs. Notice that "pear" weight is not necessarily around major organs, while "apple" weight is. Also, if your weight is in your abdomen, your back will likely be affected sooner than if the weight is distributed lower. If you're a woman with a waist measurement over 35 inches or a man with a waist measurement over 40 inches, you are at greater risk of back problems and other diseases associated with excess body fat. No matter where you fall in the fruit basket, if you're overweight, you need to deal with it. Now.

EATING TO MAXIMIZE YOUR EXERCISE

We have spent many years working with athletes all over the world and the professionals who train and care for them. Diet is an inevitable component of that work. We have the greatest respect for the wide variety of diets we encounter, but we personally adhere to a plant-based diet and nudge almost all our athletes in that direction. Your decision will be yours personally.

If you ask us how to lose weight, you're really asking us how to burn more fat. These are the components for efficient weight loss: a choice that you make; an exercise program, which we design for you; and an eating plan composed of good choices and smart portion control. Together, we will put you on your way to a lean, fit body.

We would never say that we're the ultimate authorities on diet (registered dietitians are your best bet there), but we have seen our athletes achieve medal-worthy bodies with some very simple strategies. Here are some of the best.

Keep a journal. A wise psychologist once told us, "Obsession will be served." If food is an obsession, when you eliminate that obsession, you can't replace it with something that you'll *not* do—you have to replace it with action. We have found that keeping a simple journal will do the trick at keeping your mind occupied.

Write down everything you eat, also recording what time and how you felt. If you're able to do so, use food labels and calorie counters to track your approximate calories. Several studies have found that keeping track of your daily food intake is the best predictor of success with an eating plan. Add that journal to your training log (see page 97), and you'll have a complete record of all your hard work—something to be very proud of.

Know what calories really mean. Technically, a calorie is the amount of heat needed to raise the temperature of 1 gram of water 1 degree Celsius. This is hardly useful information, but it does lead us to the purpose of calories. Muscles are like furnaces. They convert calories into fuel to rev up those furnaces so that they can manufacture energy. So to describe calories in terms of heat is logical.

Not all foods deliver the same measure of calories. Simple carbohydrates (such as sugars) and complex carbohydrates (such as starches) have 4 calories per gram. Proteins (such as meat, milk, and eggs) also have 4 calories per gram. And fat (such as lard) has 9 calories per gram. And not all calories are equal. Some (such as spinach) deliver energy and are dense in nutrients. And others (such as beer) are "empty" calories. They deliver the energy but have no nutritional value.

One pound of fat represents 3,500 calories of unused energy. If you consume 3,500 more calories than you need, you'll gain a pound of fat. If you burn 3,500 more calories than you consume, you'll lose a pound of fat. Food in, food out—it's that simple.

Phil and the Onion Rings

When I was a little guy, our family lived in San Antonio, Texas. My mom and I would sneak away from home to go on little mother-son adventures. Even when I was very young, our kitchen was stocked with only healthy food. So when my mom and I were out together, our tradition was to go to the Pig Stand in San Antonio and eat onion rings. We reveled in our conspiracy; we loved those forbidden onion rings.

My parents divorced when I was eleven. I lived with my dad. Both my parents traveled, so I seldom saw my mom. I missed her a lot.

An intermittent obsession with onion rings remained with me until only a few years ago, when I had to confront the hypocrisy of my eating fried food. I am an elite athlete. I train other elite athletes to care for their bodies. I am disciplined and educated. No detail slips by me. And yet, onion rings haunted me. After considerable thought, I realized that onion rings were a little boy's comfort food that spilled over into adulthood. They represented a special closeness with my mom. Whenever I missed her, I would go in search of onion rings. I don't even *like* onion rings.

Mystery explained. Problem solved. Now, when I miss my mom, I just call her.

Know approximately how many calories you need. As we discussed earlier, consuming too few calories slows down your metabolism. When trying to lose weight, it's smarter to inch back on calories, but not too far. If you can keep your calories high enough to prevent your metabolism from dropping into "starvation mode," you can burn through the calories you consume during your meal and then start depleting fat storage. And even better, you can kick up your metabolism with exercise to burn even more calories and deplete even more fat. Eating nutrient-rich foods gives you the energy to do that.

New dietary guidelines were issued in 2002 by the Institute of Medicine. They estimated daily energy requirements for people around age 30 of various sizes and levels of activity. We've provided that information for you in the table "Daily Calorie Needs by Height, Weight, and Activity Level." Use this as a loose guideline, as most of us are beyond age 30 and thus will burn fewer calories per day. You may be surprised just how few calories your body needs when you *don't* exercise, and, conversely, how much more you can eat when you do.

Know what food is—and what it is not. Food is fuel. Repeat after us: Food is fuel. Food is *not* comfort, although it can be comforting. Food is *not* entertainment, although it can be entertaining. Food is *not* rest, although it can be rejuvenating. Food is *not* love, although it can evoke a loving memory. Food is fuel. Nothing more.

Food as fuel provides calories for energy, nutrients to keep the body healthy, water to hydrate cells, and fiber to move it through the gastrointestinal system. Next time you're at the grocery store, shop normally and then stop right before you check out. Item by item, take a look at what you've selected. Just because it's edible doesn't mean that it's food. Ask yourself if each edible item is food that your body can use as fuel or if it's an attempt to fulfill another need that could and should be satisfied in another way. If you consistently find too little actual food among the edibles, you need to do some serious thinking about your relationship with food. You need to make some choices. (If you find yourself frequently out of control around food, talk to your doctor or dietitian about how you can best retrain yourself to think of food as fuel.)

Fall in love with the salad bar. Experts such as dietitians tell us that vibrantly colorful fruits and vegetables are great for you. The brighter and deeper the color of the fruit or vegetable, the more likely it is to be power-packed with phytochemicals—thousands of compounds that promote good health. For example, one miracle nutrient you'll find at the salad bar is folate, a vitamin that decreases homocysteine.

Daily Calorie Needs by Height, Weight, and Activity Level for 30-Year-Old Adults

Height/Weight	Women		Men	
	Active	Sedentary	Active	Sedentary
5'1", 98–132 lb	2,104–2,290 cals	1,688–1,834 cals	2,104–2,290 cals	1,919–2167 cals
5'5", up to 150 lb	2,267–2,477 cals	1,816–1,982 cals	2,490–2,842 cals	2,068–2,349 cals
5'9", 125–169 lb	2,434–2,670 cals	1,948–2,134 cals	2,683–3,078 cals	2,222–2,538 cals
6'1", 139–188 lb	2,605–2,869 cals	2,083–2,290 cals	2,883–3,325 cals	2,382–2,736 cals

Reprinted with permission from Dietary Reference Intakes © 2000 by the National Academy of Sciences, courtesy of the National Academics Press, Washington, D.C.

Cleaner House, Trimmer Waist

Exercise doesn't have to be a chore. But a chore can be exercise. We're going to give you a simple system that will knock 15.6 pounds off you in a year without your having to do anything but work around the house and yard.

Burning just 150 calories of extra energy a day will add up to 1,000 calories per week—and it will cut your risk of heart disease by 50 percent and reduce your risk of high blood pressure, diabetes, and colon cancer by 30 percent. As a big bonus, you'll also help maintain healthy bones, muscles, and joints; help control your weight by building lean muscle and reducing body fat; and take the strain of excess weight off your back.

Everyone is a little bit different and attacks a chore with different energy. If you do so with gusto, you'll burn more in an hour than someone who just "phones it in." The chores we've listed below are designed for a woman who is 50 years old, about 5 feet 6 inches tall, and of average weight (150 pounds). She is moderately fit, so she's going to fall somewhere in between high and low intensity.

Activity	Calories Burned in 1 Hour	Time It Takes to Burn 150 Calories
Chopping wood	345	25 min
Doing laundry	125	1 hr, 10 min
Gardening	345	25 min
Heavy housework	240	40 min
Heavy tool work	460	20 min
Laying tile	260	35 min
Light housework	144	1 hr, 2 min
Mopping	200	45 min
Mowing lawn	260	35 min
Plumbing	175	50 min
Preparing a meal	150	1 hr
Pushing a stroller	150	1 hr
Raking leaves	270	35 min
Shopping	155	1 hr
Shoveling snow	350	25 min
Vacuuming	200	45 min
Washing the car	175	50 min
Watching TV	60	2 hr, 30 min

High levels of homocysteine, an amino acid that circulates with blood, have been linked with heart disease, stroke, some cancers, and Alzheimer's disease. Lower that homocysteine with folate from the salad bar, and you'll reduce risks.

Another good reason to favor fruits and vegetables is that they are relatively low in calories and filled with fiber. Fiber helps control your appetite, aids digestion, and may even whisk a small number of calories out of your body before they can be absorbed. When eaten in concert with other foods, such as whole grains, small amounts of lean protein, and some unsaturated fats, it is the answer to a dieter's prayer.

Get the skinny on fat. The USDA recommends that you choose a diet moderate in all fat, but especially low in saturated fat and cholesterol. As odd as it may sound, we do need some fat in our diets. The trick, however, is to know which kind and how much, because not all fat is created equal. Here's a simple explanation.

Unsaturated fats, found mainly in cooking oils, nuts, avocados, salmon, and olive oil, are good. They supply energy and essential fatty acids, and they help absorb some fat-soluble vitamins such as A, D, E, and K. They don't increase cholesterol. Let's review: unsaturated fat—good.

Saturated fat, on the other hand, is not good. It increases cholesterol and the risk of cardiovascular diseases. This type of fat is found in fatty dairy products, fatty and processed meats, the skin and fat of

When we met Bev Browning, our coauthor, in the early 1980s, she had just begun to search for a fitness program that would fit her busy lifestyle. She decided she would take up running and train for the New York City Marathon—even before she bought her first pair of running shoes.

While an ambitious goal, running the 26.2 miles was doable for a healthy, young female, given that the race was a year away and she had the time to train intelligently and slowly. But Bev tried to do too much too soon. She thought that running would melt away the fat, but because she launched a killer training program without proper preparation, she was quickly hobbled by stress fractures in her shins and a searing pain in her left hip that translated right up into her lower back.

One thing that made her problem worse was her weight: She was overweight by more than a few pounds. She had about 30 percent body fat. The average for a woman her age and height is about 22 percent. Female marathon runners of her age and height are about 16 percent.

During our first consultation, Bev limped in with a sheath of medical records and x-rays. She knew exactly what was wrong and asked us to help her correct imbalances in strength and flexibility that she perceived were causing injuries. Also, having been humbled, she wanted a better training program.

We were glad to evaluate her and develop a workout program to promote healing, prevent further injury, and gradually ease her back into running, but there was a bigger issue to address, a delicate one. We had to tell Bev that her weight was contributing to her difficulty in ways she couldn't even imagine.

Running places demands on the entire body, and Bev's body wasn't ready to handle that kind of stress. The extra pounds were putting tremendous strain on her lower body. With every step as she pounded the pavement in running, she was hammering her hips, legs, and feet. Her spine was taking a beating. No wonder she was in such pain.

Even though Bev charged up and down the street once a day, her weight rendered her sedentary at all

poultry, lard, palm oil, and coconut oil (goodbye, movie popcorn!). Saturated fat—bad.

Cholesterol found in food tends to raise the blood level of cholesterol that naturally occurs in our bodies. An overabundance of cholesterol clogs arteries, which is not good. It's found in liver and other organ meats, egg yolks, and dairy fats. Cholesterol—bad.

Trans fatty acids tend to raise blood cholesterol. The guilty foods are those high in partially hydrogenated vegetable oils like margarine and shortening, some commercial fried foods, and baked goods. Trans fatty acids—bad.

To apply your knowledge of fats: Limit your use of solid fats, such as regular margarine, and use veg-etable oil instead, or look for trans-free margarines, such as Smart Balance. Stay away from processed meats like bacon and salami, which have not only saturated fats but also potentially poisonous additives. Try to eat two or three daily servings from the following: fish, shellfish, lean poultry, lean meat, beans or nuts, peas, and lentils. Limit your intake of organ meats and whole eggs, and when you go for dairy, choose fat-free or low-fat products.

Go sour on sugar. To most of us, sugar is a flavoring, but it's really a carbohydrate and a source of energy through calories. If you decide to eliminate sugar to save a few calories and substitute another form of sugar, like honey, you've made a mistake. The other times. Injuries didn't help. When things hurt, she automatically shut them down and avoided movement that caused pain. She didn't move as often or with as much energy as a lighter person. Or maybe she was heavy because she was sedentary.

We explained to Bev that carrying excess weight was very hard on her body, especially if she wanted to train for a marathon. Bev began to see that diet and exercise could and should go hand in hand, and that if we could lower her weight, we could increase her mileage. If we could increase her mileage, we could lower her weight even faster. And best of all, we could get her out of pain.

How Bev Got Out of Pain: We sent Bev home with a stretch rope and a program for Active-Isolated Stretching with special emphasis on her back, hips, and legs. We also made an appointment for her to meet with our dietitian, who put Bev on a healthy eating plan with slightly reduced calories spread out over all the major food groups.

Bev started dropping weight at the same time she increased flexibility and circulation to her body. In-

juries healed slowly but surely. As she became more healthy, she felt better in general. She slept better. She had more energy and confidence.

When Bev had a handle on her diet and had shed a few pounds, we reevaluated her flexibility and the ranges of motion of her joints. She had done her homework, and it showed: She was lighter, leaner, and looser. The pain in her back, hips, legs, and feet had subsided almost entirely.

Gradually, we added in Active-Isolated Strengthening. As she built muscle, she was able to burn more body fat, and she dropped more weight. Eventually, we allowed her to return to running with a regimen that was designed just for her. Weight started to melt until she was at about 20 percent body fat, a couple of points below the average female of her age and height—and perfect for an amateur marathon runner. She completed her first New York City Marathon within the year and started her own running club in Florida. Since then, our Bev has trained more than 1,000 Floridians to run the New York City Marathon!

body can't tell the difference between the sugar on your spoon and honey. For that matter, it can't tell the difference between your granulated sugar and the naturally occurring sugars in fruit and milk. It all looks the same chemically. Sugar has no nutritional benefit other than tasting great—and it adds empty calories. If you're wild for dessert, head for fruit.

Put aside your saltshaker. Sodium, the essential component of salt, is necessary for regulating fluid in your body and for maintaining blood pressure. Unfortunately, too much salt causes the body to retain fluid and raises blood pressure. Studies have also demonstrated that too much salt increases the amount of calcium excreted in urine and might in-

crease the risk of osteoporosis. Unless all the foods you eat are natural, you're going to run into salt in nearly every package, can, or jar. By reading food labels, you'll start to notice which foods really go too far (some canned soups have nearly 100 percent of your daily requirement in one serving!). Always choose the low-sodium option of your favorite brands.

Chew your food 25 times before you swallow. Digestion begins in your mouth. Chewing 25 times allows you to mix your food with saliva, an important component in the chemical reactions that break down food, particularly starches. Chewing also slows you down, so you're mindful of what you're eating, giving your brain and your fork time to catch up to each other. When your brain determines that you've had enough to eat and are full, it signals you to stop eating. If you wolf down food, you'll have too much in your stomach before the hypothalamus in your brain has the opportunity to sense fullness and transmit that information. You'll get the signal to stop eating long after you should have.

Consider vitamin and mineral supplements. One of the real challenges in cutting calories is to make sure that you still meet your need for nutrients. It's best to get all your nutrients from food, but if this is difficult, then you might want to consider vitamin and mineral supplements. (Read more about vitamin and mineral supplements on page 243.)

Break the caffeine habit. Caffeine is a powerful central-nervous-system stimulant found in hundreds of foods, beverages, and drugs. And although you may be using it to feel more alert when you crawl out of bed in the morning, you should consider cutting back. Caffeine makes it more difficult to fall asleep, decreases the time you stay asleep, and diminishes the quality of your sleep. It interferes with calcium absorption and, in doing so, increases the risk of osteoporosis. In addition, caffeine acts as a diuretic, causing dehydration.

Be smart with alcohol. Alcoholic beverages are packed with calories but almost no nutrients. Empty calories, however, can be the least of one's worries. Alcohol in excess impairs judgment and increases the risk of high blood pressure, stroke, certain types of cancers, birth defects, cirrhosis of the liver, inflammation of the pancreas, and damage to the cardiovascular system and brain. If you're going to drink alcohol, be moderate.

On a positive note, studies indicate that drinking in moderation might lower risk for coronary artery disease in men over age 45 and women over age 55.

While you're eating, don't forget to drink. Your body's fluid is a miraculous balancing act between two components: sodium (salt) and water. If your blood is too high in sodium or too low in water, water leaches out of cells all over your body and into your blood to keep it in balance.

When the cells in your hypothalamus become dehydrated, they produce a natural antidiuretic that travels from your brain to your kidneys, telling them to hold on to as much water as they can. You'll be thirsty, and yet you'll retain water. Your hands and feet will swell. You'll be uncomfortable. You'll urinate very little, and the urine will be concentrated and dark in color. Worst of all, your metabolism will begin to slow down.

On the other hand, if you are well-hydrated, water seeps back into your hypothalamus, and it stops producing the antidiuretic. You won't feel thirsty, and all will be well. All the excess water that the body doesn't need will be excreted in urine.

Shoot for 2 liters of water a day. Try to get more if you're exercising, living in a hot climate, or flying on an airplane.

Speak with a dietitian. No amount of general advice could ever compare with the personalized, tailored advice you can get from a dietitian. These professionals can take all of your vital stats—current weight, lifestyle, activity level, age, health conditions, even food preferences and eating styles—and turn them into a delicious nutrition plan that will help you achieve your goals quickly, easily, and, most important, *healthfully*. To find a dietitian, ask your physician for a referral, contact the nutrition department of a local university, look in the phone book, or write to the following organization for a list of qualified registered dietitians in your area: American Dietetic Association, 120 South Riverside Plaza, Suite 2000, Chicago, IL 60606-6995.

YOUR NEW BODY IS BORN TODAY

Hey, athlete! Yes, you! A healthy body is an energetic body. Properly fueled, you'll have enough juice in your shoes to get through even the toughest day and still have vigor to work out.

If you're overweight, and your physician has ruled out medical reasons out of your control as the cause, you now have the tools you need to put together a healthy diet and exercise plan that will get you on your way to a leaner, stronger, healthier body. Eat right, get fit, live long, and be happy!

Chapter 9

ENJOYING A PAIN-FREE PREGNANCY

Among the most gratifying experiences we've shared over the years with our athletes is when one of them becomes pregnant, and we stop training for sport or performance and start training for childbirth. We've learned so much from these women—mostly about how awe-inspiring the miracle of birth really is. But we've also learned that pregnancy can be one long, demanding endurance event, and, like other intense physical challenges, the better prepared an athlete you are, the more likely you are to ace it.

One of our most unusual moms was Claudia Malley, former publisher of *Runner's World* magazine. We had worked with Claudia for years at events and seminars for *Runner's World,* and we had even had occasion to see her in action, running in the Boston Marathon. Claudia had dropped into our New York City clinic from time to time for a tune-up, but one in particular was life-changing: Claudia came in and announced that she was expecting a child. She asked if we could help her organize her training for a successful pregnancy.

We were incredibly honored. We did extra homework to supplement our education as fast as she was advancing through dramatic body changes. We decided that our approach in training Claudia would be similar to any other athletic challenge. We planned to keep Claudia in as good a shape as possible so that she could run until it was no longer in her best interests, at which time we would all make a decision to pull her. Then we would phase her running down, while maintaining fitness to handle the stress of labor and delivery. Finally, we would work toward rapid recovery to get her back onto the road and into running as quickly as possible.

Admirable goals, to be sure. Well, at least they sounded good at the time. Although we outlined a regimen to keep Claudia one step ahead of her baby's development, we overestimated our own ability to be in charge of a pregnant athlete's body, and we underestimated Mother Nature, who actually had it all under control. All we had to do (in fact, all we *could* do) was keep mom strong and flexible. Claudia found her Active-Isolated program helped her adjust to her serious, rapid weight gain that altered her center of gravity and changed the way she carried herself. The lessons we learned with Claudia are a large part of the program we'll share with you.

When Claudia delivered her baby by cesarean section, her surgery disrupted muscles in her abdomen. Initially, Claudia couldn't lift her legs. Her doctors assured her that this was temporary, but we knew that in many ways, she'd be starting from scratch. We gave her a few days to recover from surgery and then started with small Active-Isolated stretches. Tiny movements. As we always do with our clients, we insisted on no pain and no irritation to muscles that were already traumatized.

For 6 weeks after delivery, Claudia tended to her little son and worked with us to retrain her muscles. Claudia had learned throughout her pregnancy to allow her body to dictate the workouts, and this was no different. It took some time, but she's 100 percent. She's once again running races, and, best of all, she has a beautiful child.

RELIEVING THAT LOWER BACK

Over the years in our practice, Claudia's miracle has repeated itself a number of times with our athletes and with nonathletic women who came to us for training or help with back problems after they discovered they were pregnant. Each mom presents a different challenge, but most of them have one thing in common: lower-back pain.

Years ago, lower-back pain was considered to be part and parcel of pregnancy, but today we know that biomechanical lower-back pain, which can start just before the 12th week and last as long as 6 months after the baby is born, has specific causes and treatments. We also know that if you had lower-back pain before the pregnancy, most likely it will continue. Pregnancy isn't well-known for making physical ailments better. (By the way, knowing that lower-back pain begets lower-back pain builds a strong case for getting into good shape before pregnancy.)

If you are experiencing lower-back pain, you're in good company. A little over half of all pregnant women experience it. Pregnancy is complex and can be very difficult, so why is lower-back pain the problem? And, more important, how can we get you past it?

There are a number of causes. Sports-medicine researchers tell us that lower-back pain falls into three categories, each with its own origin.

Sacroiliac joint pain. This type of pain starts in the sacrum, the triangle-shaped bone configuration where the spinal column joins the pelvis at the lower back. The sacrum feels like and looks like a solid unit, but it is, in fact, a series of joints. It appears to be solid in large part because the joints fit together snugly to act as one stable skeletal unit and are held in position by tight ligaments. But all this changes in pregnancy, when mom needs a wider pelvis. Levels of the hormone relaxin increase, signaling the pelvis to open up to cradle an expanding uterus and to allow safe, unobstructed passage of a child through skeletal structures. The ligaments relax to open the symphysis pubis, that little "separation" in the front of the pelvic bone, by widening the sacrum.

By the 14th week, when relaxin peaks, there's a noticeable shift. Bones and connective tissue that are usually extremely stable are stretched, which can be painful. Although the pain appears to originate in the sacrum, it can shoot through the buttocks, down the thighs, and all the way down to the middle of the calves. As the day wears on and mom gets tired, it seems to get worse. Of all the lower-back problems, sacroiliac joint pain might last the longest and can even outlast the baby's delivery, continuing to plague mom for several months afterward.

Lumbar pain. Nonspecific pain in the lower back, lumbar pain can have origins in bone, ligament, muscle, and tendon. During pregnancy, it could have one of several causes: rapid weight gain, an expanded uterus that moves organs out of position and changes the center of gravity, and tissues that are stretched to accommodate the expansion. To make things worse, relaxin compromises joint integrity, causing laxity. Without the tension and strength to keep the body in balance, pain-sensitive ligaments are stretched and stressed. The net effect is pain. The pain is intensified when mom is lifting something or is seated for a long time.

Nocturnal pain. This pain is often described as being like a cramp that mysteriously strikes moms at night when they should be resting. Some women experience it with sacroiliac pain or lumbar pain; some

PROTECTING YOUR BACK AS YOUR BODY CHANGES

women experience it exclusively. The source of this particular pain is not clearly understood, but a couple of theories exist. One theory is that nocturnal pain is the result of cumulative fatigue from a hard day of carrying a baby. We think this theory is probably on the mark. The supporting evidence is that a good night's sleep with rest and relaxation will eliminate the pain (until maybe the following evening).

The other theory is that nocturnal pain is caused by a mistake in positioning in bed. If an expectant mom lies flat on her back with her legs stretched out straight, the weight of the uterus can compress the vena cava—the large veins that run along the spine. In this case, the body will divert blood flow to other veins, increasing venous pressures, and this will cause discomfort. Physicians note that the compression is likely to be accompanied by nausea and dizziness that can be alleviated by shifting position to the side and getting the weight and pressure off the vena cava.

A fourth category—pain of other origin—actually has nothing to do with pregnancy. Rather, this pain may be signaling an unrelated orthopedic difficulty, injury, or illness.

It's wise to remember that things aren't always as they seem to be, especially in medicine. Back pain is tricky. Your physician is your partner in making sure that your pregnancy goes well and you stay healthy. Resist the urge to self-diagnose. Consult your physician.

EXERCISE IS GOOD FOR MOM AND BABY

Research over the past 10 years on the physical responses of moms and unborn children to exercise has significantly increased our understanding of the benefits and risks. Reassuring reports strongly suggest that exercise poses minimal risks for you and your baby and actually may make pregnancy and delivery a whole lot more pleasurable.

According to the American College of Obstetricians and Gynecologists, exercise during pregnancy, within specific limits can be very good for expectant mothers. Their research found that exercise helps you feel better; gives you energy; improves your mood and sense of well-being; eases some discomforts of pregnancy such as backaches, constipation, bloating, swelling, and fatigue; prepares you for the rigors of labor and delivery; improves your sleep; and helps you recover from childbirth more quickly. (No bowl of pickles and ice cream can do all that!)

But, please, don't use exercise to lose weight during pregnancy. Talk to your doctor about appropriate pregnancy weight parameters, based on your frame, activity level, and weight prior to pregnancy.

Modifying Your Workouts for Pregnancy

As your body changes, you'll begin to notice different ways in which your workouts need to be adjusted. One thing that's working for two is your cardiovascular system. Your oxygen requirements will be higher, so you'll be huffing and puffing sooner than before you were pregnant. Also, keep in mind that when you exercise, extra blood is deployed to your muscles and is less available elsewhere. You don't want to overdo to the point of becoming light-headed.

Surprise! You're heavier and more cumbersome

Hot Tubs Can Get You into Hot Water

As tempting as it is to climb into a hot tub to relax your back, you should seek comfort elsewhere. Hot tubs are dangerous double whammies for expectant moms. Overheating your body can be harmful to the well-being of your little one, and you run the risk of becoming dehydrated. It's easy to forget that your body is dissipating heat through sweat even when you're submerged in water. If you think warmth will help you feel better, consider a heating pad if you have your doctor's okay, or more layers of clothing.

A Note about Water

An expectant mother may experience difficulty when baby starts to get bigger and seems to be intent on taking over any space formerly enjoyed by the bladder. Additionally, mother's little angel likes to kick and has a canny knack for aiming straight for the bladder, especially when it's full. The effect is frequent and often urgent trips to the bathroom.

If this is happening to you, you might be tempted to reduce your intake of fluids. Not a good idea, especially if you're engaged in any sort of exercise program. No matter how inconvenient, you must drink water, lots of it, and often. If you feel thirsty, you're already dehydrated.

We also urge you to cut back on caffeinated drinks like tea, coffee, and some soft drinks. Caffeinated drinks are wet and satisfy thirst, but they won't do the job for you and your baby because caffeine is a diuretic.

When it comes in a tasty beverage available on every street corner, it can be easy to forget that caffeine is also a drug. In fact, some studies suggest that because caffeine passes easily from mom to the fetus, baby is affected by the stimulating effects that might influence heart rate and movement patterns, shorten gestation, and lower birth rate. Additionally, research suggests that pregnant women who consume more than five cups of coffee a day are twice as likely to miscarry. While safe consumption of caffeine during pregnancy is controversial, why risk it?

---

than you're accustomed to being. By the end of pregnancy, some women report gaining 30 to 50 pounds. That extra weight places greater stress on your joints and muscles. Your center of gravity moves forward, causing strain in your pelvis and lower back and challenging your balance. Your joints are lax, changing the way your body deals with a little extra tug or pull, and making you more prone to injury. And you may be struggling to overcome generalized fatigue. Face it, carrying a baby is hard work by day, and your sleep might be interrupted at night.

Your body might feel awkward. You might have to compensate for confusing changes. You might not get the results you expect. But exercise—even under these conditions—is good for you. Your baby is floating, suspended in amniotic fluid, and is well-cushioned from your enthusiasm. All you have to do is make sure your workout is safe. Protect your baby and yourself from extreme heat, avoid impact, eat healthy foods in sufficient amounts to supply you and your little one with plenty of nutrients, and drink as much water as you can. (Read on for more tips and guidelines on how to stay safe.)

YOUR BACK BEARS THE BRUNT OF THE CHANGES

From your athlete's point of view, your first concern will be the extra pounds that pregnancy brings—in a hurry. Not only is the weight gain a rapid one, it is carried in front of you. Your baby also displaces internal organs and puts pressure on places you didn't even know existed.

We had heard that the average weight gain is nearly 25 pounds, but even we couldn't appreciate the full biomechanical impact of that much weight carried in front of the body, with the compensations that are necessary to keep upright and maneuver through the most rudimentary movements. That is, until we were treated to a couple of hours in one of those weighted body vests designed and stuffed to get the attention of expectant fathers who need a little sensitivity training. We are both athletes and fancy ourselves pretty strong people. So you can imagine the lesson in humility we learned when, after an embarrassingly short period of time (well short of the 2-hour exercise), we were dripping wet and exhausted.

Usually, when a person gains weight, the process is a straightforward matter of increasing fat stores throughout the body. Although the distribution is not exactly even and differs depending on gender and genetic predisposition, fat cells plump up nearly everywhere, making it easier for us to handle carrying distributed weight. Weight gain through increasing fat is sometimes called creeping obesity, because it happens slowly, almost imperceptibly. The person hardly notices it and adjusts to it day by day. In pregnancy, however, the weight gain isn't about gradually plumping up fat cells all over the body. With a developing baby, it is rapid, and the distribution of the weight is centered in the uterus, low in the pelvis.

This weight in front of you places enormous stress on your back, particularly if your abdominal muscles are weak. In early pregnancy, your pelvis supports the baby's weight. But when the wee one gets big enough to bulge out in front of your hips, the pull forward is significant if you're not strong enough to use your abdominal muscles to snug the baby back into that natural cradle of your pelvis. And further, as the muscles are stretched to accommodate your increasing size, they are less able to do the work. Compensating for inability to support the weight causes that signature swayback that we commonly and affectionately associate with pregnant women.

STRETCH TO EASE YOUR BACK

We talked before about relaxin's role in softening the connective tissues and ligaments in the lower back and pelvis to widen them for delivery. As long as you're loosening up anyway, you might as well take advantage of this time to stretch and get moving. Evidence suggests that flexibility gains made during pregnancy last beyond delivery, and women who are flexible during their first pregnancy have fewer problems with joint expansion in subsequent pregnancies. Active-Isolated Stretching just might be the perfect workout to ease an aching back and get a little gentle exercise.

Before you get started, here are a few things to

POSTURE CHANGES DURING PREGNANCY

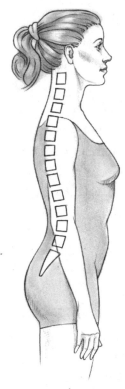

Normal posture

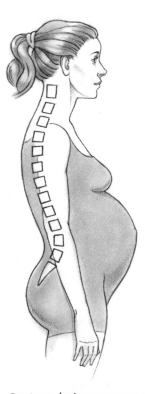

Posture during pregnancy

keep in mind for laying the groundwork for stretching during pregnancy.

Start early in your pregnancy. As your pregnancy progresses and your body changes, even things that were simple in the beginning of your program will become more difficult. Start your workout program as early in the pregnancy as possible and make small adjustments as you progress. The longer you wait to get started, the more difficult everything will be and the less likely you will stick with the program.

Actually, compelling evidence suggests that it's best to start working out *before* you get pregnant. Women who enter pregnancy with high levels of fitness have easier pregnancies, handle the stress of labor and delivery better, and recover more quickly. We want you to have a lot of fun with your pregnancy. And the more fit you are, the more fun you'll have.

Clear your program with your physician. Show him your planned workout, and get a blessing before you begin. Remember to discuss the specific stretches, the intensity, the frequency, and the duration of your workouts. Each time you visit, follow up with a progress report. Make sure your physician is advised of aches, pains, and changes in ability, such as something you did well a month ago that now seems difficult. You might be advised to scale down your exercise program or stop it completely if you have any of the following:

- High blood pressure
- Heart disease
- Pulmonary disease
- Pregnancy-induced high blood pressure

- Symptoms or a history of going into labor before the baby is due
- Vaginal bleeding or spotting
- Any compromise in the cervix, uterus, or membrane

Dress comfortably. How you dress will depend on where you stretch. Generally, we advise you to wear cool, lightweight, loose clothing that will allow you to move easily and comfortably. No tight or restricting seams or belts. Your shoes, as always, should be low-heeled, fit well, and be securely fastened. Make sure the soles of your shoes are slip-proof.

Pamper your back. After the first trimester, avoid exercises that put you flat on your back with your legs straight and extended. In this position, your uterus might compress the vena cava, large veins that run along your spine. The result might be pain, dizziness, and nausea that go along with a spike in venous pressures. The later in your pregnancy you are and the larger your uterus and baby, the more at risk you are of this unpleasant experience. It's easily avoided.

Choose a workout surface that is comfortable. We suggest a carpeted floor or a floor over which you have thrown a folded beach towel, mat, or blanket. Even your bed will work if it's not too soft. Most of the stretches we designed for you require a chair. Just make sure the chair is comfortable, supports you without slipping, and allows you to place your feet flat on the floor without strain.

Regulate the temperature. Make certain that you set the thermostat to keep you warm enough to be relaxed and yet cool enough to protect your baby from difficulties that may arise from being

When the Baby Is Born

Protecting your back doesn't stop when your baby arrives. Remember to frequently switch the side on which you carry your new baby. Always cradling junior in your left arm will cause you to overdevelop your left side and create a muscular imbalance that will put strain on your back. As the baby increases in weight, the imbalance will become more pronounced. This warning goes for dads, too.

Getting the Pressure off Your Back

Aside from doing Active-Isolated Stretching and Strengthening, you can do a number of things to help ease back pain during pregnancy. The American College of Obstetricians and Gynecologists suggests the following guidelines.

- Wear low-heeled (but not flat) shoes with good arch support.
- Ask for help when lifting heavy objects.
- When standing for long periods, place one foot on a stool or box.

- If your bed is too soft, have someone help you place a board between the mattress and box spring.
- Don't bend over from the waist to pick things up. Squat with bent knees and a straight back.
- Sit in chairs with good back support, or use a small pillow behind the low part of your back.
- Try to sleep on your side with one or two pillows between your legs for support.
- Apply heat or cold to the painful area, with your doctor's permission, and massage it.

---

overheated. Researchers caution that babies are generally safe when mom exercises—unless she is overheated. Stay out of the blazing sun, the sauna, and the steam room.

Stay alert for signals that tell you enough is enough. Pay attention to these warning signs: pain, nausea, a persistent cramp, dizziness, ringing in your ears, a racing pulse that you can't explain, a feeling of "fluttering" in your chest, breathlessness, tingling, numbness, sudden fatigue, headache, discharge of amniotic fluid or blood, a noticeable decrease in your baby's movement, or any potential symptom that your physician may have suggested earlier as being a concern. If you experience anything unusual, stop working out immediately and phone your physician or dial 911.

Expect to continuously adjust your program. Although these stretches are designed just for you, as your body changes, you might have to adjust or eliminate some stretches. As your abdominal muscles elongate over your expanding belly, they eventually separate from top to bottom along the center line of your navel. It's more difficult for you to contract them, if you can do it at all.

Additionally, later in your pregnancy, your enlarging belly might get in the way of something you'll try to do. Continue to include a stretch only if you

are comfortable. A little imagination and persistence go a long way. We urge you to keep at it.

Take 20 minutes a day for yourself. Take 20 consecutive minutes every day to stretch. Think of it not as an indulgence, but as your training—a necessary investment in the beginning of life with your new baby.

Set your pace and rhythm to lullabies. Stretching is relaxing and rhythmic, very much like rocking and in the same cadence. You have a lot of lullabies to memorize at the moment, so why not use the time you stretch to sing? With lullabies, you'll set the right pace in your workout. Just remember to breathe throughout the workout, and don't go into oxygen debt in order to hit and hold that high note, no matter how good you sound.

A STRETCHING AND STRENGTHENING WORKOUT GUARANTEED TO EASE MOM'S BACK

We'd love to see you do the full Active-Isolated Stretching and Strengthening program (see chapter 4), but a changing body needs special attention. The stretches here have been modified just for you, and the only equipment you'll need is an 8-foot length of stretch rope and ankle weights. Remember to exhale as you stretch and inhale as you relax.

MOM'S DOUBLE-LEG PELVIC TILTS

Active Muscles You Contract: Abdominals and muscles from the fronts of your hips down the fronts of your thighs

Isolated Muscles You Stretch: Lower back and buttocks

Hold Each Stretch: 2 seconds

Reps: 8 to 10

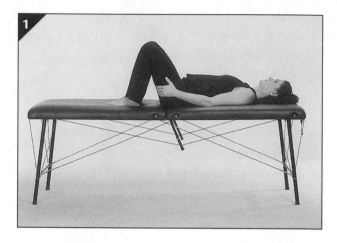

1. Lie down on your back on a comfortable surface. Pause for a moment to take a deep breath and make sure that your baby is not compressing your back. If you don't feel comfortable, skip this stretch. If you feel comfortable, bend your knees until your feet are flat on the surface on which you are lying. Place your hands behind your knees or thighs to provide a little assistance toward the end of the free movement.

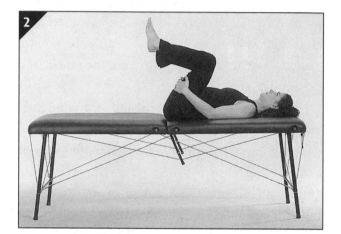

2. Using your abdominals and quadriceps, lift both your legs toward your chest, aiming your knees toward the outside of your shoulders until you can go no farther. If you feel discomfort in the front of your hips, spread your knees wider. Gently assist at the end of the stretch with your hands, but do not pull. Hold each stretch for 2 seconds and then return to the resting position. You'll feel this stretch in your lower back, but there should be no discomfort. It should feel great.

MOM'S BENT-LEG HAMSTRINGS

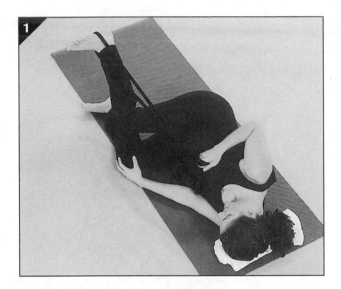

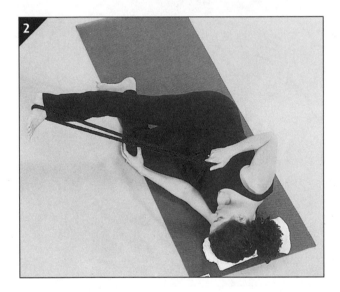

Active Muscles You Contract: Muscles in the fronts of your thighs

Isolated Muscles You Stretch: Large muscles in the backs of your thighs, just behind your knees

Hold Each Stretch: 2 seconds

Reps: 10 on the right, 10 on the left

1. Lie down on your side. Tuck a rolled towel or small pillow under your neck and head. Bend both knees to relax your back. Take your rope and hold the ends together so that it forms a loop. Slip the foot of your exercising leg (the upper leg) into the loop, positioning the loop in the arch between your heel and the ball of your foot. Take out the slack and snug it up.

   Keeping your knee bent and relaxed, bring your exercising leg up until your thigh is perpendicular to your trunk and your lower leg is parallel with your torso. Hold the ends of the rope in one hand and put enough tension on the loop to keep it from slipping away from the bottom of your foot. Put the other hand on top of the thigh of the nonexercising leg to stabilize your body.

2. Straighten your leg by contracting your quadriceps until your knee is locked. At the end of your stretch, gently assist with your rope, but don't force it. Add the slightest pressure, extending the range of the stretch just a little more. Hold for 2 seconds and then relax in preparation for the next stretch.

MOM'S STRAIGHT-LEG HAMSTRINGS

Active Muscles You Contract: Muscles from the fronts of your hips down the fronts of your thighs

Isolated Muscles You Stretch: Large muscles in the backs of your thighs

Hold Each Stretch: 2 seconds

Reps: 10 on the right, 10 on the left

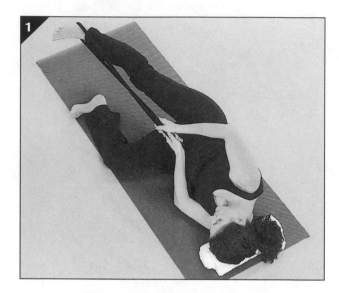

1. Lie down on your side. Tuck a rolled towel or small pillow under your neck and head. Your exercising leg (on top) should be straight. Your nonexercising leg should be bent at the knee to keep you from rolling. Take your rope and hold the ends together so that it forms a loop. Slip the foot of your exercising leg into the loop, positioning the loop in the arch between your heel and the ball of your foot. Take out the slack and snug it up. Lock your knee.

2. From your hip and using your quadriceps, bring your leg straight out in an arc toward your face as far as you can. Grasp the ends of the rope with both hands (to maintain tension so the loop won't slip off your foot) and "climb" up the rope, quickly hand over hand as your leg arcs toward your head. At the end of your stretch, gently assist with your rope, but don't force it. Add the slightest pressure, extending the range of the stretch just a little more. Hold for 2 seconds and then relax in preparation for the next stretch.

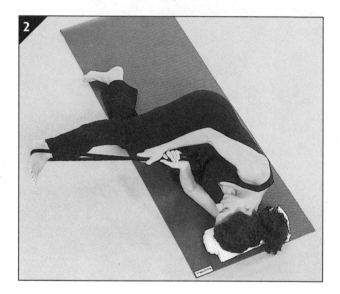

MOM'S INTERNAL ROTATORS

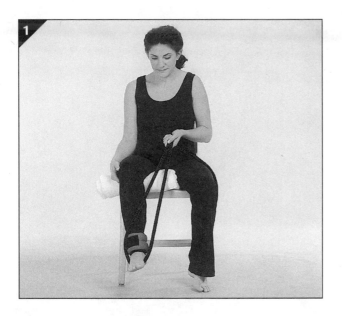

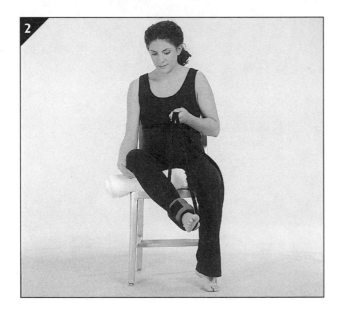

Active Muscles You Contract: Deep muscles in the buttocks that externally rotate your hips

Isolated Muscles You Stretch: Deep muscles in the top of the buttocks that internally rotate your hips, the muscles that span the hip sockets to the top of your pelvis, and the muscles that reach from the bottom front of your pelvis to the inside of your thighs halfway down your femur

Hold Each Lift/Stretch: 2 seconds

Reps: 10 on the right, 10 on the left

1. Sit somewhere from which you can dangle your legs. You might want to place a rolled towel underneath your knee to take pressure off your kneecap. Strap a light weight on the ankle of your exercising leg. Loop your rope around the arch of the foot of your exercising leg with the loose ends to the inside. Hold the rope with the hand on the opposite side of your body and gently gather it up to remove slack. Place your other hand (on the same side as your exercising leg) outside your thigh just at the knee and grasp the muscle with your thumb on the outside to stabilize your leg and to guide and control the rotation. Keep your nonexercising leg relaxed.

2. Rotate your lower exercising leg toward the midline of your body. Move from your hip. Go as far as you can. Gently assist by pulling upward on the rope to extend your range of motion. Hold for 2 seconds. As an added benefit, you'll get a good Active-Isolated strengthening of the external rotators in your hip. Relax the tension on the rope and slowly return to the starting position.

MOM'S MEDIAL HIP ROTATORS

Active Muscles You Contract: Muscles in the middle and deep within your buttocks

Isolated Muscles You Stretch: Outer hip and inner thigh

Hold Each Stretch: 2 seconds

Reps: 8 to 10 on the right, 8 to 10 on the left

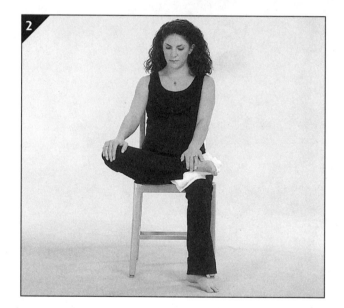

1. Sit with your back against the back of the chair. Place a small rolled towel between your lower back and the chair back. Take the foot of the leg to be stretched and place it on top of the thigh of the opposite leg, resting your ankle just above your knee. You may want to use a folded towel on the top of your thigh as a cushion.

2. Contract the muscles in your hip and outer thigh, and press your knee toward the floor. Using your non-stretching leg as a fulcrum, gently press your knee down with the hand on the same side, and stabilize and assist the stretch with your opposite hand by holding your ankle steady. Work one side at a time. Be gentle but firm. Hold each stretch 2 seconds and then return to the resting position.

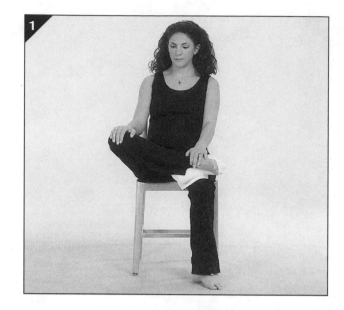

MOM'S SEATED TRUNK EXTENSORS

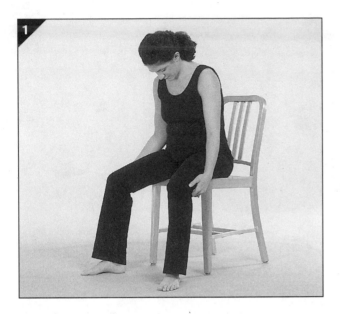

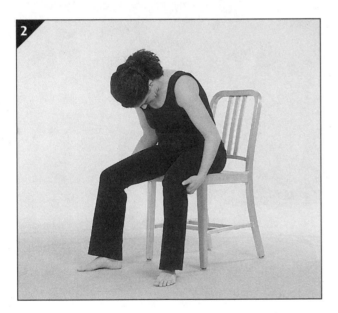

Active Muscles You Contract: Abdominals

Isolated Muscles You Stretch: Muscles that run from your pelvis to the base of your skull along the spine, and the lower-back muscles below your belt line

Hold Each Stretch: 2 seconds

Reps: 8 to 10

1. Perch on the edge of your chair with your back straight and relaxed. Place your feet flat on the floor in front of you, shoulder-width apart.

2. Tuck your chin down, as shown, and contract your abdominal muscles to roll your torso forward, until your head is as far below your knees as you can get. As your pregnancy progresses, you might have to widen the distance between your feet. Grasp the sides of your lower legs with your hands to gently assist at the end of the stretch. Pull forward gently. Don't bounce. Hold each stretch 2 seconds and then return to the resting position.

MOM'S SEATED THORACIC-LUMBAR ROTATORS

Active Muscles You Contract: Abdominals, the muscles on the sides of your chest, and the thoracic-lumbar rotators on the side opposite the exercising side

Isolated Muscles You Stretch: Muscles that run from your pelvis to the base of your skull along the spine; the stabilizing, rotating, and balancing muscles in your back and sides; and the lower-back muscles below your belt line

Hold Each Stretch: 2 seconds

Reps: 8 to 10 on the right, 8 to 10 on the left

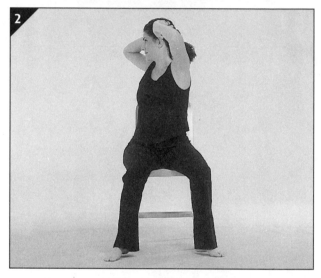

1. Perch on the edge of your chair with your back straight and relaxed. Place your feet flat on the floor in front of you, shoulder-width apart for stability. Lock your hands behind your head with your elbows out.

2. Contract your entire abdomen, including the muscles in your side, and the opposite thoracic-lumbar rotator muscles and rotate your upper body in one direction until you have twisted as far as you can go. Be gentle, but make it count. Repeat the warmup rotation four or five times in one direction until you feel loosened up and comfortable. Rotate again and hold for a moment, but this time flex your trunk forward, leading down between your knees toward the ground with your elbow. Return to an upright position. Work one side at a time, completing all repetitions.

3. Then move to the opposite side. Hold each stretch 2 seconds and then return to the resting position.

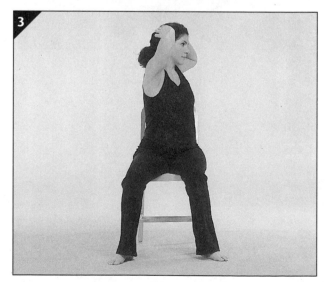

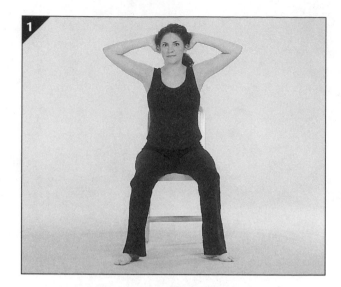

MOM'S TRUNK LATERAL FLEXORS

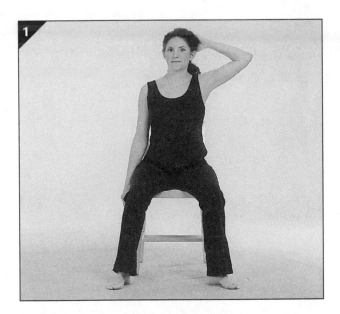

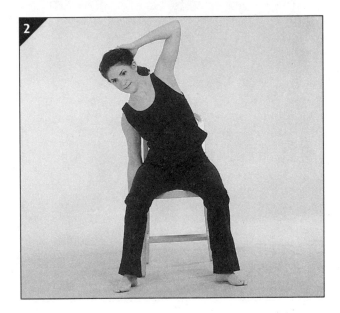

Active Muscles You Contract: Abdominals, the muscles on the sides of your chest, and the thoracic-lumbar rotators on the side opposite the exercising side

Isolated Muscles You Stretch: Muscles in your back along your spine and the muscles in the sides of your trunk opposite the exercising side

Hold Each Stretch: 2 seconds

Reps: 8 to 10 on the left, 8 to 10 on the right

1. Perch on the edge of your chair with your back straight and relaxed. Place your feet flat on the floor, shoulder-width apart for stability. Raise one arm, placing your hand behind your head with the elbow pointed away from your body.

2. Bend at the waist so that the hand of your straightened arm is lowered toward the floor. At the end of the movement, you'll feel a gentle stretch down the opposite side of your trunk. Work one side at a time. Hold each stretch 2 seconds and then return to the resting position.

MOM'S RHOMBOIDS/ROTATOR CUFFS

Active Muscles You Contract: Muscles in your shoulders

Isolated Muscles You Stretch: External shoulder rotators, commonly called the rotator cuff, and the upper back

Hold Each Stretch: 2 seconds

Reps: 8 to 10 on the right, 8 to 10 on the left

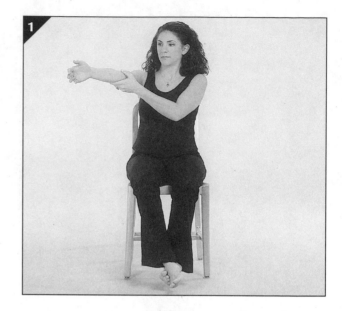

1. Perch on the edge of a chair with your back straight and relaxed. Cross your legs at the ankles, or place your feet flat on the floor, shoulder-width apart for stability. Lift one arm and hold it straight out. Lock your elbow.

2. Leading with your hand and keeping your elbow locked, move the arm straight across your chest toward the opposite shoulder. Use the other hand to give a gentle assist at the elbow at the end of the movement, as shown. Don't rotate your torso, and resist the temptation to hike up your shoulder. Work one side at a time. Hold each stretch 2 seconds and then return to the resting position.

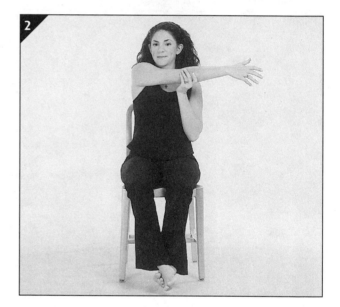

MOM'S NECK ROUTINE

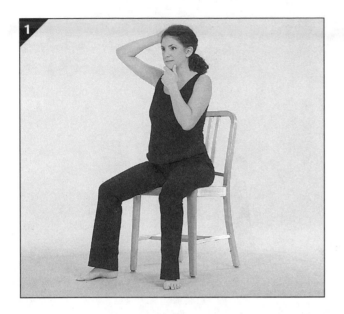

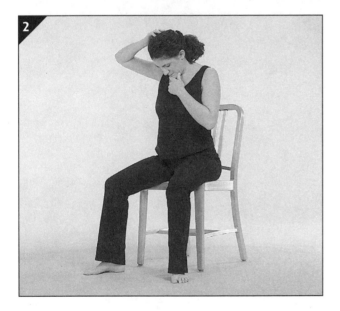

Active Muscles You Contract: Muscles in the front and back of your neck and the top of your back between your shoulders

Isolated Muscles You Stretch: Muscles in the front and back of your neck and the top of your back between your shoulders

Hold Each Stretch: 2 seconds

Reps: 8 to 10

1. Perch on the edge of a chair with your back straight and relaxed. Place your feet flat on the floor, shoulder-width apart for stability. Place one hand on the back of your head and one hand on your chin to assist the stretch.

2. Tuck your chin down and roll your head forward until your chin meets your chest, as shown. Gently assist the end of the stretch by pressing lightly at the back of your head. Return to neutral position.

(continued)

3. Now move your hands to your chin and spread your fingertips along your jawbone. Slide your head straight back until it's over your body.

4. Then roll your head straight back—chin straight up, as shown. Again you can gently assist the stretch by pressing with your fingers. Return to neutral position.

   Rotate your neck and turn your head slightly to one side and then roll it down toward your chest again. You can gently assist the end of the movement with your hands at the back of your head. Return to neutral position. Be certain to keep your shoulders down and relaxed. Hold each stretch 2 seconds before returning to the neutral positions. Repeat each stretch 8 to 10 times before moving on to the next stretch.

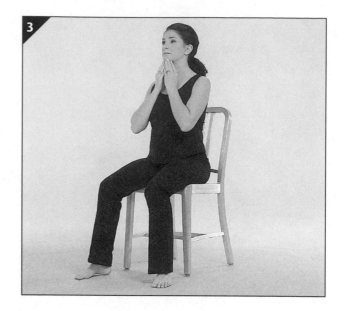

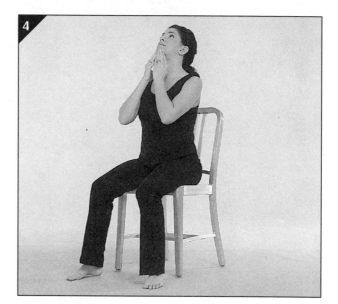

If Your Back Pain Continues

If you've tried these exercises and you're still feeling pain, your physician might suggest that you wear one of several types of braces especially designed for pregnant women to support the abdominal weight and take some of the pressure off the back. You might try prescriptive pain medications that are safe for expectant moms, bed rest, and professional physical therapy.

If back pain continues or gets worse and doesn't respond to simple attempts to get it under control, get back to your physician immediately. Back pain can be caused by preterm labor and other problems unrelated to pregnancy that need immediate attention.

GIVE YOUR ACHING FEET (AND BACK!) A BREAK

As your pregnancy progresses, your body has to adjust to rapidly changing weight. With carrying your baby low in your pelvis and to the front, your back muscles are under strain to keep you upright and counterbalance this weight and shifted center of gravity.

The other problem caused by changing weight is fatigue in your ankles and feet, and that pesky swelling that seems to be the fate of all pregnant moms as the months roll by. Sometimes the pain and discomfort can be significant.

Mother Nature designed your feet to be shock absorbers. The arches in your feet are like springs. They dissipate the vertical forces of walking and standing, and translate them into horizontal motion. When the shock absorption overloads and fails, these forces jar the ankles, knees, hips, and back. And nothing overloads the arches like a rapid increase in weight.

In our culture, women's feet are generally weakened before pregnancy by high-heeled shoes that shorten the Achilles tendons in the backs of the ankles, by sandals with no arch support, and by high-tech soft shoes that do the job of the arch instead of allowing the feet to strengthen. When we are working in Kenya, most of the women in the mountain regions don't wear shoes. All have strong ankles and arches, and when they become pregnant, they seem to have fewer problems than women in developed countries like ours. Here, "barefoot and pregnant" are too late for benefit. (Besides, "barefoot and pregnant" means something quite different in our culture, and it's not good.)

But take heart. There's a lot we can do to stretch and strengthen your feet so that you can minimize swelling and handle your increasing weight without jarring your back.

A Word about Leg and Foot Cramps

One of the best-kept secrets in sports could really come in handy for new moms. The best way to get a muscle to relax and unlock in record time is to identify the offending muscle, isolate it the best you can, and activate or contract the *opposite* muscle, assisting the stretch at the end with gentle pressure. The cramping muscle will relax its stranglehold.

For example, if you have a foot cramp that is pulling all your toes up until they feel as if they're going to break off, reach down under them and take them in your hand with your palm on the bottom of your foot. Curl your toes down against your fingers (away from the cramp) while you gently push your toes all back down. Hold for 2 seconds and release. Relax a second and then do it again.

The first time you do it, it will continue to hurt, and you'll be convinced that the action is backward. Trust us. Keep at it. In a few seconds, the cramp will be gone. The principle applies wherever you find a cramp. (Except in the case of cramps called contractions—the only way to make them release and relax is to have the baby!)

MOM'S SOLEUS

Active Muscles You Contract: Fronts of your lower legs

Isolated Muscles You Stretch: Deep muscles in the backs of your lower legs

Hold Each Stretch: 2 seconds

Reps: 10 on the right, 10 on the left

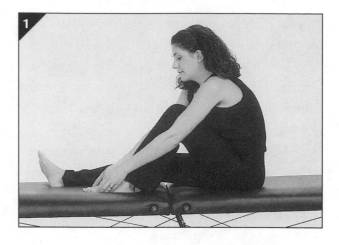

1. Sit on a flat surface. Straighten your nonexercising leg and extend it in front of you. Bend the exercising leg at the knee at a 90-degree angle and place your foot flat on the surface. Reach down, as shown, and grasp the bottom of your foot with both hands.

2. Keeping your heel flat down and pivoting from your heel, raise your foot and bring it back toward your body as far as you can go. Point your toes toward your nose. Use your hands for a gentle assist at the end of the movement. If you are unable to reach your foot for this stretch, use your stretch rope. Make a loop and place it around your foot, grasping the loose ends to stretch.

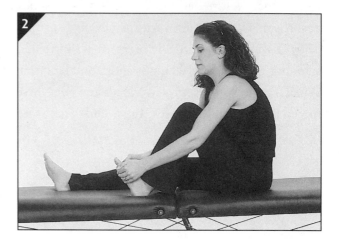

MOM'S GASTROCNEMIUS

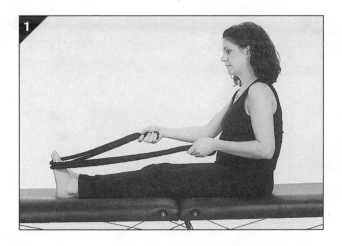

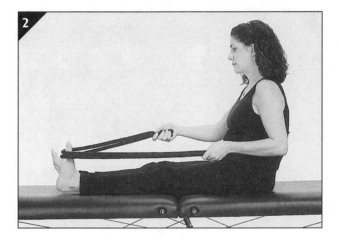

Active Muscles You Contract: Muscles in the fronts of your lower legs

Isolated Muscles You Stretch: Calf muscles

Hold Each Stretch: 2 seconds

Reps: 10 on the right, 10 on the left

1. Sit on a flat surface with both legs straight out in front of you. To get the pressure off your back, you may want to relax your nonexercising leg by bending your knee and putting the sole of your foot flat. Loop your rope around the midfoot of your exercising leg (still straight) and take each end of the rope in your hands.

2. From your heel, flex your foot back, aiming your toes toward your knee. Use your rope for a gentle assist at the end of this movement. Remember to keep your knee locked and upper body still. For an advanced stretch, you may bend forward at your hips and lean your upper body closer to your locked knee.

MOM'S ANKLE EVERTORS

Active Muscles You Contract: Insides of your feet and ankles

Isolated Muscles You Stretch: Muscles of the outsides of your feet and lower legs

Hold Each Stretch: 2 seconds

Reps: 10 on the right, 10 on the left

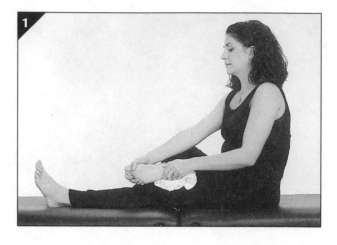

1. Sit with both legs straight out in front of you. Bring the foot of your exercising leg up, as shown, and place it on top of the thigh of your nonexercising leg, just above the knee. Reach straight down and grasp your forefoot with the hand on the side of the exercising leg; use your elbow to apply gentle pressure on the inside of the knee of the exercising leg to stabilize it. Grasp your heel with your other hand.

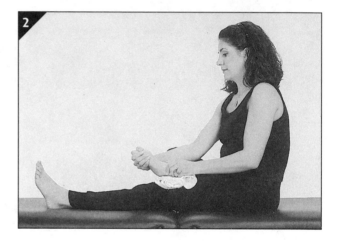

2. From the ankle, rotate your foot inward, pointing your sole up. You may use your hand for a gentle assist at the end of your stretch.

Note: You may want to use a folded towel on the top of your thigh, under the ankle of your exercising leg.

MOM'S ANKLE INVERTORS

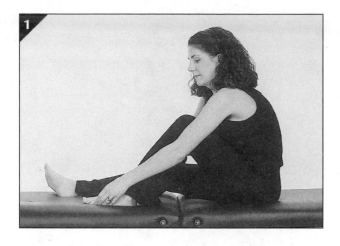

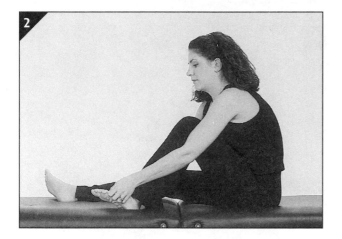

Active Muscles You Contract: Outsides of your feet and ankles

Isolated Muscles You Stretch: Muscles of the insides of your feet and lower legs

Hold Each Stretch: 2 seconds

Reps: 10 on the right, 10 on the left

1. Sit with both legs in front of you. Bring the foot of your exercising leg up toward your buttocks by bending your knee. Keep the heel of your exercising foot on the surface.

2. Grasp your midfoot with both hands. Rotate the foot to the outside, using your ankle. Point your sole out. Use your hand for a gentle assist at the end of your stretch.

MOM'S LOWER-LEG TRIPLE PLAY

Active Muscles You Contract/Strengthen:
Lower legs

Isolated Muscles You Stretch: Lower legs and ankles—front, inside, outside

Pace of Stretch: Up slowly, pause, down slowly

Reps: 10 on the right, 10 on the left—can work simultaneously

Equipment: Tube sock, light ankle weight, rolled towel

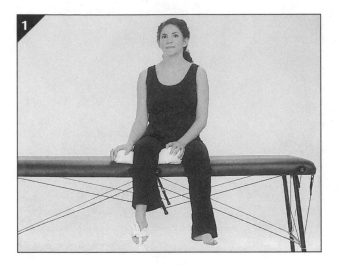

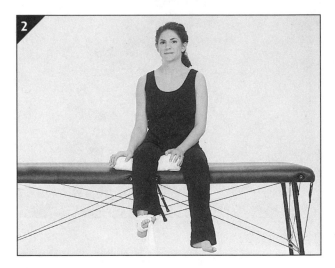

This exercise will help reduce swollen legs and feet.

Stuff a 1-pound ankle weight into the toe of a long tube sock. Tie the sock onto your exercising foot by dangling the weight under the ball of your foot and threading the sock between your big toe and the toe next to it. Make certain to have plenty of sock left to loop around your foot. Continue to wrap by looping the end of the sock around the outside of your foot, under your arch and back up over the top of your foot. Fasten it securely by tying under the top wrap.

1. Sit up straight and contract your abdominals to stabilize your torso. You might want to place a rolled towel underneath your knees to take pressure off your kneecaps and reduce stress on your back. Slightly separate your knees and feet. Point your toes down straight to the floor, as shown. Now, slowly raise the front of your foot until your heel is down and your toes are up as high as you can get them. You'll feel the stretch in the outside of your lower leg and the top of your foot. Pause and then slowly return to the starting position (toe pointed down).

2. Maintain the same basic position. Sweep your foot up and toward the midpoint of your body, pointing your big toe to the ceiling. It's a diagonal movement. You'll feel the stretch in your arch and the inside of your lower leg. Pause. Then sweep your foot back down until your big toe is pointing straight to the floor.

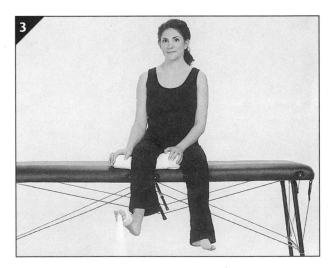

3. Then continue the sweep up and to the outside as far as you can go. You'll feel the stretch in the outsides of your ankle and lower leg. Slowly return to the starting position.

MOM'S TOWEL PULLS

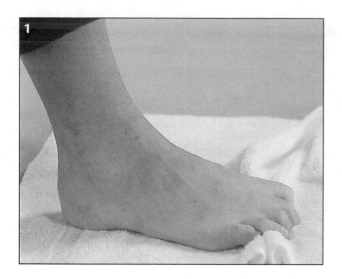

Active Muscles You Contract/Strengthen: Medial arch of foot

Isolated Muscles You Stretch: Lower legs, feet, and ankles

Reps: 10 on the right, 10 on the left

Equipment: A towel

1. For this exercise, you need to have a smooth floor so that your towel will slide easily. First, lay the towel out on the floor in front of a chair. Put the short end of the towel against the legs of the chair and spread the towel length in front of you. Sit in the chair with your back straight and your bare foot flat on the edge of the towel. Work only one foot at a time. Without moving your heel, contract all your toes to bunch up the towel and draw it toward you, as shown, until you have done 10 repetitions of toe contractions or run out of towel.

   Straighten out the towel and turn it sideways, so that the length of the towel is now against the legs of the chair. Put your heel on the towel. Starting with your little toe, contract all your toes to tightly draw up the towel and sweep it toward the midline of your body. The mental imagery we use is that we're bringing the little toe under the foot to meet the big toe, and we're going under the floor to do it in a U-shaped arc. Without moving your heel, continue to gather and sweep the towel across the floor in front of you until you have done 10 repetitions or run out of towel.

   Finally, straighten out the towel, but leave it sideways. Keep your heel on the towel. Starting with your big toe, contract all your toes to tightly bunch the towel toward you and sweep it away from the midline of your body. The mental imagery we use is that we're bringing the big toe under the foot to meet the little toe, and we're going under the floor to do it in a U-shaped arc. Without moving your heel, continue to gather and sweep the towel until you have done 10 repetitions or run out of towel.

Chapter 10

STANDING TALL AGAINST OSTEOPOROSIS

When Dolores White shuffled into our clinic, she was a fragile woman, stooped over with a dowager's hump that thrust her head forward and forced her face down. Her waist was nearly nonexistent, and her steps were small and unsure. She used a walker. Her son was at her side, guiding her.

The contrast of this woman alongside the dancers and athletes who frequent our clinic was startling. She said frankly, "I haven't always been like this, you know. I was once just like they are. I could run and dance. This hump wasn't always there." She said that she had once stood as tall as we do and that she wished she could live her life over again. "I would have done some things differently," she lamented. Her biggest regret? Not knowing the consequences of neglecting to take calcium and stay active.

The consequences to which Dolores was referring were osteoporosis and the cascade of physical problems that plagued her as her body became more fragile and shut down. Osteoporosis has caused vertebral fractures in her upper spine, resulting in that painful and debilitating dowager's hump.

Osteoporosis used to be called the silent killer, but there's nothing silent about osteoporosis anymore. The press and the medical profession are succeeding in getting the word out, and on account of effective prevention, earlier detection, and advances in medication, it's less a killer than it once was. But it's still dangerous.

The treachery of osteoporosis (literally, "porous bones") lies in decreasing bone mass, which increases the risk for fractures, especially in the hip, spine, and wrist. When left unchecked, osteoporosis quietly, insidiously steals bone mass until a person is so fragile that a deadly fracture can occur just by moving the wrong way. Of the 25 million Americans who either have or are at risk for the disease, 80 percent are women. The dangers are significant: 40 percent of all women will have at least one spinal fracture by the time they are 80 years old. These postmenopausal women's diminished estrogen levels rob them of their protection and leave them vulnerable.

Yet the disease is largely preventable, chiefly through regular exercise (such as the Active-Isolated Stretching, Strengthening, and Cardio program) and a diet rich in calcium and vitamin D. Doctors also are optimistic that medications will improve in the future and that detection methods will become less expensive and more widely available.

And for those who have osteoporosis, its destruction can be slowed or halted. We helped Dolores arrest osteoporosis with Active-Isolated

Stretching and Strengthening, and she now walks without even a cane. She has reclaimed her independence and enjoys life again. (Last we heard, she had gone back to school!)

A little education can help you halt osteoporosis in its tracks. First, let's look at where it comes from.

WHAT'S HAPPENING IN YOUR BONES?

Bones are made up of calcium and proteins. Cortical bone is the hard outer part of the bones, and trabecular bone is the spongier part on the inside, more like a honeycomb of bony plates.

The spongy trabecular bone is most vulnerable to the disease because the normal process of bone replacement changes with age, which makes the bones porous, brittle, and fragile. The National Osteoporosis Foundation reports that osteoporosis is not a normal part of aging; instead, it's the result of not achieving and maintaining good, strong bones throughout a lifetime, starting when you're very young.

From birth until early adulthood, bone is constantly replacing itself. At any given time, 5 to 20 percent of your skeleton is rebuilding. Then, at about age 35, you reach your peak bone mass, and the dynamic process of rebuilding begins to slow down. At this point, bone loss exceeds production. Calcium absorption also declines, and your body's ability to manufacture vitamin D diminishes.

In women, when menopause factors into the equation and estrogen levels decline or drop completely, the body loses even more of its ability to absorb calcium, a process dependent largely on estrogen that is no longer present. The result is that a woman can lose up to 35 percent of her cortical bone mass and 50 percent of her trabecular bone over her lifetime.

If bone loss is severe or continues over a long period, the bones become too fragile to withstand everyday physical stress, and they fracture. The more bone mass you start with, the more you'll be able to maintain as this loss occurs.

Unfortunately, osteoporosis has no obvious symptoms. A fracture may be the first signal that things are going wrong. The first bones to weaken are usually those in the spine, which is composed largely of trabecular bone. As osteoporosis advances—most often between ages 50 and 70—the spine can undergo a series of deformities and actually collapse, eventually reducing a woman's height by as much as 8 inches. A spine weakened and made fragile by osteoporosis can fracture and collapse unexpectedly from the most seemingly ordinary activities, such as opening a car door or brushing teeth.

The second most common fracture is that of the wrist. Most broken wrists are the result of falls, where women have extended arms to break their impact on the ground. Although these breaks heal fairly easily, broken wrists are good warning signs that trouble is brewing.

Fractures of the hip—or, more accurately, the upper part of the thigh (the femur)—are the most dangerous consequence of osteoporosis. Although these fractures can be the result of falls, they also appear to occur spontaneously. Hip fractures can be very dangerous, because healing requires prolonged bed rest, and confinement to bed can cause potentially lethal secondary conditions, such as pneumonia or blood clots.

ARE YOU AT RISK?

Women with low levels of estrogen face the greatest risk for osteoporosis. That includes not only women who have reached menopause naturally or surgically but also women who earlier in life had delayed or irregular menstruation. Other risk factors include the following:

A family history of osteoporosis. If your grandmother and mother had osteoporosis, chances are good that you will, too. Heredity is responsible for 70 percent of peak bone mass; the remaining 30 percent is up to you.

Chronic disease. Some chronic diseases that alter hormone levels and affect the kidneys, lungs, stomach, and intestines—such as end-stage renal disease—increase bone loss.

Age. As a natural part of the life cycle, bone loss increases with age.

Fractures after age 50. Breaks that aren't the result of hard falls or blows may be the first signal that bone health is declining. It's better to be evaluated before you have a fracture, but every fracture—especially if there was no obvious cause—should be a warning.

Insufficient calcium. The National Institutes of Health Consensus Development Council recommends 1,500 milligrams of calcium per day for women over age 50 who are not taking estrogen replacement therapy, and 1,000 milligrams per day for women over age 50 who are taking estrogen.

Inadequate exercise. One study reported that women who were very active had a 6 to 8 percent increase in bone mass, compared with a 0.25 to 2 percent increase in less active women.

Overexercising. Exercise—especially load-bearing exercise—is important, but overdoing it can impair bone building. Studies show that some female athletes with low body fat are unable to store sufficient estrogen and can even stop menstruating. Once estrogen levels drop, women are at risk for osteoporosis. You want to keep your body fat higher than about 16 percent—although most of us won't have any trouble with that, as the average fit woman's body fat percentage is between 20 and 25 percent.

Smoking. This nasty habit changes the liver's metabolism of estrogen, making it less biologically active. Women who smoke actually enter menopause a year or two earlier than nonsmokers. Also, there is conclusive evidence that cigarette smoking inhibits bone cell formation.

Excessive use of alcohol. As few as three drinks per day fill you up with empty calories and impair your ability to make good choices regarding food, which can contribute to poor general nutrition, including low intake of calcium and vitamin D. Alcohol also inhibits the liver's ability to absorb calcium and to activate vitamin D. Without access to these vital nutrients, osteoporosis sets in.

Body build and race. Women who are thin, small-framed, Caucasian, or Asian are statistically at greater risk.

Prolonged use of certain medications. The aluminum in some antacids can bind to phosphorus and lower its levels, which would cause your body to excrete more calcium. Other medications having this effect include thyroid hormones, anticonvulsants, steroids used for asthma or arthritis, certain diuretics, tetracycline, and long-term use of the anti-tuberculosis drug isoniazid. Your physician will help you determine which medications put you at risk.

MEASURING BONE MASS

The problem with diagnosing osteoporosis is that it is sneaky. No symptoms rear their heads until the first bone breaks. Where this disease is concerned, it's always better to err on the side of caution and take action early. When you turn 45, ask your physician to evaluate your bone mineral density, especially if you have one or more of the risk factors. Several radiographic methods are available for assessing bone density. All are painless, noninvasive, and safe, and most are readily available to you and covered by insurance.

While useful in spotting a fracture, an x-ray is not sufficient to diagnose osteoporosis. A bone has to be more than 30 percent deteriorated before it possibly shows up in an x-ray. Scanners are far more sensitive and give you a running head start at diagnosis and treatment. They also can predict your chances of fracturing in the future if you do nothing to mitigate the effects of bone loss. And they can give you periodic updates on how well you're doing to get osteoporosis under control and keep it there.

Two types of scanners are used in imaging. Central scanners measure density in the spine, hip, and total body. Peripheral scanners measure density in the finger, wrist, kneecap, shin, and heel.

Central scanners include the following:

■ Dual energy x-ray absorptiometry (DXA) is an improved, faster form of dual photon absorptiometry, measuring bone in the lower arm, spine, and femur with low radiation exposure. It can be used to scan the entire body.

- Dual photon absorptiometry (DPA) is a method to assess cortical and trabecular bone mineral in the spine and hip, and total bone mass. It assesses the lower spine and adjusts for soft tissues. It is accurate, but bone spurs, aortic calcifications, and arthritis may give false readings. DPA delivers low doses of radiation. It is used infrequently.

- Quantitative computed tomography (QCT) gives the radiologist a cross-sectional view of the vertebrae, allowing accurate measurement of the trabecular bone mineral content. This sensitive indicator of early osteoporotic changes is a little more expensive than the previously mentioned methods and delivers a little more radiation.

Peripheral scanners include the following:

- Single photon absorptiometry (SPA) is an inexpensive method that is used to assess cortical bone mineral in skeletal appendages. SPA delivers low doses of radiation at the wrist.

- Radiographic x-ray (RA) uses an x-ray of the hand and a small metal wedge to calculate bone density.

- Single energy x-ray absorptiometry (SXA) measures the wrist or heel.

- Peripheral dual energy x-ray absorptiometry (pDXA) measures the wrist, heel, or middle finger and compares those readings to normal readings of someone your age, gender, and size, and to the normal readings of someone like you at optimal peak bone density.

The results of your test will give you and your physician information that will assist you both in making decisions regarding healthy bones.

PREVENTING BONE LOSS THROUGHOUT YOUR LIFE

For the past few decades, the best lifelong prevention for women has been a three-way approach: estrogen, a good diet, and plenty of exercise—especially load-bearing exercise. Recent research about supplemental hormones indicates, however, that estrogens need to be approached with caution.

In younger women, hormones—including estrogens—are in perfect balance. As a woman ages, however, estrogen levels drop, signaling the end of menstruation and childbirth years. Unfortunately, the drop in estrogens also reduces the body's ability to remodel bones. For postmenopausal women, estrogen is one of two drugs approved by the FDA for the prevention of osteoporosis. Essentially, estrogen slows bone loss by acting directly on the bones, preserving mineral. It also blocks some bone-dissolving hormones and helps activate vitamin D, which in turn enhances calcium absorption. Estrogen increases collagen as well, a substance that helps form new bone tissue. The "bone mineral age" of a woman who takes estrogens is on average 10 to 12 years younger than her biological age.

But there's a problem. A big one. A major study of the effects of hormone therapy (HT) on women ages 50 to 70, run under the auspices of the National Heart, Lung, and Blood Institute of the National Institutes of Health (NIH), was halted 3 years early when preliminary results demonstrated that the risks for the study group on combined HT—specifically conjugated estrogens—outweighed the benefits.

The main goal of this trial had been to see if hormone therapy would help prevent heart disease and hip fractures and to examine the effect of HT on breast cancer. Researchers discovered small but significantly increased risks of breast cancer, coronary heart disease, stroke, and blood clots for the group of women on HT. While the benefits of hormone therapy did include a decrease in vertebral and other osteoporotic fractures with HT use, NIH officials concluded that the risks were significantly high enough to justify stopping the study for public health reasons and for the sake of the women who participated. If you are taking HT solely for the prevention of osteoporosis, you and your physician might consider stopping it, because other medications exist that can help prevent osteoporosis and fractures and that appear to carry fewer risks for breast cancer. (See "Damage Control" on page 232.)

Although estrogens might not be right for you, you still have other things to try for healthy bones.

A good diet. A diet rich in calcium is a valuable weapon against osteoporosis. Calcium keeps the bone replacement process in balance so that your body stores more than it loses in waste. Low-fat dairy products, such as fat-free milk and low-fat yogurt, are good sources of calcium, as are leafy green vegetables (except spinach), nuts, tofu, and fish. But if none of those sounds appetizing, many fortified foods will do, including some orange juices, breads, dairy, and soy milks.

Calcium (and vitamin D) supplements. As we stated before, you'll want to shoot for 1,000 milligrams (if you're over age 50 and take estrogen) to 1,500 milligrams (if you're over age 50 and don't take estrogen). Because the body can absorb only about 750 milligrams at once, physicians recommend dividing the doses: half in the morning, and half in the evening.

Choosing the Right Calcium Supplement

When you first step up to the shelf in your local pharmacy to choose a calcium supplement, you'll be dazzled by the selections . . . and confused. It's important that you select the calcium that's right for you.

Not all supplements contain the same amount of elemental, or pure, calcium. Some forms of calcium are more bioavailable than others—meaning that they are quickly dissolved so that your body can easily use them.

If you want to conduct a comparison test of the calcium you're considering so you'll know how easily the mineral will dissolve, simply drop one tablet into room-temperature vinegar and stir every 5 minutes. The U.S. Pharmacopeia (USP), a nonprofit organization that sets standards for medications, reports that at least 75 percent of the calcium should dissolve within 30 minutes. If it doesn't, the tablet contains little bioavailable calcium and is probably not of much use to you.

If you don't have that kind of time, here's our handy list of a few calcium supplements, listed in order of percentage of elemental calcium.

- Calcium carbonate (Tums, Os-Cal 500, Caltrate, Alka-Mints). With 40 percent elemental calcium, this is the least expensive, dissolves quickly, and is the most concentrated tablet. It is absorbed best with food.
- Calcium phosphate (Posture). Although it has 31 percent elemental calcium, this is one of the least soluble and least bioavailable.

- Calcium citrate (Citracal, Solgar). With 21 percent elemental calcium, this dissolves the fastest and is best absorbed on an empty stomach.
- Calcium lactate (TwinLab). Though this dissolves more reliably than calcium carbonate, with 13 percent elemental calcium, it will require taking more tablets to get a good result. It's not advised for women who are lactose intolerant.
- Calcium gluconate (Roxane, LifeScript). With 9 percent elemental calcium, this dissolves more reliably than calcium carbonate, but because it contains less elemental calcium, getting the best result will require taking more tablets.
- Bone meal, dolomite, oyster shell. Avoid these unless your physician directs you to take them. They are high in calcium but potentially contaminated with toxic metals and generally not recommended.

Calcium absorption is improved by vitamin D, so make sure that your supplement also contains some of this important nutrient. Calcium is also hard for your body to absorb, so rather than take all your calcium at one time, you'll increase absorption if you take 750 milligrams twice a day with food. And if you suspect that calcium is causing digestive upset—constipation, bloating, or gas—be sure to wash it down with plenty of water.

(See "Choosing the Right Calcium Supplement.")

Calcium, no matter how you get it, is boosted by vitamin D, which is activated by the liver and kidneys. Your body manufactures vitamin D naturally, with the assistance of ultraviolet sunlight. Getting your daily requirement takes only 10 minutes of exposure a day, but it's very easy for your levels of vitamin D to get too low, especially if you can't get outside very often during daylight hours. Some studies also suggest that the older we are, the more difficult it is for the body to translate sunshine into activated vitamin D. So why take the chance of getting low in D?

Between age 51 and 70, the daily requirement for women is 400 IU; after 70, you need 600 IU. One of the best sources of vitamin D is fortified milk, but you'll have to drink four 8-ounce glasses every day. That might be difficult to do, so be sure to get a little bit of sun and take a supplement. That way, you'll get all you need.

Exercise. If you already have osteoporosis, there's no question that you're more fragile than you used to be, but you can still work out. Just go easy, and talk to your doctor about any necessary precautions.

Exercise is crucial for keeping muscles toned so that a fall is less likely or at least less severe. Some research suggests that load-bearing exercise such as walking or weight lifting stimulates bone formation by triggering the same kind of remodeling that would occur with stress and rest.

Load-bearing exercise places the resistance of weight on bones. But as the body adjusts to load, the exercise that was once beneficial to your bones can suddenly becomes less so. Take walking, for example. At first, your bones—from your feet to your back—work against gravity and the weight of your own body, and all your bones benefit and remodel. But as you grow fitter, the bones become used to this load. Gravity and the weight of your own body will no longer challenge them. It's up to you to keep your routines challenging to your bones by mixing up your activities or by progressively increasing the work your body has to do. The key is to continuously create resistance, enough to make your bones—and the rest of you!—feel challenged.

If you don't have osteoporosis, load-bearing exercise is a great way to make sure that you'll never have it. Experts agree that, no matter what activity you select, it should be fun, so you'll be more likely to stick with it.

In many cases, women who have begun experiencing some of the more unpleasant symptoms of osteoporosis—such as a dowager's hump—will stop doing exercise because of pain or discomfort. If this is your situation and you want to begin slowly, we recommend the following four exercises to start you off. Do these for 2 weeks, and you're certain to feel your back and hips loosening up. Once you feel better, you can start the full Active-Isolated program.

If you have begun experiencing symptoms of osteoporosis, try these four stretches.

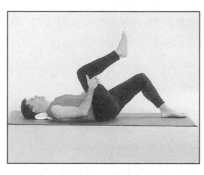

1. SINGLE-LEG PELVIC TILTS
See complete instructions on page 39.

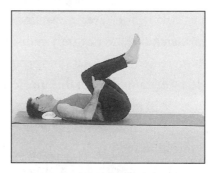

2. DOUBLE-LEG PELVIC TILTS
See complete instructions on page 40.

(continued)

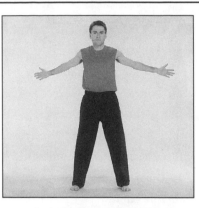

3. PECTORALIS MAJORS
See complete instructions on page 53.

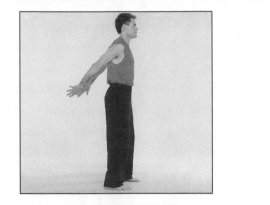

4. ANTERIOR DELTOIDS
See complete instructions on page 54.

DAMAGE CONTROL

Prevention goes a long way, but if bone demineralization has begun, several medications other than estrogen are available to slow down or even halt the loss.

We include this information here as an overview of your pharmaceutical options. Of course, the best place to find out which drug (if any) is right for you is your doctor's office.

Alendronate (Fosamax). A member of the bisphosphonate family, this drug is FDA-approved for women and men. Bisphosphonates stop or slow bone breakdown of osteoporosis but don't slow the buildup of new tissue, so they allow the bone to "catch up" with the natural remodeling cycle. These medications are probably more effective than estrogen in slowing and preventing bone loss, especially if your risk factors are unusually high. In research trials, alendronate not only reduced bone loss but also increased bone mass in the spine and hip. Taking 10 milligrams daily of this medication reduces fractures by 50 percent.

One problem is that alendronate is absorbed through the intestine and can be irritating. Because of that, you must take it with 6 to 8 ounces of water first thing in the morning on an empty stomach, and you must stay upright for at least 30 minutes to keep it from irritating the esophagus. Other side effects might include musculoskeletal pain, nausea, heartburn, and abdominal irritation. The other reservation about alendronate is that, once taken, it sticks to the bone—probably for life. Although researchers think that it is unlikely to be harmful, no one knows for sure.

Alendronate is approved for treatment or prevention of osteoporosis caused by prolonged use of steroids and glucocorticoid medications in both men and women. A once-a-week form is now available, and it might be just as effective as the daily dose but with fewer side effects.

Risedronate (Actonel). At a dose of 5 milligrams a day, this drug, also a bisphosphonate medication, slows bone loss, increases density, and reduces the risk of fractures. Like alendronate, it has to be taken with plenty of water first thing in the morning, and you may not eat, drink, or take any other medications for an hour. Some side effects include upset stomach, nausea, vomiting, diarrhea, and headache. Like alendronate, it is approved for use by men and women for the treatment or prevention of osteoporosis caused by prolonged use of steroids and glucocorticoid medications.

Raloxifene (Evista). One of the new designer estrogens known as selective estrogen receptor modulators (SERMs), raloxifene is taken as a pill once a day to prevent bone loss and increase bone mass throughout the body, especially in the hip and spine.

Raloxifene, along with calcium and vitamin D, appears to reduce the risk of first spinal fractures by about 55 percent within 3 years. Women who have already suffered one spinal fracture appear to reduce their risk of subsequent fractures by 30 percent, although there's no proof yet that hips are as well-fortified.

Like estrogens, raloxifene appears to reduce blood lipids, thereby reducing risk of cardiovascular disease. But unlike estrogens, it does not appear to increase risk of breast and uterine cancers. In fact, researchers are suggesting that raloxifene reduces the risk of breast cancer by 76 percent among postmenopausal women who use it.

Raloxifene doesn't reduce the incidence of hot flashes—and might make them worse. Side effects appear to be few, although SERMs have been associated with some deep vein thrombosis. Because SERMs are relatively new on the scene, long-term effects of raloxifene are not yet known. Speak to your doctor for more information.

Calcitonin. Marketed as Calcimar, Cibacalcin, and Miacalcin, this protein hormone used to be available by injection only, but it now comes in a nasal spray. Calcitonin is a naturally occurring hormone that regulates how much calcium is in the body and how bone metabolizes it. If you are a woman more than 5 years beyond menopause, taking calcitonin may inhibit the breakdown of your bone and increase your spinal density, but it may be of little benefit to other bones. Women who use it, however, report that it also reduces pain associated with fractures.

Unfortunately, while none of the delivery methods is that pleasant, the nasal spray may win out. The spray might cause a runny nose, but the injections might trigger an allergic reaction, flushing of the face and hands, rash, nausea, and the need to urinate frequently.

Parathyroid hormone. This hormone, taken in a daily injection, stimulates bone growth by building new bone faster than old bone is broken down. In a recent 21-month study involving 1,637 women, those who received the injections had up to 13 percent more bone in their spines than those taking a placebo. They also reduced their risk of new spinal fractures by up to 69 percent.

MAN-TO-MAN TALK: OSTEOPOROSIS IN MEN

While osteoporosis is considered to be a woman's health hazard, the truth is that 2 million American men have it, and 3 million more are at risk. One-third of all hip fractures are endured by men, and, of these cases, a third will not survive more than a year. Clearly, this disease is a killer, yet a diagnosis of osteoporosis remains commonly overlooked among men. Part of the problem is that men have larger, stronger bones than women. When evaluating simple fractures in men, or even while doing annual physical examinations, doctors traditionally have not been quick to consider the possibility that osteoporosis could be setting in. We hope that's changing.

The causes of osteoporosis in men are similar to those in women: a low peak bone mineral density when they were younger and excessive bone loss as they age. Like women, if men don't have a good base before they start to lose mineral density, then the onset of osteoporosis is certain. Diagnosis is also the same: If you notice a little loss in height, a change in your posture—head forward and a slouch—or sudden back pain with no real explanation, osteoporosis could be the culprit.

Risk factors are also similar to those of women, with a couple of additions: Osteoporosis in men can be caused by insufficient levels of the sex hormone testosterone, especially if undiagnosed and never balanced. And Caucasian men are at greatest risk, although all ethnic groups are vulnerable.

In order to protect yourself, heed this advice from the National Osteoporosis Foundation: Get treatment for medical conditions that cause bone loss, stop smoking, drink only moderately, get active with load-bearing exercise, take 1,200 milligrams of calcium a day if you are over age 51, and make sure that you either have plenty of exposure to the sun or take at least 400 IU of vitamin D every day.

At this time, alendronate and risedronate are the only two medications from a class of drugs called bisphosphonates approved by the FDA for treatment of osteoporosis in men, mainly for steroid-induced osteoporosis. But even though medications are not as available for men as for women, you have other options to consider.

Your physician might suggest testosterone replacement therapy. Both genders have the hormone estrogen, and it's thought that testosterone contributes to the circulating levels of estrogen in men. As a man ages, and testosterone decreases, so does the estrogen. By increasing the naturally diminishing levels of testosterone, it might be possible to increase the levels of circulating estrogen and slow bone loss. A simple blood test can determine testosterone levels and tell you for sure if you're a little low.

Another medication your physician might suggest is calcitonin, which has been used for a long time in women to slow or stop bone loss. It may relieve some pain of fractures, if they've already occurred. Your physician might administer it as an injection or send you home with a nasal spray.

Besides adjustment in medication, osteoporosis is treated exactly the same in men as women. Because many men have grown up in a tradition of sports and physical prowess, it's hard for a guy to think in terms of his body being fragile, but it is . . . for now. You have to take it easy, and tuck your ego in.

If you're gung ho, back off the weight and the impact of exercise, and add duration. It's possible for you to enjoy building strong, flexible, and balanced muscles, knowing that stronger bones will follow. When we work with osteoporotic men, we subscribe to the "less is more" school of thought. Stick to the programs in this book, avoid injury so that you can stay in the game every day, and you'll be surprised.

OSTEOPOROSIS PREVENTION HAS A BRIGHT FUTURE

Physicians expect that within the next decade better medications will be available to prevent and treat osteoporosis. Some of the most promising include bisphosphonates and activated vitamin D, but keep in touch with your physician to talk about the latest advances.

While you're waiting, start by scheduling regular bone scans, eating a calcium-rich diet (including supplements), taking enough vitamin D or spending 10 minutes in the sun every day, and enjoying the exercise program that will help build bone and prevent falls. We want you standing tall, for life!

Chapter 11

LIMBER BACK, YOUTHFUL BODY

Over the years, we've worked with many of our clients from the time they were world-class athletes, through their retirement from competitive sports, and into their later years as recreational masters athletes. Watching them tackle some of the challenges of mounting years has completely redefined the way we think of aging.

Forget the images of rocking chairs and shawls. We've seen marathon runners and rock climbers discover that retirement gives them the time to enjoy themselves that they never had while they were in the workforce. We've seen desk jockeys who, once they've hung up their office stripes, suddenly realize their athletic passions.

Yet, for all this activity, even our best masters athletes will admit to you that age has slowed them down a bit. Almost all of them have noticed that, as they have aged, they have gotten a little shorter. Edward Benzel, M.D., of the department of neurosurgery at the Cleveland Clinic in Ohio, a neurosurgeon who specializes in the spine, puts it quite simply: As we age, our human bodies settle.

Some scientists say that we are programmed to age, that our bodies contain some sort of internal regulators or cellular level "switches" that signal a specific moment past which we begin to age and decline. Others think that we age because of cellular error, due to either normal wear and tear or damage done to specific cells by chemical or physical failures.

Well, here's the Wharton Theory of Aging: It happens. It's part of the cycle of life. What counts is how you deal with it—which is why we're here.

HOW YOUR BACK AGES

The limit of the natural life span and how we can expand it is a hotly debated topic. Many experts believe that the maximum that can be achieved with healthy humans is about 120 years of age. Others believe this upper level can be expanded to 150 or slightly more. Regardless of the upper-limits issue, the fact is that it's very possible to keep older human beings more active and alert in their final years.

Of particular interest to us in our discussions of the back is that cells shrink when we age and "settle," as Dr. Benzel says. The gelatin-like centers of the disks in your spine condense, and you become a little bit shorter. While your spine shortens—even just a small amount—the ligaments and tendons that surround the bones might not shrink at the same rate. When you're younger, those connective tissues support and hold everything tight and in alignment. But when the spine shortens and the connective tissue does not, the spinal column literally becomes loose. It becomes easier to throw your back out or suffer other aches and pains. Also, without their plump cushions, your disks are less effective as shock absorbers.

Normal activity brings about an acceleration of wear and tear on the bone, even causing jagged edges called bone spurs. As the bone spurs get worse and expand, they can cause a narrowing of the spinal canal and the spaces between the vertebrae. Before you know it, you could be suffering nerve impingement and some loss of function. People who experience this describe it as first an awareness of pressure, then pinching, then pain.

Can this deterioration or "settling" be avoided? Apparently not. It's part of the natural process of aging. When researchers examine a vertebra from a young person, by all accounts, the interior of the disk is firm and whole. When they examine a vertebra from an older person, the interior of the disk, as one researcher described it, is like "sawdust and crabmeat." (While we laughed nervously at her graphic description, we asked, "Always?" She answered solemnly, "Always.")

Before you slam this book shut and run for cover, believe us when we tell you that there's a lot you can do to make sure you're well and healthy with a strong, flexible, comfortable back throughout your later years.

STAY STRONG, LIVE LONG

Richard Sprott, Ph.D., formerly of the National Institute of Aging, is blunt about what he believes can be done about aging. "When it comes right down to it, life is a crapshoot. You come into this world with a set of genes, and you don't know what they are. You can make some guesses based on family history, but you don't really know what your genetic susceptibilities are. You make some choices and hope it works out for the best."

We are here to make sure that the choices you make are the right ones, for although we cannot stop the inevitable march of time, we can certainly rewind your clock.

As we age, we lose muscle mass—about 1 percent per year after age 30. Not only do the sizes of the individual cells decrease, the total number of muscle cells diminishes. This phenomenon is called sarcopenia. Researchers are not certain why it happens, but they suspect the combined effects of several factors. Reduced levels of physical activity, declining testosterone in men, declining estradiol in women, declining growth hormone in both genders, an aging central nervous system, a reduction in the synthesis of muscle proteins, and poor diet all contribute to the decline.

But scientists tell us that it's no longer acceptable to blame aging for a decline in fitness. Rather, it's the other way around: A decline in fitness accelerates aging and certainly accounts for many of the "symptoms" we associate with aging.

It's not uncommon for a sedentary man to go from 18 percent body fat at age 20 to about 38 percent by age 65. Women are capable of even worse. They can go from 23 percent at age 20 to almost 44 percent by age 65. These increases in body fat alone can put a human being at risk for type 2 diabetes, high blood pressure, stroke, and heart disease.

When a person retires to a rocking chair and winds down normal activity, he or she loses muscle tone. This weakening makes everything even more difficult, sending the person into a downward spiral. Without minimal fitness, a loss of function, balance, and flexibility occurs. Falls are more common. But, again, there's *plenty* you can do to help make sure you never experience debilitation.

In the past, you may have asked yourself, "Oh, why put in all the effort if aging is inevitable?" If living a longer, healthier life is not enough of an incentive, just remember that good muscle tone, strength, and flexibility are critical to maintaining independence. It's a matter of "use it or lose it." So, let's use it!

MAINTAINING THAT CRITICAL MUSCLE MASS

Fitness is defined as a combination of good health, flexibility, strength, endurance, and cardiovascular vitality. To be honest, no one component is more important than any other, but strength training is the only way to build muscle mass. In fact, studies of masters athletes (over age 60) who regularly engage in aerobic exercise and have done so for a long time tell us that although these masters are leaner and healthier than their sedentary counterparts, they have the same amount of muscle mass and strength. The only way to build muscle mass is to lift weights, no matter what your age.

Studies have found that the density of the lower spine and thighbone in postmenopausal women who strength train is much higher than in their sedentary counterparts. While other methods of preventing bone loss, such as medications and calcium, are effective, none has the additional benefits of strength training. The fit women not only improved bone mass but also added muscle mass, strength, balance, and an overall sense of well-being that goes with being active and confident. And exactly the same holds true of men.

The good news is that it is never too late to begin a fitness program, especially one that involves strength training. Indeed, a landmark study on nursing-home residents conducted by the Jean Mayer USDA Human Nutrition Research Center on Aging at Tufts University and the Hebrew Rehabilitation Center for the Aged, both in Boston, revealed that flexibility and strength improved significantly in older people in their eighties and nineties who participated in an exercise program. Study recruits were people whom doctors characterized as "frail." After lifting weights just 3 days a week for 6 weeks, the residents had increased their strength by 180 percent. Their average walking speed increased by 48 percent. Two threw away their canes. And one was able to rise from his chair without pushing off from the chair arms for the first time in memory.

Amazing, tremendous; all hail the power of exercise! But here's the cautionary part of our tale: At the end of the 6 weeks and all their success, the residents returned to their sedentary lifestyles. After 4 weeks, they had lost more than 30 percent of their strength in a rapid reversal of all the good that

had been done by exercising. The amazing turns terrifying! Here's a compelling case for getting off—and staying off—your duff no matter how old you are.

FLEXIBILITY: THE FOUNDATION OF SENIOR FITNESS

At any age, but particularly as we get older, flexibility is the key that unlocks all the other components of fitness. If you can get your body to move, you can put in place the other workout pieces—strengthening and cardio work—providing that you are medically able to participate. The Chinese say, "You are as young as your spine is flexible." We would add, "and strong."

The Active-Isolated Stretching routines you'll find in our exercise section (see pages 98 to 101) are the perfect way to begin. Most of the stretch routines can be accomplished from sitting or reclining positions, so the program may be started slowly and gently if you're not used to working out or if you have physical limitations.

Stretching requires no special equipment except your stretch rope. You don't need special clothing. And you can do it almost anywhere. And the benefits of the Active-Isolated method are many.

- To elongate a muscle (the antagonist), you must fire the opposing muscle (the agonist). The effect is a relaxed, lengthened muscle and a slightly strengthened opposing muscle.
- The rhythmic action of your routine pumps blood throughout the area you are stretching.
- Your heart works a little harder, and you breathe a little more deeply—exhaling on the extension phase and inhaling as you relax the position.

Indeed, from your first workout—without even having to get out of bed—you could be isolating and exercising muscles, elongating and strengthening muscles and connective tissues, expanding the ranges of motion if your joints, getting your heart rate up, and slightly enhancing your cardiovascular fitness.

This gentle method is the best way to slide into an exercise program. Like busting up a logjam one log at a time, removing little "jams" starts things moving. Once a few things start to loosen, real progress can be made.

The more you do, the more you are able to do. Add the strength component of the program when you're ready, and then eventually start the cardio training. Before you know it, you'll feel better than you thought possible.

EXERCISING FOR THE LONG HAUL

What's the best excuse men use, because of late-in-life back problems, to get out of lifting or hauling?

"It's an old football injury."

While the remark is often made tongue in cheek, it is more than likely true.

Some sports cause early back injuries that will plague a person throughout a lifetime. One European study cited weight lifting and soccer as sports that contribute to accelerated spinal degeneration. These sports' excess strain and impact were most likely the cause of the injuries. In the United States, we'd probably add football and rugby to the list of culprits.

But aside from a chronic injury, exercise doesn't appear to have any adverse effect on the back in later life—in fact, just the opposite. Athletes who have been active throughout their lives age far more gracefully than their sedentary counterparts. Top athletes often enjoy vigorous exercise and activity long past retirement from competition. Researchers believe that the continued training protects these athletes from spinal problems commonly associated with age. One of the German Olympic Team physicians, Fritz Niethard, M.D., is studying aging athletes to determine how and why they function so much better than sedentary people. "To have a better Volkswagen," he says, "we must study the Formula One machine."

If You Want to Start Slowly

If it's been a while since you worked out, and you want to ease into the Active-Isolated Stretching program, we have two stretches that will unlock your pelvis, relax your back, lengthen your stride, and show you what's possible in a few life-changing minutes of easy effort. Follow the instructions for preparations in chapter 4 on page 36, then get yourself started with these two favorites.

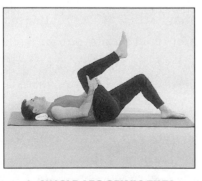

1. SINGLE-LEG PELVIC TILTS
See complete instructions on page 39.

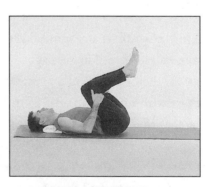

2. DOUBLE-LEG PELVIC TILTS
See complete instructions on page 40.

Let's not wait until all the scientific data is in. We know that it's true that a lifetime of activity and fitness leads to successful aging. Here are some ways to make sure all goes well.

Make It Safe

If you've been sedentary for a while, you should start physical activity slowly. Exercise at short intervals (5 to 10 minutes) and gradually build up to your desired level. Work out gently, with no straining. Remember that *some* exercise—even if it's a brief session with small movements—is better than none at all. You'll soon be up to speed.

Clear it with your doctor. Take this book to your physician and talk to her about your plans. If you are on medications that affect your blood pressure or heart rate, make sure your doctor explains what will happen when you start working out, so you'll know what to expect. Discuss risk factors, illnesses, and injuries that might make it necessary for you to start slowly or modify or skip an exercise. If nothing else, this conversation will be a great way to get a baseline physical report—a "before" profile so that you can compare the stunning results of "after."

While we believe that everyone at any age will benefit from exercise, some people should start slowly and with small movements. If any of the following conditions or situations pertain to you, make sure that your physician clears you to participate in this program.

- Any chronic disease, such as diabetes, or a family history of chronic disease
- Smoking
- Obesity
- Any new undiagnosed symptom of illness or injury
- Abdominal aortic aneurysm
- Critical aortic stenosis
- Chest pain or discomfort
- The feeling that your heart is skipping, racing, or fluttering

- Blood clots
- Infections or fevers
- Shortness of breath
- Acute deep-vein thrombosis
- Hip or back surgery
- Unexplained, undiagnosed weight loss
- Sores on your feet or ankles that will not heal
- Swelling in your joints
- Pain or limping after you've fallen
- Bleeding or detached retina, recent eye surgery, or laser treatment
- Hernia

Take your time. A few small movements will get you there, especially if you've been inactive for a while. If you push a workout, you risk getting injured or so seriously fatigued that you'll have trouble showing up for tomorrow's session. Just as getting out of shape took some time, getting back into shape will not happen overnight. But remember, you'll experience remarkable progress in just one workout, even if you stumble through every exercise and cut the workout short. Plus, the effects are cumulative. Small gains in strength and flexibility will build into larger ones. You're moving!

Don't ever hold your breath. This concern is particularly important if you're straining during the strength exercises, which causes a spike in blood pressure that could be problematic for you. Keep breathing: Exhale as you bring the weight up, inhale as you let the weight down.

Be sure to drink plenty of water. If you wait to drink until you feel thirsty, it's too late. Thirst is a symptom of dehydration, not some early-warning system to let you know that it's time to drink. Staying hydrated is especially important as we grow older. Researchers tell us that our ability to discern thirst is compromised as we age. In later years, we must rely on intellect and good planning a little more than we did when we were young—otherwise, we can be deceived into thinking that we're hydrated.

Also research demonstrates that, as we age, the ability to regulate fluid balance in the body can be affected by a downturn in kidney efficiency. This inability to regulate fluid balance can be made worse by some chronic diseases associated with aging, such as cardiovascular diseases and high blood pressure.

No need to worry. Just know that no matter how thirsty you are or are not, it's necessary for you to drink at least eight glasses of water a day—about 40 ounces. Because your sense of thirst might be impaired, you might want to put drinking on a schedule to make sure you get enough liquid.

Although we suggest that you drink at least eight glasses of water a day, you may substitute any other liquid except alcoholic or caffeinated beverages. (Both alcoholic and caffeinated beverages are dehydrating, so don't count them in your eight glasses. If you're going to drink them, do so in moderation.) Those liquids could be milk or diluted juice or a decaffeinated beverage.

Follow instructions specifically. They're designed to keep the strain off your back. We've spent our entire careers studying athletes and clients with varying degrees of ability and disability. Your workouts are engineered to work muscles—one or a few at a time—in small movements organized in very specific sequences that activate muscles and unlock joints when they're ready.

The key words here are "small movements." You'll find the work easy and effective beyond your imagination if you follow the instructions. You might not be able to carry a stretch to its full range or lift a weight at first. Just do the best you can with each stretching and strengthening exercise.

Most important: Don't skip around. Do everything in order. Little by little, you'll see real results.

Avoid painkillers *before* exercise. Pain is a useful tool for evaluating your body. Masking it can give you false information, which could lead you to bad decisions. While using painkillers can make you more comfortable so that you can keep moving, using them to mask a profound pain and let you "push through" can lead to injury. We had a client who regularly took ibuprofen before exercising to mask the pain of a stress fracture in her pelvis and let her continue to train for and run marathons—with disastrous and long-term consequences. Her career ended because of bad judgment.

Make It Realistic

The biggest downfall we see among people starting to exercise, or getting back to it after a long hiatus, is to have grand illusions that can be dashed immediately. Know that this is a journey that will yield rewards at every stage, as long as you're patient and pragmatic about your expectations.

Make your goals attainable. That way, every workout will be a success and make you feel great. If it's been a while since you worked out, just focus on showing up every day and "stepping up to the line." Look at every workout as a step ahead of where you were. It's taken you a lifetime to lose the high level of fitness you once had. You're working now to regain the integrity of your body, to learn how to use it again, and to teach it that you're going to put it back to work. Everything else will fall into place in its time.

Take it easy, but take it! The advice to "take it easy" that we get from loved ones as we get older may be well-intentioned, but not necessarily in your best interest. In our vocabulary, "take it easy" means work hard but avoid pain at all costs.

Follow the instructions for the exercises specifically; they're designed to keep the strain off your back. If something hurts, stop. The adage "No pain, no gain!" is simply untrue. Pain is nature's gift to you. We humans are neurologically wired to perceive pain and remove ourselves from the source of that torture in a split second, without thinking.

If you experience pain in a move, you've gone too far, and you're damaging something. At any age, damage and the accompanying injury will slow down a fitness program, but recovery is even slower as we get older. Muscles and connective tissues are not as elastic. Bones might be a little more brittle. A measure of caution is not only prudent but also necessary. Go slowly and gently. But go.

Don't forget to rest. When you feel exhausted, drop back the routines or just skip a day. Rest will allow your body to rejuvenate, refresh, and rebound. You'll be able to get right back to the workout when you're ready.

Rest is valuable for athletes of all ages—and especially true for the older athlete. Because recovery is a little slower, you'll need to give yourself extra time. We tell our older athletes that their bodies respond to training progressively, not aggressively. You have to give the neural pathways a chance to "remember" how to move, and you have to give your muscles a chance to work up to the demands you're now making. It takes time. If you overdo it, you risk injury, which could sideline you even longer. We would rather have you in the game. Just make sure that you come back to working out.

Make It Convenient and Fun

You could know every benefit of exercise in the world, but unless you make it convenient, your other responsibilities may conspire against you. One trick is to make sure you're having a blast—not many people would go out of their way to avoid having fun.

Ditch the job, but keep the calendar. The fun of retirement is that our schedules suddenly become a lot less rigid. Sometimes, schedules disappear completely. For some, this newfound lack of structure leads to a complete breakdown in discipline—and unexpected stress. Suddenly, it's hard to get anything done, including a workout.

If you find yourself always putting off exercise, try doing your routines first thing in the morning, after a gentle warmup. Many of our clients have told us that getting it out of the way first thing helps them

feel as if they have really accomplished something by 8:00 A.M.!

Work in minisets. Fit the activity into your life as easily as you can. For example, it's okay to break the workouts into small segments. Ten minutes of exercise three times a day will get you to 30 minutes. With our programs, you don't need a special space or lots of equipment, so you can easily find places that are perfect for you—on your rec room floor in front of the TV, in your sunny backyard, even on the kitchen floor while you're cooking dinner.

Tell yourself that you have to go "play." It's a shame that we call exercising "working out." This phrase cues the brain to think of it as work. Nothing could be further from the truth. This is your time to play. Find things you enjoy and then share them with your family and friends. Exercise is not meant to be a drudgery. Approached with the right attitude, it will bring you a world of joy.

EATING FOR ENERGY AND LONGEVITY

A balanced diet is just as important for you as for any of our athletes. The trick is to make sure you get everything you need, because as we age, we tend to have a problem opposite to one in our younger years: We tend to eat *less*. Sometimes this happens because we gradually lose some of our sense of taste.

Taste is dependent on two things: sense of smell and number of tastebuds. The first strike of aging comes to our senses: All senses diminish with passing years. Then, from age 40 to 50 in women and from age 50 to 60 in men, the number of tastebuds diminishes. And each remaining tastebud also begins to atrophy, further compromising our ability to taste.

The first sensitivities to go are the ability to discern salt and sugar, followed by bitter and sour. The result is that food doesn't taste as good and isn't as interesting. Also, the aging mouth produces less saliva, causing dry mouth and making digestion a little less efficient than when we were younger.

Fight Free Radicals with Antioxidants

You've heard a lot about free radicals. Free radicals are molecules in the body, usually of oxygen, that have lost an electron. Whereas most molecules have their electrons in pairs and are balanced, the free radical has only one and is unstable. Because the natural order of the universe is for electrons to be in pairs, the free radical goes in search of electrons to steal. They are like evil, little bandits that careen through the body, looking to raid the other molecules. When they find one, they attack and snatch an electron. The hapless molecule that has been raided is crippled and can no longer function properly. It can even die. If this sounds terrifying, realize that free radicals are unavoidable. If you want to see them in action, cut open an apple, let it stand, and watch it turn brown.

Free radicals in the human body form in the lungs and enter the bloodstream through metabolism. By damaging cells in the lungs and oxidizing cholesterol to form plaque in the arteries, free radicals are thought to contribute much to the process of aging in individual cells and, as a consequence, of the entire human mechanism.

If free radicals are indeed a factor in the aging of cells, then it is possible that antioxidants might help mitigate that damage. They are your body's warriors and protectors. Antioxidants combine with free radicals to neutralize them and convert them into harmless waste products. Some antioxidants actually repair damaged cells. The key antioxidant vitamins are C and E, and beta-carotene. Beta-carotene is converted by the body into vitamin A. Antioxidants are naturally abundant in vegetables, fruits, and nuts. A good rule of thumb is that the deeper the color of the plant, the more likely it is to be rich in antioxidants. (Additionally, green tea is a great source.)

We are always happier when you get all your nutrients from food, but a simple, inexpensive supplement might put you on the winning side.

Copy this cheat sheet and take it along to the grocery store to stock up on the richest sources for these important antioxidants.

Vitamin C		Vitamin E	Beta-carotene
Asparagus	Oranges	Almonds	Cantaloupe
Broccoli	Papaya	Cereals fortified with E	Carrots
Brussels sprouts	Potatoes	Hazelnuts	Collard and mustard greens
Cantaloupe	Red peppers	Spinach	Commercial vegetable juices
Commercial	Spinach	Sunflower seeds	Kale
vegetable juices	Strawberries	Vegetable oils	Mangoes
Cranberries		Wheat germ	Peas
Kiwifruit		Yams	Pumpkin and squash
			Spinach
			Yams

Eating just isn't as much fun, so meals tend to be smaller and less frequent. Consequently, it's increasingly difficult to get all the nutrients that a healthy body needs. Studies of aging are particularly focused on a decrease in protein intake, because one of the effects of inadequate protein is an accelerated loss of muscle, where protein is stored.

When you are stressed, have an infection, or are consuming too little protein, the body draws on stored protein in muscles to keep organs functioning. Although it's not clearly understood why, when you strength train, your body is able to store more protein, even if you aren't eating enough. The more protein you have on reserve, the better able you are to maintain muscle mass. The more muscle mass you maintain, the stronger you are, the more protected you are from osteoporosis, and the more calories you burn. The more calories you burn, the more food—of all types—you can eat. What a wonderful cycle! Ask your doctor to recommend an appropriate number of protein servings per day, based on your age, gender, weight, and any persistent health conditions you may have.

Sadly, no exercise on earth can help save your sense of smell or your tastebuds, but you can still do your best to get the nutrition you need. While we suggest that you get all your nutrients from food, we live in a real world—we know that it's some-

times not possible. In order to stem the tide of muscle loss, in addition to getting an adequate amount of protein, be sure to take a multivitamin formulated for mature adults every day. Good-quality, inexpensive vitamin and mineral supplements abound. And frankly, some vitamins are more difficult for the body to absorb from food after age 50. Taking supplements greatly increases your chance of benefit.

Experts suggest that taking a single multivitamin/mineral supplement is a good idea, because vitamins and minerals work together in very specific proportions. If you aren't sure about what you need and how much, it's smart to let an expert arrange the combinations for you. Just follow the dosage instructions on the label.

What about Joint Health Supplements?

You may have heard about "joint health" supplements that contain glucosamine hydrochloride, glucosamine sulfate, or a combination of glucosamine sulfate and chondroitin sulfate. If the claims are true, backs could theoretically be made more stable and, therefore, more comfortable. This promise is particularly attractive to people who have osteoarthritis and other degenerative disk diseases that cause pain and dysfunction. Let's take a look.

Glucosamine sulfate. Found naturally in the connective tissues of the body, glucosamine sulfate is responsible in large part for cartilage's ability to provide buffering and gliding of bone against bone without friction. When taken orally, it's absorbed easily and moves straight to the cartilage within a few hours. It boasts unique anti-inflammatory properties, and research suggests that when taken orally, it may stop the erosion of cartilage, soothe the inflammation, and promote regeneration of cartilage.

Glucosamine hydrochloride. This supplement has been less studied than glucosamine sulfate, but it

appears to be as effective. It has the advantage of more rapid absorption.

Chondroitin sulfate. Although it has been less studied than glucosamine sulfate, chondroitin appears to have all the same properties: It may stop the erosion of cartilage, soothe the inflammation, and promote regeneration of cartilage. It is also found naturally in cartilage.

These supplements are available in capsules and pills and do not require a prescription. Although these supplements have not been widely studied in the United States, they have been in use in Europe since the 1960s and appear to live up to their claims.

A word of caution: If you choose to take these supplements, make sure your physician knows and has given you a green light. Glucosamine may cause upset stomach, heartburn, or diarrhea. Glucosamine sulfate also appears to increase insulin resistance, so people with diabetes, beware. And people on blood thinners need to avoid chondroitin sulfate.

FOR GOODNESS SAKE, STOP SMOKING

We know that smokers are tired of hearing about lung cancer and heart disease, but there's yet another insidious side effect of smoking. For reasons not yet fully understood, smoking deteriorates the spine.

Researchers from Johns Hopkins University in Baltimore discovered that a history of smoking, high blood pressure, and coronary artery disease are risk factors for atherosclerosis, or clogging and narrowing of the arteries. No big secret here, right? The shocker is that these same risk factors are also significantly associated with the onset of lower-back pain and degenerative disorders of the disks between the vertebrae. Additionally, researchers have linked high cholesterol to the development of lumbar spondylosis, or degenerative osteoarthritis in the lower spine.

While studies continue, inarguable evidence suggests that injury and degeneration of the lower back are caused by damage to the vascular structures of the disks and joints—and that damage is caused by atherosclerosis and smoking. Although the exact mechanisms of the links between back pain and smoking are still unclear, every physician we've spoken with regarding spinal health has emphatically stated that any person with a back problem has to stop smoking. Now.

STAYING SAFE ON YOUR OWN

Studies tell us that falling poses a serious health problem for adults over 65 years old and is a leading cause of accidental death in adults over 75. One out of three will take a tumble. Even if there's no injury, once having fallen, an older person is statistically more likely to fall again.

Sometimes, it doesn't matter if the second fall never happens—the fallen senior may just live in constant anticipation of it happening, abandoning life in the fast lane and proceeding with caution. When activity is suddenly limited to the safe and secure, life can tend to wind down unnecessarily.

Without resorting to packing yourself in cotton batting, you can do plenty to avoid falls. In fact, people of all ages can benefit from a few tips for preventing a stumble and tumble.

Stay fit and healthy. Keep bones healthy with calcium and vitamin D. Keep your weight under control. See your physician regularly for thorough checkups that include screening for osteoporosis and a comprehensive review of all your medications. Exercise regularly. It's never too late to start, but it's always too early to give it up.

See your eye doctor regularly. He can make sure your glasses are the right prescription. And be sure that both your regular glasses and your sunglasses are the same prescription. The Framingham Eye Study reports that vision impairment is the cause of 18 percent of hip fractures from falls annually.

Be a good housekeeper. Keep your house clutter-free, and make sure the areas where you walk are wide and clear. Immediately wipe up spills on the floor. Wet spots are slick and invisible and quickly forgotten until you slide across the kitchen. Polish floors with nonslip floor wax. Keep your bed linen simple so that you won't get tangled up in it as you try to get out of bed.

Slip-proof your home. Make sure your carpets, rugs, and bath mats are skid-proof and flat on the floor. No curling edges on which to trip. No slippery bottoms on which to slide. Put skid-proof adhesive strips or a textured rubber tub mat on the bottom of your tub or shower stall. Make sure towel racks are secured tightly to the bathroom wall, so that if you need to hold on to one, it will support your weight. If you have steps or stairs, make sure they're in good shape, skid-proof, and well-lit with light switches at both the top and bottom.

You want to look slick, but your clothes shouldn't be. Wear shoes and slippers that are in good shape and fit well. If you have shoelaces, keep them tied. Wear shoes that are flat or low-heeled and have thin, skid-proof soles. Select clothing that is easy to put on and take off without having to be a gymnast, and make sure that wearing it allows you free and easy movement and doesn't get in your way.

Let there be light. As we grow older, we need to consider upping the wattage on our lightbulbs and increasing the number of area lamps. Make sure your environment is well-lit and that you have easy access to plenty of light switches. Install night-lights everywhere you might wander in your home after bedtime. Keep flashlights in every room. Keep a flashlight in your car. Take night-lights with you when you travel.

Train your pet. Encourage your furry friend to refrain from jumping on you unexpectedly or scurrying under your feet as you move. If you have a real scholar on your hands, try to train your pet to return toys to a basket or a box, rather than leaving them dangerously scattered on the floor all over the house, or to fetch small items for you, so you don't have to bend down and reach. Yes, even cats can be taught.

Hang on tight. If you stand on a chair to reach something, make sure it's stable and not wobbly. If you can't work with someone spotting you, scout a sturdy shelf or knob to grab in case you start to feel unsteady (*before* you climb up on the chair). If you climb a ladder, make sure it's firmly and securely stabilized at both ends. A helper can brace the ladder and protect you from slipping. If you're unsteady at heights, invest in an extension "grabber" for reaching and gripping small items above your head. Install grab bars in your bathroom: at the toilet, in the shower, and in the tub.

Manage winter. If you live in snow country, keep snow and ice off your porch, steps, walks, drive, and sidewalks—anywhere that you will walk. If you must walk on slippery surfaces (or surfaces that appear to be), ask for assistance. Most people will be glad to lend you an arm, but choose your companion wisely—no sense in two of you taking a tumble! If you must navigate alone, try to choose a route that is bordered by stable things onto which you can lean or cling.

Keep alcohol under control. Avoid drinking alcohol to the point that you're tipsy. Not only will you be off balance, your judgment will be impaired. Not good.

Stay in communication. As we grow older, we tend to be alone more than when we were younger. Establish regular contact at least once a day with someone who will check on you if you don't check in. Keep a phone in every room of your house. Carry a cell phone. Invest in the emergency panic button that goes along with your security system, and keep it handy.

Stay in the game. Action breeds action. Sure, things may take a little bit longer. They may even be a bit more difficult. But in the end, your life is worth it. Stay active.

In the words of Robert Browning, from his poem "Rabbi Ben Ezra" (1864):

Grow old along with me!
The best is yet to be,
The last of life, for which the first was made . . .

Part 5

Stress and Slumber

Chapter 12

PUTTING TENSION BEHIND YOU

In the dark days that followed 9/11 and the attack on the World Trade Center, we, like all New Yorkers, struggled to find a way to help our city stand up and fight back, to heal a gaping wound that was kept raw by fear and exhaustion. As did most New York City businesses, ours fell silent, so we had time to join the massive volunteer effort. Our offering was therapy for weary workers.

We turned our attention toward a fire station in East Harlem, Engine 58, Ladder 26, affectionately known as the Fire Factory. We selected this station because it is home to our lead therapist Tom Nohilly's brother-in-law, Jimmy Cody, and it seemed right to rush to help family. Another reason was that the Fire Factory responds to more calls than any other house in the world. They are hammered under even the most ordinary circumstances, but 9/11 would add an unbearable burden to their workload for a long time. Perhaps most taxing, they were grieving for their dead and searching for missing friends and fellow firefighters in the twisted, smoldering rubble at Ground Zero. Their lieutenant was missing. Jimmy had been appointed to replace him.

We could do nothing at Ground Zero, but we could do a little for the men who struggled to deal with it every day. Ultra-Lite donated 10 massage tables, and we organized a small army of therapists who worked at the Fire Factory from September 2001 through January 2002. With the chief's blessing, we set up right in the station. We stayed as focused on our jobs as they were on theirs, all of us on a tender, unspoken mission.

Rarely did any of our team have the luxury of an uninterrupted hour of treatment with a firefighter, but between bells that signaled scrambles to the truck and polite apologies, we helped them relax their bodies with the same techniques we use to get elite athletes onto Olympic tracks and ready for medal-winning performances. And now, we share our methods with you.

Keeping the body operating at peak efficiency through stress features two components: first, physically preparing for the immediate demands, and second, overcoming the fear and tension that can take an insidious toll on the body, especially the back.

WHY DOES TENSION ATTACK THE BACK?

If you ask most people what happens when they tense up, they'll tell you what you already know: We carry our tension in a small zone of pain right between our shoulder blades up to the base of our necks. But why does tension take up residence in this very specific place? Theories abound.

Tension can be emotional. Tension in the back is directly related to state of mind. Instinctively, when we're upset, we curl up. One theory holds that this curling might be an adult version of the fetal position, in which we might feel a little safer, or that we're trying to protect our hearts from hurt. Another suggests that we are folding in our energy to guard chakras—vortices of energy thought to exist in key points in the body.

Regardless of why, that curled-up posture takes a lot of effort, straining and fatiguing the muscles in your upper back and neck. The longer you despair, the more strained and tired those muscles get. And worse, the muscles in the front of your chest will begin to shorten, pulling you even lower. It's no accident that we refer to an unhappy person as being *down.*

We're going to tell you something shocking: Unhappy people are prone to injury and illness. Nearly 80 percent of all the physical problems we treat are related, directly or indirectly, to tension and pressure. When faced with a client who falls into this majority, we go ahead and make friends, because we know we're going to be together again. No matter what we do to unlock the body or how successful we are in restoring function, sooner or later, this client is going to come back unless he gets a handle on life. We aren't saying that getting happy will guarantee you a lifetime of health and injury-free fitness, but it helps. Big time.

Tension can be physical. The emotional aspect of carrying tension between the shoulder blades is not the only culprit. Fitness, or lack thereof, plays an even bigger part.

When your back is in pain, your abdominal muscles are the suspected cause. Weak abs cause your pelvis to be unstable, so your back—all the way from your sacrum to your skull—has to compensate to keep your body balanced and erect in posture, sort of like a gyroscope. But without the assistance of supporting abdominal muscles, your struggling back becomes a very unstable gyroscope.

While the problem originates at your pelvis, it qualifies as full-blown disaster by the time it reaches your head. Weighing in at 8 to 12 pounds, the head is heavy. When your abdominals are weak and your back is struggling to compensate, that heavy head pulls your spine forward. Shoulders follow suit as the front of your shoulders foreshorten and collapse. This sag may be subtle at first, but it doesn't take long for your upper back, designed to stabilize, to become fatigued from trying to support weight. It will short out. A strong, fit body ensures that all your muscles are doing their jobs and that they are sparing your back from having to compensate.

Tension can be postural. People can even make tension between shoulders worse by postural mistakes. When you sleep on your side with a pillow that fails to support your head and neck, you collapse your lower shoulder, folding it toward your chest and straining the muscles in your back for hours. When you work at a desk, you sit and put all action in front of you, so that you reach out and down toward the desk—and your upper back is stressed. When you drive, you reach forward and up to steer—and your upper back is stressed. When you eat, your plate is on the table in front of you, so you reach down and toward it—your upper back is stressed.

In fact, there's a *lot* you do to stress your upper back. If you switch positions frequently and keep your back relaxed and moving, there's usually no problem. Problems can start when you are sedentary and still and you sustain stress for long periods of time. Add personal tension to biomechanical mistakes and long-term fatigue, and you have a knotted, cramped upper back.

Case Study: Harry Stetz

Harry Stetz is a successful Miami mortgage broker and a wonderful guy. He came to us with a frozen shoulder and midthoracic spine pain from having a bus door accidentally close on him. He had been trapped until someone could pry it open and release him.

He had tried traditional therapy, but it didn't work—in fact, things were getting worse. We were able to use Active-Isolated Stretching to unlock his cervical spine, and then we started working lower. But we could sense a terrible fear.

As we would touch him, he would recoil. Emotions are powerful, and somehow, in some way that we can't explain, the body stores them on the cellular level. It's not uncommon in deep-muscle massage to press our hands into someone and cause an explosive emotional release or trigger the recollection of a long-forgotten memory of pain and sorrow or fear. We've had to stop work and let a person cry it out, or sit and hold hands for a while. It's one of the mystical links—between mind and body—that we can't prove. We just know it's there.

Our working on Harry's back was bringing up sudden memories of being trapped and severely beaten as a fearful child. We had to stop and let him deal with it. He had been storing pain, injury, and fear that were locking up his back and probably had little

to do with the injury. Or maybe the severity of the injury was exacerbated by being trapped by a bus door and its close association with being beaten. We'll never know.

How Harry Got Out of Pain: Although the pain was in his upper back, Harry's shoulder was locked and his neck was painful. We started unlocking his neck through stretching very gently and slowly. Very slowly. We did soft semi-circumduction and neck rotation, lengthening his neck extensors.

When his neck released through stretching, his shoulder let go. We were able to begin stretching his shoulder. Again, gently and slowly. Muscular work was occasionally interrupted by his need to share a memory or work through an emotional trauma. We would talk. As we released his muscles, he began to release his hurt. We don't know how or why this happens, but we do know that when Harry acknowledged and healed the hurt of his childhood, his back stopped hurting. And we got his shoulder unlocked.

When he was flexible from doing his Active-Isolated Stretching, he was able to add strengthening. We put a special emphasis on his upper back and shoulders. He felt better immediately, but every day got even better. In 3 weeks, he got his arm over his head and could put his shirt on without assistance.

YOU CAN'T AFFORD TO IGNORE TENSION-RELATED BACK PAIN

Stopping tension-related pain in its tracks is very important. While many back problems originate in that upper-back zone, they don't necessarily stay there.

Back problems beget back problems. Just when you thought you couldn't be more locked up and incapacitated, this pain sneaks down to your lower back to hobble your step, creeps up your neck to inflict a world-class tension headache, or radiates down your arms in an exhausting ache or a shooting pain.

When those muscles between your shoulder blades become fatigued, they begin to shut down in a process that is a little like strangulation. The area becomes *hypoxic,* or deprived of oxygen as blood flow is slowly squeezed off when tissues constrict. This condition presents a double whammy, because not only does blood carry oxygen to the muscles so they can function properly and thrive, it also helps carry away metabolic waste generated when the muscles fire. When metabolic waste, like lactic acid, accumulates, you experience cramping—your body's alarm signal that you've moved beyond fatigue and are segueing into full-blown injury. It doesn't take much longer before signals from your brain through nerves to the muscles are cut off and a debilitating, painful loss of function follows.

Up to the point of hypoxia, you might have recruited blood flow to the area by reducing the swelling and getting yourself moving. Now it's too late for an easy way out. Your muscles can't pick up the signals they need to fire. You'll have to get serious now—and that means getting rid of that tension. Luckily, we have the answer.

GET OUT OF PAIN FAST: EIGHT QUICK RELEASES

The quick-release techniques we developed for elite athletes and refined in the Fire Factory between bells are the same ones you'll find here. These can be done at your desk or even standing right in front of another person, who won't be able to tell that you're stretching.

Quick releases are not exactly exercises. They don't constitute a workout. They're fast, subtle moves, which are powerful and effective. Because they fly below the radar of conventional fitness, we call them "stealth health."

This series is *not* a routine. These small moves that release tension can be done individually, in any order. Whenever you feel tension in your back, just move quickly to release it. Just as you scratch an itch, you release a tense muscle.

You'll get the most out of these movements if you remember the basic principle of releasing tension: All muscles work in pairs. When one muscle contracts and shortens, another must relax and lengthen. One muscle is activated; the opposite muscle is quieted and relaxed into a stretch. This action allows more circulation of blood and oxygen. So when you have a spasm or cramp between your shoulders from tension, it makes good sense to relax it by activating opposite muscles.

For example, when the muscles on the left side and back of your neck are in spasm (which they always are when your upper back is locked), you'll want to fire the opposite muscle group on the right side and front of your neck. By repeatedly activating the opposite muscle group in a sort of pumping action, the muscles in spasm are isolated and quieted. Further, they are gently stretched, which begins the all-important restoration of circulation. Continuing further down in a tension lock are the upper back extensors. To isolate and relax them, we have to activate the opposite muscles on the front side of the body, which are the pectoralis majors in the chest. The key is movement.

If you're looking for a rhythm to which you can pace these movements, the mantra is "Let it go, feel the flow." Recite it a few times, and you'll understand the rhythm.

ROLL YOUR SHOULDERS

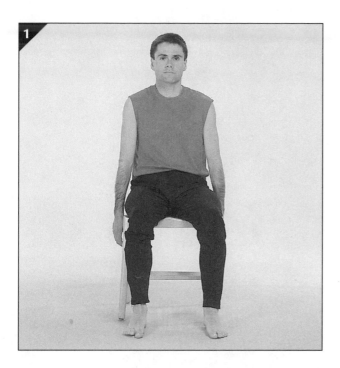

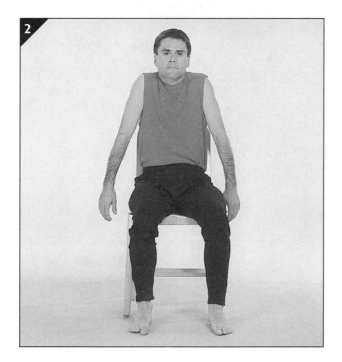

Active Muscles You Contract: Inner group of muscles that steadies and controls your upper back and the connection of your shoulder

Isolated Muscles You Stretch: Outer group of muscles that steadies and controls your upper back, your chest, and the connection of your shoulder

Hold Each Stretch: 2 seconds

Reps: 10 forward, 10 backward

1. Sit in a chair with your back straight. Let your arms relax as you dangle them straight down. If the arm of the chair is in the way, move forward. It's better to sit back, however, so that your tailbone is directly underneath you.

2. Roll your shoulders forward, up, around, and back. Breathe in as you come up. Breathe out as you roll back. Lead with your hands and keep your shoulders from hunching. Keep your head up and in alignment with your spine. Pause between movements, relax your neck, and repeat.

Note: When you roll your neck, you might hear noises that sound like grinding and gristing. Don't worry, your neck isn't broken. This normal sound is synovial fluid as it moves within bursa between bones. Or you might be hearing the disruptions in smooth flow caused by very small muscle adhesions. You might even hear a tendon or a ligament flipping. Your skull magnifies all sound, and your ear picks up this sound from the inside. Don't panic. Everyone generates these sounds, and no one but you can hear them. And as you continue, they will lessen.

ROLL YOUR NECK

Active Muscles You Contract: Nothing specific. This is a warmup.

Isolated Muscles You Stretch: Nothing specific. This is a warmup.

Hold Each Stretch: 2 seconds

Reps: 10 to the right, 10 to the left

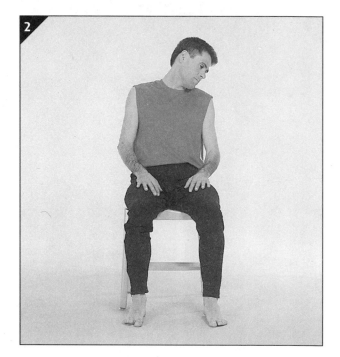

1. Sit in a chair with your back straight. Relax your shoulders. Tuck your chin in. Roll your head toward your shoulder—around and up. Inhale on the upward roll.

2. Hold for 2 seconds and then start the roll toward your opposite shoulder. Exhale as you pass through the midpoint of your chest on your way to the other side. How far should you go? To normal range of motion, when your chin is parallel to the floor and your eye hits neutral plane. Don't tilt your head back. Don't continue the roll past where you're comfortable or past your shoulder. Roll back and forth.

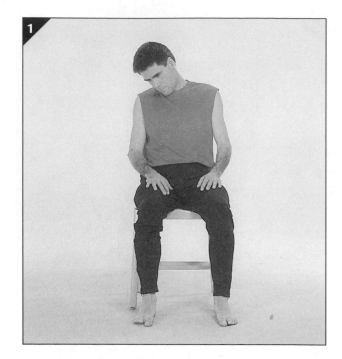

Note: When you roll your neck, you might hear noises that sound like grinding and gristing. Don't worry, your neck isn't broken. This normal sound is synovial fluid as it moves within bursa between bones. Or you might be hearing the disruptions in smooth flow caused by very small muscle adhesions. You might even hear a tendon or a ligament flipping. Your skull magnifies all sound, and your ear picks up this sound from the inside. Don't panic. Everyone generates these sounds, and no one but you can hear them. And as you continue, they will lessen.

RESET THE BACK OF YOUR NECK

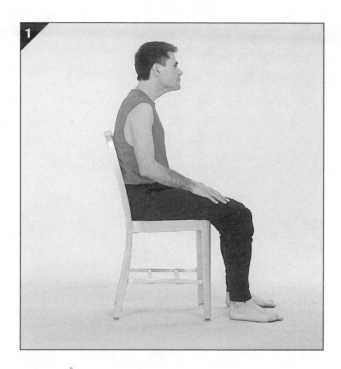

Active Muscles You Contract: Muscles in the back of your neck

Isolated Muscles You Stretch: You're resetting your upper cervical vertebrae.

Hold Each Stretch: 2 seconds

Reps: 10

1. Sit in a chair with your back straight. Face forward and relax. Glide your head straight forward, as shown, with your chin parallel to the ground, as though your head were on a rail or a track. You're about to reset the upper cervical vertebrae at the base of your skull. When your head is as far forward as you can go, lead with your chin and gently roll your head back until your nose is in the air. Try to elongate the front of your throat. Hold for a moment.

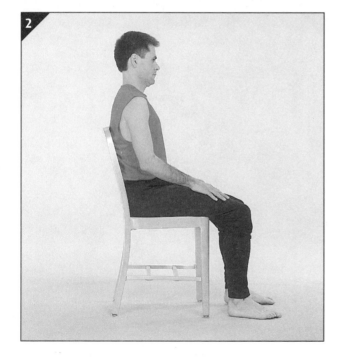

2. Return to neutral position. Glide your head back until it's in alignment with your spine. Hold. And then glide back out again to repeat the lifting and lengthening.

RELAX THE SIDES OF YOUR NECK

Active Muscles You Contract: Muscles in the side of your neck (flexors)

Isolated Muscles You Stretch: Muscles in the opposite side of your neck (flexors)

Hold Each Stretch: 2 seconds

Reps: 10 to the right, 10 to the left

1. Sit in a chair with your back straight. Your head and neck should be in alignment with your spine.

2. Lower your ear to your shoulder as you exhale. Slowly bring your head back up as you inhale. Do all 10 on one side before moving to the opposite side. Finish this stress buster with shrugging your shoulders quickly up to your ears as far as you can. Quickly relax your shoulders and let them drop. Do this three times in rapid succession.

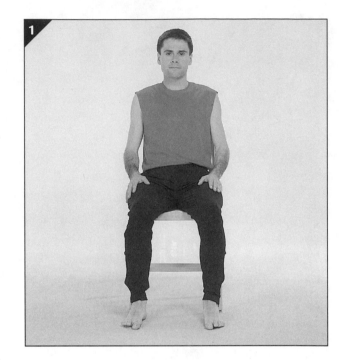

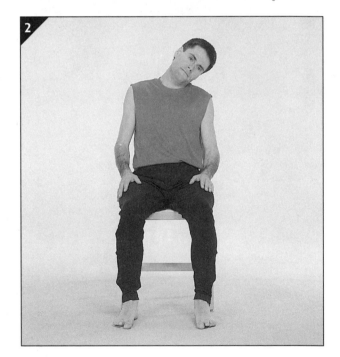

PROMOTE NECK ROTATION

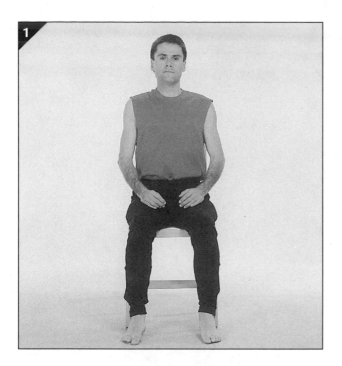

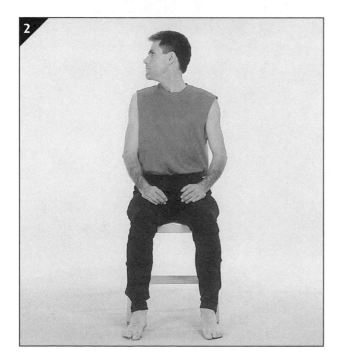

Active Muscles You Contract: Muscles in the side of your neck (rotators)

Isolated Muscles You Stretch: Muscles in the opposite side of your neck (rotators)

Hold Each Stretch: 2 seconds

Reps: 10 to the right, 10 to the left

1. Sit in a chair with your back straight. Your head and neck should be in alignment with your spine. Elongate your neck and bring your head up, as though the crown of your head were attached to a helium balloon. Try to feel light. Keep your chin parallel to the ground.

2. Keep your shoulders forward. Turn your head straight to the side until your chin is over your shoulder. Exhale as you turn. Lead with your eyes. Hold for 2 seconds. Inhale as you return to neutral and then rotate again to the same side. Do 10 to the right, then 10 to the left. How far should you go? Well, this depends on you, but it should not hurt. And no matter how far you go on the first rotation, you can be assured that the last one will be a little farther.

RELEASE THE SIDE
AND BACK OF YOUR NECK

Active Muscles You Contract: Muscles in the front of your neck

Isolated Muscles You Stretch: Muscles in your upper shoulders at the base of your neck, including trapezius muscles

Hold Each Stretch: 2 seconds

Reps: 10 to the right, 10 to the left

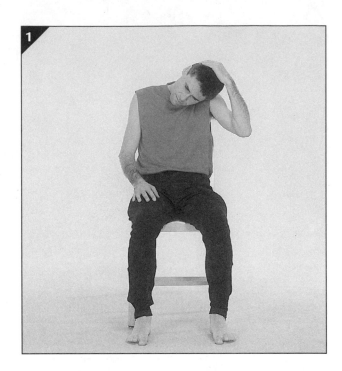

1. This move is a little bit obvious, so if you don't want people to know you're stretching, this one is out. Sit in a chair with your back straight. Your head and neck should be in alignment with your spine. Turn your head to the right to a 45-degree angle. Then drop your head forward, bringing your left ear toward your chest. Place your hand on the top of your head and gently press to get the most out of the stretch. Hold it for 2 seconds. Do all 10 on one side before moving on to the opposite side. When repeating this movement, keep your head in rotation as you return to neutral position. You can keep your head at that 45-degree-angled position. Also, please note that momentum is going to want to take your trunk down with your head, so you'll have to concentrate to isolate the head and neck movement from the torso.

STRESS AND SLUMBER

STRETCH THE BACK OF YOUR SHOULDER

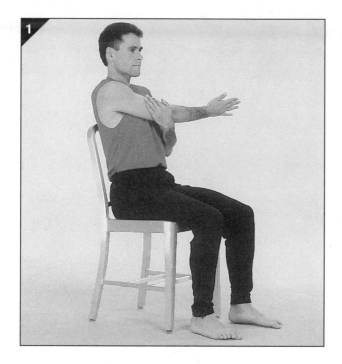

Active Muscles You Contract: Muscles in the front of your shoulder

Isolated Muscles You Stretch: External shoulder rotators

Hold Each Stretch: 2 seconds

Reps: 10 on the right, 10 on the left

1. You can do this one from either a seated or standing position. (This one isn't too subtle, but its benefit is worth the potential embarrassment if someone catches you doing it.) Simply lift one arm, with the elbow locked, and raise it straight across your chest toward the opposite shoulder. Use the other hand to gently assist and get the most out of the stretch. Hold for 2 seconds and relax. Return your arm all the way to neutral. Relax a moment. Do all 10 on one arm before moving on to the other arm.

STRETCH YOUR WHOLE BACK

Active Muscles You Contract: Abdominals, muscles on the sides of your chest, and the thoracic-lumbar rotators on the side opposite your exercising side

Isolated Muscles You Stretch: Muscles that run from your pelvis to the base of your skull along the spine, and the muscles throughout your back and sides that stabilize your torso and help you maintain balance and change direction

Hold Each Stretch: 2 seconds

Reps: 10 to the right, 10 to the left

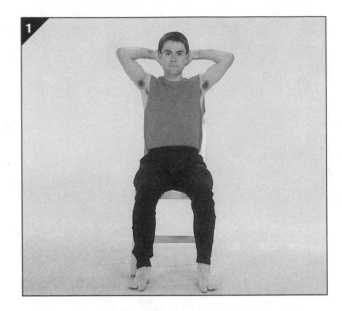

1. Like a few of the others, this stretch is obvious but worth the effort. Sit in a chair with your back straight. Your head and neck should be in alignment with your spine. Lock your hands behind your head, with your elbows pointed straight out. Tuck your chin down very gently.

2. Rotate your upper body to the side as far as you can twist. Do this three times, trying to go a little farther each time.

3. When you're warmed up, on the third rotation, rotate, hold, and then flex your trunk forward, leading your torso down toward the floor with your elbow. That elbow should dip between your knees. Hold for 2 seconds and return to upright by unwinding the rotation so that you're facing forward again. Repeat this rotation and dip 10 times on one side before changing to the opposite side.

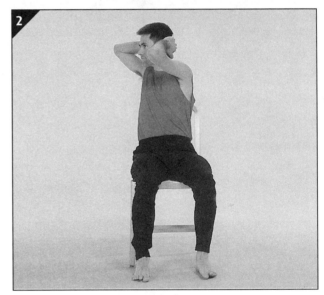

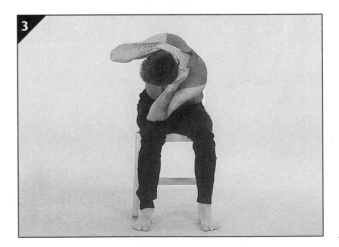

OTHER FAST TENSION RELEASERS

Quick releases are great, but they may not work for everyone, every time. Here are some other quick fixes that can help in a hurry to lessen the tension in your back.

Ice it. When your shoulders are locked up, people usually head for the hot-water bottle or heating pad. It's easy to get fooled into thinking that because heat feels good and relaxes you, it's doing the job. Besides, ice is initially uncomfortable. We'll even admit that the first few seconds can take your breath away. We advise our clients to tough it out, however.

When you're battling a cramp between your shoulders, ice reduces swelling and promotes circu-

---

How Tight Are You?

Most of us lack body awareness. You may not know what's "normal" flexibility and how much you can improve with a simple program. We recommend that you start a fitness program by acquainting yourself with your body and your back. Only by knowing where you start will you have any sense of progression toward your goal.

Instead of the standard sit-and-reach test, which is not an accurate measure, we suggest three other ways to evaluate your flexibility.

Let's check your back. Sit on the floor with your feet flat on the floor and your knees flexed. This posture takes the hamstrings out of commission so that you can isolate your back. Actively contract your abdominals, bend at the hips, and draw your torso down a little bit, pointing your head toward the floor between your feet. Don't bounce to get there. Draw yourself down slowly. It doesn't matter how long you can hold it.

If you can roll your back forward and still get your head past your knees, your back is fairly flexible. If you can get your head anywhere past your midshin, your back is very flexible. If you can't get your head down to your knees, you have work to do.

Here's another hint that your back is tight: If you can't sit upright in this position without putting your hands back on the floor behind you, you have a *lot* of work to do.

Now, let's check your calves. Stay seated on the floor. Put your legs straight out in front of you. Bend one knee and draw your foot toward your buttocks with the bottom of your foot flat on the floor. Bending at the hips, lean forward over the straight leg. Reach down and take the ball of your foot in your hands. Keep your heel on the floor and pull the ball of your foot toward your torso. You want to get a 15-degree range of motion on the ankle by drawing your toes to your nose.

If you can't reach your foot, the calf is too tight. A tight calf means a tight hamstring, which means that your hip rotators and glutes are having to overcompensate and are shortened. We always point out that no back is an island. It's all connected. If your calf is tight, your back will follow. You have some work to do.

Finally, let's check the flexor muscles in your back along your spine, and the muscles in the sides of your trunk. Stand with your feet slightly apart and your knees slightly bent and relaxed. With both arms at your side, contract your trunk at the waist and slide the palm of one hand down your thigh, bending sideways from the waist without shifting your pelvis. Stand back up, then slide that palm down the front and the back of your thigh. You should be able to get your fingertips just below your knee from all threre angles. The less able you are to hit that target, the less flexible your lateral trunk flexors are. You have work to do.

---

lation. The body is designed to run extra blood to areas that are cold. (That's why your nose turns pink when you're out in the cold.) You need that blood flow to remove metabolic waste and reoxygenate your muscles. Additionally, ice numbs the skin and reduces pain so that you'll feel less guarded about moving your back. The more you move, the better off you'll be.

Ten minutes is sufficient to numb the skin and recruit healing blood flow, but not long enough to cause damage to your skin. If you're still in pain after the first application, try icing the site every hour on the hour. Three times should yield good results, but use your own judgment. (In serious injury of a professional athlete, we've maintained a 24-hour schedule, but this is rarely necessary.)

Ice can be applied directly to a painful site for 10 minutes. If you don't have a conventional ice pack, take a paper cup and fill it with water. Freeze it, and peel away about an inch of the cup's top to expose the ice. As the ice melts, keep peeling. Hold the ice by whatever is left of the cup to keep your fingers comfortable, and massage your back with the exposed end. If you can't reach your back and have no one to help you, place ice in a plastic bag, put it on the floor, and lie down on it.

Or use a sealed bag of frozen peas and drape it against your back. The pack stays neat because the frozen peas are sealed up, and the bag conforms to the contours of your body. You can reuse your bag of peas by refreezing it.

Treat it with over-the-counter analgesics. Sometimes the fastest remedy is the tried-and-true pill. A number of over-the-counter analgesics or painkillers can help take the pain out of a tension backache.

Try "floor tennis." You can sometimes work out tension between your shoulders by lying on a tennis ball. Place a tennis ball on the floor, then lie on it, positioning the ball just outside the point of tension, not on the spine, but in the depression on either side of your spine, between your vertebrae and your shoulder blade. Relax your weight down on the ball very slowly. Keep your knees bent so that you can lift your pelvis off the floor and glide back and forth with the weight of your upper back on the ball. It's a sort of self-massage done upside down.

This massage feels great as long as you don't roll the ball directly under your spine. You'll be putting painful pressure on the vertebrae, where there's no muscle to benefit from massage. Roll as long as you enjoy it or until the tension releases. If you can't get the tension to release within 10 minutes, move immediately into a full Active-Isolated Stretching routine, and see if the combination of floor tennis and a stretch rope does the trick. Our bet is that you'll be all right before you know it.

Shrug it off. One interesting theory holds that muscles have cellular memory. They "know" where they're supposed to be and how they're supposed to feel. Assuming this is true, it's possible to lead a muscle quickly into pain and tension in order for it to access its cellular memory to recoil and rebound back into comfort, back into its perfect state of being. In other words, you are using your body's memory to quickly, dramatically demonstrate to it that pain is very wrong and then, following that moment, letting your body show you what will make it right.

The action is painful, yet simple: tense and release. Hunch your shoulders up as high and as tightly as you can lift them. Exhale as you bring your shoulders up. Hold for a few seconds. Let it hurt, hurt, hurt! Then inhale completely as you quickly drop your shoulders down. Breathing deeply is very important because you need oxygen in your blood to help your muscles fire properly and to help carry away the metabolic waste from a fatigued muscle that has been in a full clinch. The body uses the "sigh" to release tension naturally. If you don't feel like engineering a few deep breaths, just sigh the

CASE STUDY: SAM ZOMBER

Sam is a businessman in New York City who spends most of his time in a high-stress job, hunched over a desk with a phone to his ear. When we met him, he had had two knee surgeries that had made walking difficult. As his mobility wound down, Sam gained weight. His left knee was still swollen and painful, his left hip was inflexible, and he walked slowly and painfully with a distinct limp, made worse by excess pounds. But his biggest complaint was that his back hurt. It was constantly fatigued. He was in terrible pain and was occasionally seized by a screaming spasm.

Sam's knee injury was wreaking havoc. We immediately identified the weakened knee as the culprit. When the knee is weak, the thigh is strained and the hip flexors have to compensate. When the hip flexors compensate, the pelvis is thrown out of alignment and strains the lower back. A knee injury usually moves right up the chain of mystical links, but Sam's also moved *down* the chain to his ankle. Remember, the body is a fully integrated system. When one part falters or fails completely, it sets off a chain reaction of compensations and imbalances. And although we can usually identify the obvious injury as the lowest and weakest link on that chain, sometimes the injury works its mischief right on down the line. In Sam's case, his left ankle was frozen in a muscular fusion from misuse, disuse, and compensation.

How Sam Got Out of Pain: Before we could strengthen Sam, we had to unlock him, so we started on stretching exercises just like those in this book. When we had restored range of motion to the joints of his body, we added strengthening. Although we helped Sam learn to stretch and strengthen a back in spasm, we made sure that he was diligent about everything below the belt from his hips all the way down to his ankles. We also worked to strengthen his abdominals, so they could support his back. The net effect was that when we balanced his gait and tightened his midsection, his back stopped hurting. He walks now with very little limp and carries a stretch rope.

---

same way you always do. Repeat until you feel the tension relax.

Breathe deeply into relaxation. Our friend Andrew Weil, M.D., believes that tension is the culprit in many cases of illness and injury. As the director of the program in integrative medicine at the University of Arizona College of Medicine in Tucson, Dr. Weil devotes a great deal of time to training his patients to relax, body and soul. We share techniques.

As we've told you, when you're tense and upset, you jack your shoulders up and carry that tension in your body. When you're relaxed and serene, you don't do that. Thus, it stands to reason that personal serenity would do much to prevent or mitigate tension in one's body and, more specifically, in the upper back between the shoulders.

Achieving a peaceful state of mind might be as easy as practicing Dr. Weil's Yoga Breath. Get comfortable and close your eyes. Breathe through your nose, one nostril at a time. Start with the left nostril by blocking the right. Inhale to a slow count of four. Hold to a slow count of seven. Exhale to a slow count of eight. Switch sides. Block the left, breathe with the right. Switch sides again.

Do this four times per side. Imagine with each breath that you are filled with energy and that your muscles are relaxing, lengthening, strengthening, and getting organized—fiber by fiber.

Drink more water. The human body is largely water. When you are dehydrated, healthy cells that are usually plump and juicy dry out and shrivel up. Their composition and function are disrupted. They don't slide as easily against each other, and, in fact, they actually shred. If your upper back is tight because you're tense, and you're also dehydrated, you'll exacerbate the damaging effects of the tension on your muscles. Make sure that you drink plenty of water. As an added benefit, you'll feel better in general if you stay hydrated.

Not only should you drink throughout the day, you should plan to hydrate before, during, and after every workout. Plain water is good, but some athletes prefer sports drinks that hydrate as well as replace electrolytes lost in sweating and carbohydrates such as glucose, sucrose, fructose, and glucose polymers. They can help boost energy immediately. Some experts believe it is best to drink water before your workout to hydrate you, and the sports drinks later, during your workout, when your body needs the carbohydrates and is prepared to handle and use the sugars you're taking in. Plenty of good sports drinks are on the market. Because results and reactions vary with individuals, you need to test them during training. By the way, studies indicate that no matter what you drink, it will absorb more quickly from your stomach and into your cells if you drink it cold.

Be sure to rest. When you're tired, you droop and keep the muscles in your shoulders and upper back in tension. The more tense and in pain you are, the less likely you are to get good rest. The less rested you are . . . well, you get the picture. This cycle of pain and exhaustion is a catch-22. An exhausted person can't hold posture properly. Muscles don't fire properly. Fatigue erodes everything in your body, mind, and spirit.

Rest. You'll be amazed at how breaking the cycle can help ease the tension from your shoulders.

Sleep in the right position. When you sleep on your side without proper support for your head and neck, your head drops down. With your head dropped, the shoulder on which you're resting will collapse forward toward your chest, compressed under the weight of your body, and blood flow to your shoulder becomes constricted.

This position throws your body into automatic contraction, with the center of gravity balanced on your hip and folded shoulder, which strains your upper back. If you hold this position all night, the constriction and tension will take a toll. Either get a pillow that supports your head and neck, keeping them in alignment, or sleep on your back.

We also recommend that you avoid sleeping all night on your abdomen, with your head turned to one side, propped up on a pillow. This position hyperextends the neck and causes fatigue. (See page 277 for our recommended sleep positions.)

WE ALL "KNEAD" A LITTLE HELP FROM A FRIEND

Nearly every human who has ever worked in an office has been spontaneously recruited to be a massage therapist. We have all grabbed a friend behind his neck and kneaded those upper-back muscles with our thumbs to relieve a searing spasm. Why do we all know how to do it? Because we all seem to need it at some time or another. Let us show you how to do it right. Not only will you help your friends, you'll be the most popular person in your group.

MASSAGE 1

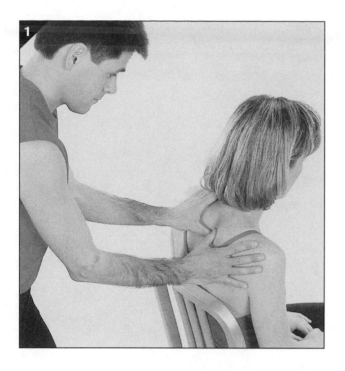

1. Have your friend sit in a chair. Stand behind her. Place your palms on top of her shoulders resting your fingers over the shoulder and your thumbs on the muscles between the shoulder blades. These are the levator scapulae and upper rhomboids. You squeeze, pressing the shoulders with your thumbs, while your friend contracts her shoulders, like an exaggerated shrug. Hold for 3 seconds. Let go as your friend relaxes. Repeat. As you squeeze and release, this will resemble a kneading motion. How hard should you squeeze? Firmly. You want your friend to feel gentle awareness, but not pain. Continue until your friend is a puddle.

This tension reliever can be expanded if your friend has a specific point of pain and tension. Once you've helped relax the middle of the upper back, keep your fingers lightly and high on the shoulders, but slide your thumbs down over the "knot," as shown. Press firmly and gently for a few seconds. Release. Do this several times or until the tension lets go. How will you know that you've released the tension? Either you'll feel the muscle relax under your thumbs, or your friend will start breathing again and say, "Ah-h-h."

MASSAGE 2

1. Have your friend sit in a chair. Stand behind her. Have her roll forward and down from her hips, aiming her forehead to her knees. When she's fully curled down, put your thumbs on either side of her spine.

2. Have your friend slowly roll back up as you slide your thumbs firmly up her back. Each of you will determine the rhythm and the intensity of the pressure. Advance your thumbs up only 6 to 8 inches by the time your friend is fully upright. Don't move your thumbs. Have her curl down again and then roll back up as you advance your thumbs up another 6 to 8 inches. Continue this progression until you've reached the base of her skull.

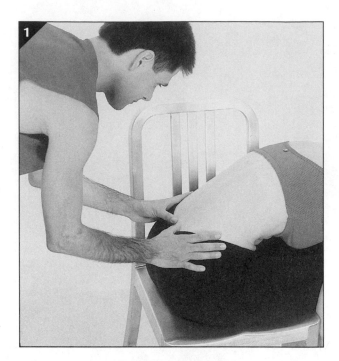

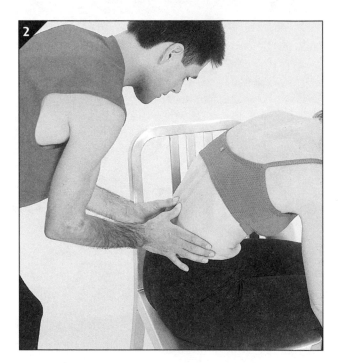

STRESS AND SLUMBER

MASSAGE 3

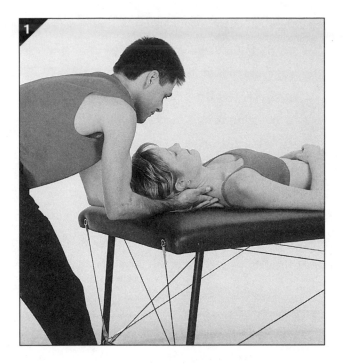

1. (This one requires that you have trimmed nails and are wearing no jewelry.) Have your friend lie flat on her back. Position yourself just above the top of her head. Cup your palms together with the palm of your dominant hand on top, facing up. Have your friend lift slightly so that you can slide your cupped palms under her back before she relaxes her weight down onto your hands. Rest your friend's head on the upturned insides of your forearms. Contract your fingers until they're positioned over the muscles to one side of the spine. Draw your hands toward you, pressing your fingers into the muscles as you slide. Run from the shoulder blade to the top of the shoulders three times on each side of the spine.

On the third pass, uncup your hands and put one hand on each side of the spine. Slide your fingers continuously from the back up the neck as your friend tucks her chin and lifts her head.

Then using gravity and the weight of your friend's head in your palms, knead the base of her skull with the tips of your fingers in short, firm, gentle strokes.

Finally, lock your fingertips under the base of her skull and gently, firmly pull toward you as she exhales. Do this to the count: "Pull, two, three, four. Release, two, three, four." We joke with our clients, telling them that we almost never actually disconnect a head—but beginners do need to be cautious. Nothing should *ever* hurt.

Mike Frankfurt is an attorney in New York City with a busy practice and an even busier life. He's on the board of the New York Road Runners Club and is cofounder of the Armory Project. As a former top competitive all-American cross-country runner in college, Mike expected to be able to maintain a top level of fitness and energy throughout his life. And there was no reason for any of us to believe that this was anything but possible.

But the demands of his career had thrown tension right into his lower back. His shoulders were locked up in a searing knot at the base of his neck. He had used running—the passion of his life—to keep him in top physical shape and to diffuse the tensions of the day, but his running began to falter. With the dogged discipline of a lifelong athlete, Mike continued to run frequently, but his pace slowed to a labored walk. He was in constant pain. The less he could run, the less he could work off tension. The more tension he carried in his back, the more pain he had and the less he could run. It was a vicious cycle that was about to have disastrous results.

How Mike Got Out of Pain: Fortunately, he sought our help. We unlocked him in one visit with a full Active-Isolated Stretching routine. The back spasm abated immediately. He worked hard to repair the damage and restore full and balanced range of motion. It took a few weeks of daily workouts. When he was ready, we introduced strengthening. The programs we used are identical to those in this book. Today, we're great friends and work out with him frequently, and when he's on his own, he is an ardent practitioner and advocate of Active-Isolated Stretching and Strengthening. He keeps stretch ropes at home, in his car, at the office, at his summer cottage, and in his suitcase. He is never without the means to relax the tension in his back. And he's back to running.

About knots: As you massage, you'll notice knots. In your partner, they feel like small, firm lumps within soft, smooth muscle fibers. In yourself, they feel like ignited charcoal embedded under your skin.

Acutely painful to the touch, knots are adhesions—sort of like scar tissue—that are caused when the muscle is microscopically torn. Muscles are fibrous, like bundles of rubber bands. When a few of these fibers are injured and tear, they recoil into snarled disruptions. As they try to heal, they reconfigure out of their smooth pattern. The torn ends of the individual fibers stick together (adhere) in a disorganized knot, like a scar.

You don't have to suffer trauma for it to happen; fatigue or overuse can cause a little tear in muscle fibers. In fact, it's pretty common. In areas that are used heavily or have generous blood flow, a microtear is no big deal. But in an area like the upper back, where blood flow is less generous than other areas of the body and easily impeded, microtears cannot heal quickly and easily. They develop into adhesions, or the knots we all know so well.

To break up these adhesions and restimulate blood flow, gently and firmly massage the knot. The muscle fibers will eventually relax and smooth out; the adhesion will loosen and let go. Eventually, the knot will disappear along with the acute pain.

The more fit you are, the less tension you'll carry in your body. The less tension you carry, the easier and faster fitness will come to you. Letting go of a lot of unnecessary strain will allow muscles to respond to training and restore your vital energy. Enjoy!

Chapter 13

NOW I LAY ME DOWN TO SLEEP

Our appointment book had only the name Rick Dawson and the words "back problem" scrawled in red ink and underlined for emphasis. We thought little about his visit that afternoon, but when he got to our office, it was obvious that his back problem might be the least of his worries.

In fact, the back injury was a fairly minor muscle strain. Far more significant was the fact that Rick Dawson couldn't speak in full sentences. And what he did say was whispered and hoarse. Not that we ever pay a bit of attention to fashion, but even we noticed that his clothes were mismatched and his hair looked as if it had been styled with a weed trimmer. He couldn't make eye contact with us. He rubbed his face continually in an obvious attempt to clear the cobwebs. Clearly, this man was on the verge of some sort of breakdown. These symptoms could *not* have been the result of such a minor muscle strain.

We were right . . . and wrong. Although his back was bothering him a little, it was sufficient to keep him awake at night. And therein lay the problem. A few sleepless nights had turned a strong, competent, capable, grown man into a crazy person. It wasn't the first time we had seen it, and it wouldn't be the last.

Gerald Rosen, M.P.H., M.D., a sleep expert from the University of Minnesota, reports that his research

has identified the specific skill levels most vulnerable to fatigue: motivation, creativity, judgment, decision-making processes, and interpersonal harmony. All pretty key skills to function well in today's society.

No matter what else is going on in a client's life, sleep makes all the difference between getting on top of a problem and throwing in the towel. That's why we want to talk about sleep and how important it is and give you our program for a blissful, restorative, pain-free rest.

SLEEP CAN BE A PAIN IN THE BACK

In the grand design of all things, sleep is the way the human body heals and restores. Even Shakespeare wrote in *King Henry IV, Part 2*, "O gentle sleep! Nature's soft nurse . . ."

If you can't sleep because your back is bothering you, you're not alone. Fifty-six million Americans experience pain-induced sleeplessness an average of 8.5 nights a month, and they sleep fewer than 5 hours on those awful nights. And the pain that the majority of those folks experience is back pain. It's the number one culprit, followed by headaches and muscle pain. And to make matters even worse, some medications used to ease an aching back also disrupt sleep.

If your back is bothering you, it's likely you will not

sleep well. Researchers who study pain management tell us that falling asleep is the toughest part. You would think that clearing that hurdle and finally drifting off would assure a restful night. But even if you manage to get to sleep, one toss or turn the wrong way can cause pain that awakens you as suddenly and surely as the rude jolt of an alarm clock. If you can't get comfortable enough to drop back to sleep, or if it happens more than once a night, the net effect is a brutal, restless sleep. In the morning, you emerge from between the tangle of sheets, exhausted and angry—so not only is your back aching, but you spend the day emotionally drained, mentally dulled, and cranky. Being tired will exacerbate your perception of pain, making it noticeably less manageable, and change the energy with which you carry your body, further aggravating your back. But there's more.

Under normal circumstances, your body uses the time you've spent horizontal to enjoy a reprieve from the effects of vertical gravity on your back—and the time you've spent asleep to refresh and rejuvenate on a cellular level while your metabolism is slowed. Deprived of those opportunities, your body's ability to heal is diminished. It takes only a few nights of disturbed sleep, or no sleep at all, for some serious erosion in body, mind, and spirit to set in.

We have studied sleep and integrated it in a very deliberate way into every training and rehabilitation program we supervise. We've learned that if you are going to take successful control of healing, you have to take control of sleeping. This begins with understanding why sleep is beneficial, how it works, and how you can get good at it. Then, because we live in a 24-hour-a-day society that values constant activity into the wee hours and regards resting as slacking, we have to teach you to be unapologetic about hitting the sack.

WHY DO WE NEED TO SLEEP, ANYWAY?

All scientists agree that sleep is essential to life. Indeed, laboratory animals that are deprived of sleep eventually die from it. But no one is really certain why sleep is so necessary.

There are a few theories, probably all of them valid to some extent. Combined, they provide the truth.

The Adaptive Theory: Sleep improves an animal's chances of survival, especially when sleep habits are appropriate to an environment and protective. Animals sleep when they don't have to compete with a greater number of animals for territory and food. An example of this sleep schedule adaptation is the bear that sleeps through the winter so that she doesn't freeze to death or starve when food is scarce.

Perhaps by simple evolution and natural selection, we are alive because of our sleep schedules. For all of us, nature imposes the need to sleep when we have the least access to food and, more important, when we are most vulnerable to danger. In fact, from even our earliest childhood bedtime rituals, we acknowledge that sleep time is a time of danger and vulnerability. The most common bedtime prayer is "Now I lay me down to sleep, I pray the Lord my soul to keep. If I should die before I wake, I pray the Lord my soul to take." Clearly, dying is on someone's mind every night. It's best that we pull the covers over our heads.

The Energy Conservation Theory: Animals with high metabolisms sleep more than those that burn calories more slowly. Sleep allows them to conserve energy for bursts of activity necessary for hunting and overcoming prey. This makes sense because we know that the body directs extra energy into healing when the back is injured, and as a consequence, there is a biological imperative for extra sleep.

Programming-Reprogramming Theory: Rapid eye movement (REM) sleep increases as unimportant information is apparently dropped from memory and essential information is stored permanently. This theory is supported by studies of infants, who are processing new information at a rate more rapid than at any other time in life and who sleep longer and experience the most REM sleep. Even adults who are studying and processing new information tend to experience an increase in REM sleep. We also know that when an adult is deprived of REM sleep, his ability to think creatively and solve

Are You a Lark or an Owl?

The intricate ways in which all organisms negotiate between day and night, or light and dark, are called circadian rhythms. In humans, our brain perceives a "day" to be between 24.5 and 28 hours, so we are heavily reliant on clocks and cues like meals or work schedules to tell us where we are in the time continuum, so we'll know when to sleep and when to wake.

No matter how we adjust our responses, our understanding of the circadian rhythm is linked to light. Within the rhythm, our wakefulness and alertness are preferences established early in life. "Larks" are people who are more active in the early-morning hours; "owls" are more active at night. Sometimes knowing which you are can help you adjust your schedule to be more productive, to take advantage of those hours that are peak for you. For example, knowing when you're at your very best and in the highest energy will help you plan your workouts. Seize the moment for yourself: "Larks" will benefit most from a morning workout, and "owls" will enjoy the night.

problems is significantly, measurably diminished.

A drop in estrogen also diminishes REM sleep. Perhaps this explains why women right before menses sometimes experience drops in cognitive function and mood swings that emulate depression. This also might explain why after menopause and estrogen loss, some women complain of feeling "dulled." Certainly, a correlation exists between estrogen loss and these symptoms, but it's interesting to think that a drop in REM sleep might be the defining factor.

The Restorative Theory: This one is our favorite. In sleep, the body restores itself. Neurotoxins are neutralized, cells divide, tissues synthesize, and growth hormones (essential for healing) are released during non-REM sleep. Athletes, children, and young people, all of whom are physically active, spend more time in the deepest sleep stages than inactive people do.

As we said, no one knows for sure exactly why, but we all understand that we must sleep. We need it for our mental, emotional, and physical well-being. So we might as well get good at it.

MASTERING THE CYCLES OF SLEEP

Although we think of sleep as being the absence of activity, nothing could be further from the truth. In fact, from a neurological standpoint, sleep is an outrageously dynamic process. Scientists categorize sleep in five stages, each repeated as many as five times during the night. As night progresses and if there are no disruptions, each cycle gets a little longer.

Stage 1. This is the light sleep into which you descend as you first nod off. Some people call this the "twilight." Maybe you're still vaguely aware of your surroundings, still attuned to a television program. If someone turns off the television while you are in stage 1, you might awaken to the change in sound in the room. Your muscles begin to relax. Your brain waves are irregular and rapid.

Stage 2. As you drop more deeply into sleep, you enter stage 2, a time of deeper relaxation. Your heartbeat and breathing slow. Your brain waves are larger, with intermittent bursts of electrical activity called sleep spindles.

Stages 3 and 4. These are the deepest sleep stages. Now someone could turn off that television, and you would not be aware of it. Your brain produces large, slow delta waves. Your breathing and heartbeat slow even further. Your muscles relax more deeply. The world is quiet for you for about an hour. Dreams are more common here than in stages 1 and 2. If you're going to walk or talk in your sleep, now would likely be the first incident of the night.

Stage 5. The sleep most of us know best—rapid eye movement, or REM, sleep—occurs at this stage.

It is so designated because researchers can observe twitching and tracking of the eyes, as if the sleeper is watching something happen. In fact, that's exactly what's going on, because it is here in REM sleep that we dream most vividly. In fact, our brain waves are very similar to those we exhibit when we're wide awake.

The first time you enter REM sleep, you might be there only 5 minutes. Eventually, you'll cycle out of REM, to return again later. Later cycles can be up to an hour. Researchers tell us that we spend a quarter of our sleep in REM sleep, dreaming.

SETTING THE STAGE FOR SLUMBER

People who lived back in the days before electricity slept more than we do today. Our ancestors organized their lives in accordance with the rhythms of the seasons and sunrises. They would go to sleep when the day was literally done: when the sun had gone down and the fire faded into glowing embers in the dark. The temperature of the room would drop, cooling the air. Bodies, physically tired from a day of hard work and full from an evening's meal, would slow metabolically. People would curl up into their blankets to sleep. Hours later, at sunrise, light and warmth would gently, naturally raise metabolism and stir people to get up, rested to face another day, and hungry.

Today, in sharp contrast, we have pushed back the darkness to create a 24-hour society without day or night. At night, we create day. We flip on a light, jack up the thermostat, order a pizza, and continue to work and play in total darkness. Day is even more indistinguishable. We can turn it into night. We can turn off lights, block out the sun with shades, lower the temperature of the room to frosty with a simple command, and drop into soft, fragrant sheets to sleep at high noon. No problem.

But all this efficiency, flexibility, ingenuity, and joy come with a price, for although times have changed, human need for sleep has not. Most of us are so out of touch with the natural rhythms of the universe and our own bodies that we are sleep-deprived to some degree.

According to the National Sleep Foundation, compared with people a century ago, people today get an average of 20 percent fewer hours of sleep per night. And we've each added a full month per year to the time we spend working and commuting to and from work. Here are a few ways you can counteract these changes to get the sleep you need.

Turn your bedroom into a sacred space. The room should have only two purposes: making love and sleeping. If you are using your bedroom for any other activities, put an end to them now. No television. No computer. No bill paying. No library filled with adventure novels. No foosball table. Nothing that excites the imagination or provides a distraction. The space should be serene and well-ordered.

Create a tranquil environment. Your bedroom should be peaceful. If you are disturbed by outside noises—like the street sounds of New York City right outside our windows—consider investing in an electric fan or a sound generator, a little electronic device that produces white noise. These sound generators are widely available and inexpensive, and they produce a wide range of sounds: ocean waves, crickets, babbling brooks, rainstorms, wind, the clickety-clack of a moving train, and so forth. It doesn't matter what you listen to as long as it drones softly and lulls you to sleep.

Incidentally, these little sound generators are great for travel. They allow you to take the familiar sound of your own bedroom with you, no matter where you go.

Adjust your thermostat. Although scientists suggest that you'll do better if your bedroom is a little cool and you can snuggle into the covers, it's entirely up to you. We're not trying to influence you, but the golden number is 60° to 65°F (16° to 18°C).

The trick is to find a temperature you like and stick with it. Avoid extremes whenever possible. A very warm room will signal your body metabolically that it's time to get up. A very cold one will cause you to tighten up muscles. You might sleep, but you'll awaken exhausted and sore. Find the middle ground.

Keep your bedroom as dark as you can get it while still feeling safe. Don't apologize if you need a little light. If the room is too dark for your personal sense of safety and causes you to feel insecure, you'll be on guard all night and will not sleep well. The room doesn't have to be pitch black, just darkened to the point where your human instinct to sleep when it's dark is triggered.

Sleep in a comfortable bed. We're not just talking about clean sheets and a firm mattress. We also expect you to control every variable of the environment. We once had an athlete with continuing sleep difficulty even after several meetings, so we went through a step-by-step review of his plan. He was doing everything right, he insisted. In fact, even his dogs were sleeping better. "Dogs?!" Yeah, he puzzled. His four golden retrievers were really enjoying the new bedtime program and were a whole lot less restless all night than usual.

Fatal flaw revealed. He was doing everything right—and then piling four snoring, sprawling, scratching, twitching dogs on top. (Just as a note, he didn't have to kick his dogs out of bed. He traded his double bed for a king-size one.)

Go to bed within 1 hour of the same time every night. This includes the weekends. If you stay awake too long, you'll find yourself, ironically, frustratingly, too tired to fall asleep. If you go to bed too early, you'll not be sleepy. You'll lie awake and toss and turn.

Gradually decrease your exposure to bright light. Throughout the course of the evening, in the hours leading up to bedtime, gradually dim the lights. When we are around low light, our natural instinct is to wind down our day and to move toward rest. Bright light is neurologically stimulating and signals that it's time to get up. If you gradually turn off the lights in your house and keep the lights low in your bedroom, your brain will signal you to relax.

Cool off. Wear lightweight clothing, if anything at all. Even if you've taken a warm bath to relax, take a few extra minutes to dry off, allowing the water to evaporate, which will drop your skin temperature a little.

Cut off your caffeine in the very early evening. If you still have trouble falling asleep after doing so, back up the cutoff to late afternoon. If you still can't sleep, back it up to the middle of the afternoon. Shortly, you'll find the magic cutoff time: no caffeine after it, or you're rattled all the way past bedtime. Remember, caffeine is not only in coffee and tea but also hidden in chocolate and some medications. Be aware.

Cut off or limit alcohol consumption in the evening. Some people think that a glass of wine will relax them and help them sleep. It may, but it also interferes in their ability to get into and stay in deep sleep, where the benefits of rest are the greatest.

Avoid nicotine. This stimulant delays sleep. Of course, we have other issues with it, but that's another book. Please don't smoke. Not before bed. Not ever.

Avoid napping if you're not used to it. A quick snooze might seem like a good idea at the time, but it will certainly interfere with your ability to fall asleep later and stay that way. Unlike eating, sleeping is not as effective if it's parceled out over the course of 24 hours. For most of us, it's best done all at one time. There are people who are great at napping and enjoy tremendous benefits, but you have to try it and decide for yourself. (For more information, see "The Art and Science of Napping" on page 277.)

Go to bed tired. This one is tricky because there are several kinds of fatigue: mental, emotional, and physical. Any one of the three is sufficient to trigger your need for sleep, but you will sleep better if you are *physically* tired.

In the grand design, humans were built to toil all day and sleep all night. In today's culture, we work, but we don't expend a great deal of physical energy. You might feel wasted by bedtime, but your body—tethered to a desk all day and driven home in a car and then plopped in front of a television set all evening—simply isn't tired out. You need to get some heart-pumping, butter-burning, blood-rushing, sweat-inducing exercise some time during the day on a regular basis in order to command good sleep. You'll be stunned by the difference it makes.

Be aware of your exercise schedule. Pay attention to the timing of exercise in relation to your ability to sleep, and adjust your workout schedule if it interferes with your ability to settle down. Most scientists recommend that you exercise early in the day, suggesting that rigorous activity in the late evening stimulates you too much to allow sleep. But frankly, this has not been our experience. Often, the

Do You Need More Sleep?

You might think that you're getting enough sleep, even when you're not. (Remember, when you have a sleep debt, your judgment might be impaired!) Here's a short self-test suggested by Peter B. McCullagh, director of the North Florida Regional Medical Center Sleep Disorders Center in Gainesville, Florida. If three or more of these statements describe you, you might need to hit the sack for more hours and more quality and consistency in those hours. If your sleep debt is extreme, seek professional advice.

- I don't feel refreshed after a night's rest.
- I frequently feel tired.
- I forget things.
- People remark that I look tired.
- I am cranky, irritable, and short-fused.
- I have trouble concentrating, especially on quiet projects.
- I sit through meetings, lectures, and sermons, but I can't tell you what was said.
- I am completely reliant upon my alarm clock to get up in the morning. I hit the snooze button more than once.
- I feel lethargic until I've had more than one cup of coffee in the morning.

- I have trouble calculating numbers.
- I snore so loudly that I disturb my bed-partner . . . or the neighbors.
- I sometimes daydream or "zone out."
- I keep the volume on my car radio so loud that it startles me when I first turn it on.
- I fall asleep when I'm bored or relaxed.
- I sometimes awaken myself with a single loud snore.
- I have to keep my room or office cool in order to stay alert.
- I often awaken in the morning with a headache.
- I am sometimes inexplicably weepy.
- I sometimes have difficulty getting my thoughts organized.
- I fall asleep in under 5 minutes after I go to bed.
- It takes me longer than 15 minutes to fall asleep after I go to bed.
- When I'm driving, I sometimes realize that I've covered miles without being aware.
- On my days off, I sleep longer than I do when I am on a work schedule.
- I sometimes need to nap to get through the day.
- Naps don't really refresh me.

only time we have to exercise is late at night, after our last client has left the clinic. We've found that a hard workout dissolves away the tensions of the day, tires us out physically, and allows a better night's sleep. We would say that you have to do what works for you. Simple experimentation will quickly yield an answer.

Establish a little bedtime ritual. The brain is very adept at picking up cues and getting the body ready to react. The ritual doesn't need to be elaborate, just predictable.

Make a list of things you do right before you go to bed, simple and unremarkable things like "I put out the cat, put on my pajamas, brush my teeth, and turn off the light." If you are consistent night after night, your brain is conditioned to recognize the ritual and wind your body down to prepare for bed as you start to advance through the list. It knows what's coming, even if you don't consciously think about it. If you bounce into bed without preparation and clear intention, then your brain is likely to wonder, "What are we doing here? Should I start the winding-down sequence now, or is something else happening?"

Have a bedtime snack high in carbohydrate. Hunger pangs and a growling stomach will keep you awake. We suggest carbohydrates, because they raise the levels of tryptophan, an amino acid that triggers the production of serotonin, the neurotransmitters in your brain that cause sleepiness. You might want to rethink Grandma's recipe for warm milk and honey by pouring out the milk and keeping the honey. The protein in the milk inhibits the uptake of tryptophan and doesn't really help much.

Keep the snack light: a few crackers, a rice cake. Speaking of cake, be careful of chocolate when in search for bedtime snacks. Hidden caffeine will defeat the purpose.

Finish your mental tasks. Do all you can do to wind up your day so that you can go to bed with a clear conscience. L. L. Colbert, the former president of Chrysler Corporation, said, "When I've had a rough day, before I go to sleep, I ask myself if there's anything more I can do right now. If there isn't, I sleep sound."

Fretting is useless. Sleeping isn't walking away from your battles. Sleeping is preparation. If you are wrestling with a challenging problem that threatens your ability to sleep, decide to deal with it in the morning, when you are rested and prepared to do battle again. Give yourself permission to sleep so that you'll be better able to think creatively and energetically.

Get some sun today. Studies suggest that exposure to natural light during the day contributes to the body's ability to make the most of sleep. In fact, it's thought that the benefits of exercise in the broad light of day are greater than exercise in an enclosed gym. We aren't saying that you have to buy a deck chair and move your computer to the roof of your building, but we are suggesting that you poke your nose out the window once in a while.

Wind it down. It's a rare person who can step away from engaging activity and flop into bed to fall asleep immediately. Many of us need to wind down at the end of the day, when activity requires no "output" from us, no participation required of us except presence. Try reading or watching a little television or listening to music.

Get your partner on board with matters regarding sleep. Everything you do to get a good night's sleep can be undone by a partner who either differs in opinion or practice. Cooperation makes all the difference in the world between success and a sleepless night.

Do some stretches before bed. Once you've set the stage for slumber, doing some gentle, rhythmic stretching releases tension and puts you on track for a good night's sleep. Here are some quick stretches that we use to relax us right before bedtime.

If you're having trouble sleeping, try these four stretches before you get into bed.

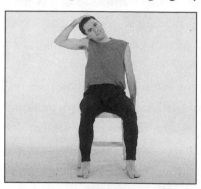

1. NECK LATERAL FLEXORS
See complete instructions on page 62.

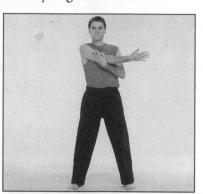

2. ROTATOR CUFF 1
See complete instructions on page 57.

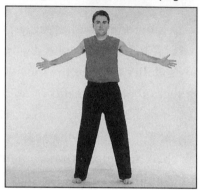

3. PECTORALIS MAJORS
See complete instructions on page 53.

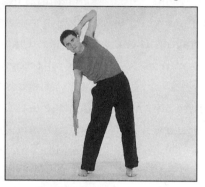

4. TRUNK LATERAL FLEXORS
See complete instructions on page 51.

Now, hop into bed and get horizontal. Move to the final two relaxers.

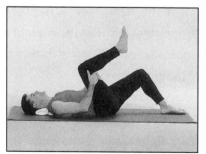

1. SINGLE-LEG PELVIC TILTS
See complete instructions on page 39.

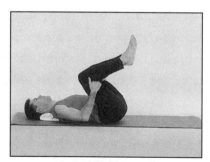

2. DOUBLE-LEG PELVIC TILTS
See complete instructions on page 40.

SLEEP POSITIONS THAT TAKE THE STRESS OFF YOUR BACK

A few years ago, Phil was hit by a car in Kenya and returned to the United States with fractures that needed to be set. His consulting orthopedist in New York, Dr. Marvin Gilbert, sat down to discuss Phil's new challenge of living in casts.

One of the concerns he wanted to cover was how Phil would sleep. We asked if he had any recommendations. He said, "I always tell my patients to find any position that's comfortable and sleep that way." It was simple, good advice. We pass it along to you.

As a side note, we have clients who have slept in chairs while their backs were healing. But for the purposes of this discussion, we're going to assume that you'll be sleeping in your bed. Unless your physician suggests otherwise, you need to experiment until you find a position that feels good. Here are a few tips.

Consider a firm mattress. "Firm" does not mean "concrete slab," but the mattress should support your body comfortably. Old, soft mattresses might have sentimental value, but wallowing down into a mire of lumpy feathers and foam will cause you to tense and "guard" a tender back out of alignment. If you simply cannot give up an old favorite, consider sliding a full sheet of plywood between the mattress and box spring.

Sleep on your back or your side. You might be more comfortable when your spine is aligned as closely as possible to its natural curves. We urge you to try to stay off your stomach, not just because it puts your spine into a sort of concave arch, but because you have to spend the night with your neck rotated, face to the side, to keep you from suffocating. This puts added strain on your neck and cervical spine.

If you choose to sleep flat on your back, you might consider putting pillows under your knees and your neck to take some of the tension off your lumbar spine. If you choose to sleep on your side, we suggest you put pillows between your knees and under your neck to keep the tension off your lower back and pelvis.

Many people use body pillows, which are the length of your torso. No doubt they developed when pillow company executives remembered that many of their customers enjoy "spooning" with their partners: sleeping belly to back with the top leg thrown over the partner's body. Not only are body pillows almost as comforting as a hug, they take the tension off your lower back and pelvis. Additionally, they give you something against which to "lean" so that you can find the right position, lock it in with your body pillow, and relax.

Consider a pillow that supports your neck. Traditional pillows, although wonderfully fluffy and soft, do very little for vertebral alignment. They either lift your head, arching your cervical spine to the ceiling; fail to support your head at all, arching your cervical spine to the floor; or get it just right for most of the night. You have a one-in-three chance of sleeping without strain.

You and your physician might determine that you would benefit from a firm cervical pillow that is sculpted of a single piece of foam and shaped like a roller coaster (see "The Cervical Sleep Pillow" on page 278) as opposed to the traditional pillow that is pliable, stuffed with fluff, and shaped like a muffin (most of the night). A cervical pillow rises to conform to your neck and then forms a trough to cradle your head. If you were to take an x-ray of your spine while you were using this pillow, you would notice that the vertebrae are in straight alignment. Some people do very well with them.

THE ART AND SCIENCE OF NAPPING

Although researchers suggest that sleep is most effective when it's done all at one time, napping boasts several powerful arguments. Napping reduces your sleep debt during those times when you're falling behind, and a nap before an upcoming late night is like putting money in the bank—you can get a little ahead.

If you're a veteran napper, you're in good company. Famous inventor Thomas Edison slept little during the night, but disappeared from his lab during the day to enjoy little siestas. Winston Churchill slept in the afternoon for 2 hours to help him cope with the stress of leadership during the war. Albert Einstein declared that naps refreshed him and helped him be more creative. John F. Kennedy, Ronald Reagan, and George W. Bush all have napped without apology.

Another big fan of naps is Phil Wharton. Between

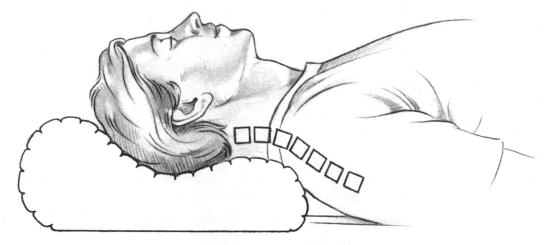

The cervical sleep pillow helps align your vertebrae throughout the night.

being a competitive marathon runner who trains hard every day, a therapist with an around-the-clock on-call schedule, and a New Yorker with a taste for the good life—plays and museums, Knicks games, new restaurants, and Central Park all demand his attention—Phil needs all the rest he can squeeze in.

Before you get winded trying to picture a day in the life of Phil, you need to be aware of very small blocks of time that are mysteriously "booked" in his day planner. These blocks of time are merely gone—unavailable for appointments, unexplained, and un-apologized for—and what he does during those stolen moments is nap.

Phil has the ability to settle down in the midst of pandemonium, slow his breathing, quiet his thoughts, close his eyes, and nod off. He can do it in a crowded room, in a moving cab, or standing up. One friend who particularly admired this skill admitted that he at first thought Phil was so perennially exhausted and sleep-deprived that he had no choice but to drop off. But Phil chooses when and where he sleeps, because he understands sleep's value in refreshing the mind, restoring the spirit, and healing the body.

The need to sleep is set in large part by an internal clock in our brains called a suprachiasmatic nucleus, which controls the natural rhythms of our bodies and is "programmed" for two distinct periods of sleepiness during a 24-hour cycle. The most significant is between 3:00 and 5:00 in the morning, when we are the least alert and our heart rate, breathing, and temperature are at their lowest. The other period of sleepiness is between 3:00 and 5:00 in the afternoon.

If you, like many people, assumed that the classic "afternoon slump" was caused by a high-carbohydrate lunch and an extra glass of sweetened tea, think again. It's the suprachiasmatic nucleus telling your brain that it's time to sleep. It's no accident that many cultures have organized lifestyle around a late-afternoon drop in energy. Businesses close. People rest. It's siesta time.

Perhaps the best example of using naps to improve performance comes from the Kenyan marathon runners. Kenyans dominate the marathon so completely that the running world now regards them as mystical, even superhuman. "How do they do it?" is the question on the mind of every runner who finishes second and third, right behind a wiry, grinning Kenyan.

Besides their closely supervised training; their work with the best athletic, dietetic, medical, and rehab people in the world; and, all modesty aside, their use of Active-Isolated Stretching and Strengthening, the Kenyans have a secret: They nap. When they're not running, eating, chatting, or tending to a little chore, they're horizontal, restoring their energy. We know the strategy works because they're able to sustain the intensity and duration of a training regimen that appears to be nearly beyond human capability.

What about us mere mortals? We could all benefit from the recovery power that napping boasts. Mark R. Rosekind, Ph.D., who led the Fatigue Countermeasures Program at the NASA Ames Research Center at Moffett Field, California, is an advocate for napping to improve alertness. At NASA, he and his team studied the effects of planned 40-minute naps on pilots in the shuttle cockpit. With a nap, the pilots' performance improved 34 percent and their alertness increased by 54 percent. Based on what we know from this study and others like it, here are a few tips for getting the most out of your nap.

- Set the stage the best you can for quiet and relaxation. You don't want to be distracted or disturbed.
- Sleep no more than 45 minutes, so you can awaken quickly. Nap any longer, and you'll have trouble shaking out the cobwebs.
- If you have more time or perceive that you have a larger sleep deficit to fulfill, extend your nap to about 2 hours so that you will be more likely to go through an entire sleep cycle. Cutting the cycle short after you're deeply asleep—beyond 45 minutes—will result in disorientation when you try to wake up. Not only that, but you'll have a tough time returning to full function.
- If you're looking to nap in an airport or train station, drop onto the floor in an out-of-the-way corner. Try to get up against a wall and wear a hat to protect your head from whatever might be on the carpet. Carry-on bags, when properly pummeled and pounded into shape, can be pillows for your head and neck, and props for your feet.

- On airplanes and trains, the best naps are horizontal. If you have access to two or three seats, put the armrest up. Rest on your side with your back against the seat backs and your knees bent, head toward the window, feet toward the aisle. Grab a pillow to support your head and neck, and align your cervical and thoracic spine.
- If you must nap in a seated position, try a cervical support pillow shaped like a large, soft horseshoe. Place it behind your neck and put your seat back in a reclining position, to keep your head from rolling. Travel versions of this pillow are inexpensive, lightweight, and inflatable, and they pack easily.

HOME REMEDIES FOR A SLEEPLESS NIGHT

We know that when your back hurts and you're ragged from tossing and turning, desperate measures can seem tempting. Good judgment can get clouded. But if you're having trouble sleeping and decide to do something about it, slow down and use your head. When you're suffering from back pain and you're under the care of a physician, it's likely that he has already prescribed painkillers. They'll help you relax to fall asleep and stay that way. If you are still having trouble sleeping, do *not* self-medicate on top of prescription medications. Call your physician and have a heart-to-heart chat.

Try relaxation techniques. Achieving a peaceful state of mind might be as easy as practicing Dr. Andrew Weil's Yoga Breath. Get comfortable and close your eyes. Breathe through your nose, one nostril at a time. Start with the left nostril by blocking the right. Inhale to a slow count of four. Hold to a slow count of seven. Exhale to a slow count of eight. Switch sides. Block the left, breathe with the right. Switch sides again. Do this four times per side. Imagine with each breath that you are filled with energy and that your muscles are relaxing, lengthening, strengthening, and getting organized—fiber by fiber.

Another favorite of ours is to imagine yourself in a hammock between two trees. Peaceful. Swaying back and forth. Back and forth. Deeply relaxed. More

How Much Sleep Do You Need?

We all require different amounts of sleep at different stages of our lives. Infants and children need quite a bit; the average requirement for adults is about 7.5 to 8 hours. Once we hit 60, we sleep a little less and increasingly poorly because our sleep is frequently disrupted.

These generalizations aside, your body is biologically programmed to need a specific amount of sleep just for **you.** Here's a scientifically proven trick to decoding that secret for yourself.

Next time you have a few days off, try not to schedule anything in the evening or morning. Cut loose all discipline and "go with the flow" where sleep is concerned. Set the stage for good sleep. Ignore external signals that it's time to go to bed, like the end of a favorite television program. Put away any clock that allows you to count the hours between the sheets or that announces your wake-up call. Just go to bed when you're sleepy and get up when you wake up.

This process may take a couple of days because the first night's sleep might be a matter of making up sleep deficit. You might need a bit more than "normal," and it could take a few nights to get in the groove.

After a couple of nights, pay close attention to that moment you feel the need to go to sleep and the moment when you wake up, then do the math. Now you know how many hours of sleep you need, and when your body wants them. You might be surprised to realize that your body wants to go to bed earlier and awaken earlier than you have been.

If studying your own sleep cycle sounds simple, it's actually not. For some, it takes going camping or being otherwise cut off from the external cues of artificial scheduling before they can do this kind of study. Once you have the number of hours your body needs, don't cast it in stone. Keep in mind that the need fluctuates along with your fatigue levels. If you are an office worker who spends a Saturday playing in a tennis tournament, then on Saturday night, you can count on having to sleep a little longer than usual. If you're ill, you'll need more sleep. If you're injured—as in a back injury—you'll need more sleep. Healing takes energy. Energy has to be recharged by sleep.

---

relaxed with every sway. Now eliminate the trees. You're still in the hammock, swaying back and forth. Back and forth. Even more deeply relaxed. Now eliminate the hammock. You're still swaying back and forth. Back and forth. Profoundly, deeply relaxed. Before long, you'll be lulled into sleep.

Take aspirin or NSAIDs. Aspirin and nonsteroidal anti-inflammatory drugs (NSAIDs), such as ibuprofen, can serve a couple of purposes. Taken properly, they can reduce pain and inflammation by blocking the production of prostaglandins (chemicals that cause inflammation and trigger transmission of the pain signal to the brain). And, most important, when you feel comfortable, you'll sleep a little better.

A few of words of caution: Pain is your body's way of communicating clear messages to you about the status of an injury. Don't use over-the-counter painkillers to mask pain that you and your doctor need to be evaluating and using for information. NSAIDs have possible side effects of which you need to be aware: nausea, indigestion, diarrhea, and peptic ulcers. Aspirin can cause clotting disorders, prolonged bleeding, colitis, gastrointestinal disorders, ringing in the ears, and aggravation of asthma, hives, and gout. Both interact with other medications. Be careful.

Break out the heating pad. Usually, we recommend ice for treating injury by reducing swelling, slightly numbing, and promoting blood flow, but an aching back at bedtime presents an unusual challenge. Low in subcutaneous fat and rich with nerves, the back muscles sometimes tense up when they're iced—especially if you're trying to do it yourself. The better solution might be to warm the back and relax it.

Take a hot bath. If you don't have a heating pad, you might achieve the same relaxation with a hot, but not scorching, bath. Be careful getting into and out of the tub. One slip will jar a back that's already in trouble.

For added comfort, roll a towel and tuck it under your neck. If you plan to spend a long time in the tub, keep a plastic bottle of cold water within easy reach and keep drinking. Heat causes you to sweat. Sweating causes you to dehydrate, but you might not notice if you're already wet.

Consider antihistamines. Antihistamines such as Benedryl are used to combat cold and allergy symptoms and to relieve itching. But one of the serendipitous side effects of an antihistamine is that it causes drowsiness. For this reason, many hospitals use them to relax patients who need to be gentled into sleep. Even a low dose will do the trick. The quality of sleep is pretty fair. Read the package instructions and follow them to the letter. Also, be sure that you time the dose carefully. Once you've taken it, your day is done. No more operating heavy machinery for you.

Look into over-the-counter sleeping aids. If you read the package carefully, you might notice that over-the-counter sleeping pills are largely a combination of aspirin and antihistamine—not a bad combination for a sleepy person with an aching back. Generally, they have been found to be safe for healthy people, but their effectiveness may vary. Avoid them completely if you plan to end your evening with a glass of wine or any other drug. Follow package instructions very carefully.

Sample some herbal teas. In recent years, we've noticed an increasing number of herbal teas targeted toward sleep. In fact, their packaging is so restful that just seeing it on the shelf causes us to yawn. We can see no real harm in drinking these teas, but the FDA doesn't regulate their production. Use caution and do your research—if you trust the company, drink the tea in moderation.

Look into botanical supplements. Several nutritional supplements are thought to calm the nervous system and support sleep. Among them are valerian, passionflower, kava kava, and skullcap. Just as with herbal teas, we urge you to do as much research as you can before taking an unregulated botanical, which may have potential drug interactions. Over the years, we have encountered enthusiasts who swear by them, but clinical research is still lacking. Without it, we can't endorse or recommend.

Consider melatonin. Melatonin is the nutritional supplement that came to fame when shift workers and jet-lagged travelers touted its ability to "reset" the internal clocks for sleeping off natural schedules. While some evidence suggests that it's effective under some circumstances, research results continue to be conflicting.

Marketing has overshadowed doubts cast by clinical testing. Manufacturers usually suggest that the dose for melatonin is 3 milligrams, an amount which produces blood levels of 10 to 40 times greater than naturally occurring levels. This can't be good, now can it? Also, although it is used widely and happily throughout the rest of the world, it remains unapproved by the U.S. Food and Drug Administration. Without regulation, purity and potency are inconsistent here. Buyer, beware. If you want to try it, you can find it in health food stores.

DOCTOR-ASSISTED REMEDIES FOR A SLEEPLESS NIGHT

Our consulting pharmacist, Melissa Fox, Pharm.D., points out that when everything you have tried fails, your physician might be able to help. She has compiled a list of medical protocols available to promote sleep.

Professional relaxation techniques. Relaxing will reduce tension and pain, and give you some tools for easing out of discomfort and into sleep. Among the most respected relaxation techniques are hypnosis and biofeedback.

Hypnosis is a technique through which a trained therapist helps you achieve deep relaxation so that your thoughts are clear and you're more open to suggestion. When it's used for back-pain-related sleep problems, the therapist will discuss controlling pain and learning how to relax on your own at bedtime.

Biofeedback therapists use equipment that monitors involuntary physical states such as tension and temperature. Training to change your states, and being able to see the immediate results of affecting those states, allow you to manage them on your own.

Benzodiazepines (Ativan, Xanax). These medications are in a class called hypnotics, meaning they relax. They work by kicking up the activity of a neurotransmitter (GABA) that calms brain activity and promotes muscle relaxation. They shorten the time it takes you to get to sleep, increase the total time you're asleep, decrease the number of times you're awakened, and improve sleep quality.

Configurations vary, so your condition will dictate which of the benzodiazepines your physician might consider. People develop tolerances fairly quickly, so this medication might be effective for no more than a few weeks and may cause "rebound insomnia" and other unpleasant symptoms when the patient stops taking it. For this reason, coming off benzodiazepines will be closely supervised by a physician.

These medications are not advised for people who have sleep apnea or a history of substance abuse, or women who are pregnant. Also, patients may not drink alcohol, even the day after using long-acting benzodiazepines.

Imidazopyridines (Ambien). Like benzodiazepines, these medications are hypnotics and work by kicking up the activity of GABA, which calms brain activity. But unlike benzodiazepines, they don't promote muscle relaxation. In every other way, they are similar in their ability to produce and support sleep. They work quickly and are usually gone from the body within 5 to 10 hours if the patient is healthy and has no drug interactions that might prolong the effects.

Tricyclic antidepressants (Elavil, Endep). It's not uncommon for a physician to prescribe tricyclic antidepressants for a patient who is not depressed, because this medication improves sleep—reducing the time it takes to fall asleep and improving the quality. In some patients, improved sleep has been linked to reports of reduced aches and pains. Also, tricyclics are not particularly habit forming. Stopping the drug is not likely to produce unpleasant symptoms or rebound insomnia.

Anxiolytics (BuSpar). These sedatives are used to treat anxiety but are also known to promote and support sleep. While they don't interact with alcohol, anxiolytics may require patience; they can take up to 3 weeks to take effect.

Barbiturates (Nembutal). These drugs have a relaxing effect but are used infrequently to treat insomnia because it's easy to build up tolerance. Your doctor would have to increase the dose to achieve consistent results. Also, they can be addictive. Too long on a barbiturate means possible symptoms of withdrawal when the patient quits.

Part 6

Pain-Free Solutions for Everyday Situations

Chapter 14

YOUR HEALTHY BACK AT WORK

When we began our practice, our clients were professional and Olympic athletes, dancers limping in from the Broadway stages, and movie stars needing to be trained for roles too physically demanding for them to handle. Our appointment book looked like a Who's Who of the sports and the entertainment industries.

When we worked with one of these people, it was always an urgent situation. Careers were at stake; thousands of dollars were on the line. We had to get our clients up and performing without a minute to lose.

Then something amazing happened. We had a friend who was a typist with severe lower-back pain. She asked if we could get her out of pain and train her to sit in her chair so that she could type all day.

We had never thought of training someone to sit still. In fact, it seemed ludicrous to us. But we love this woman and agreed to evaluate her. Her nickname for herself is "The Typing Troll," because she sits hunched over a keyboard for hours on end. All the musculature in her body was perfectly conditioned to support a seated posture for marathon lengths of time, but she was sadly out of shape with imbalances and weaknesses almost everywhere. She had no endurance.

We had worked only with athletes and performers—how could we train someone to sit still?

We considered the challenge carefully. She had a special skill for which she was uniquely conditioned. But other things were going wrong physically. She was in pain. Was it possible that we could fill in all those gaps and turn her into a lean, mean typing machine?

We were sure that our methods of flexibility, strength, and cardio work would be effective—if we could find a way to scale back the intensity and duration of each workout so that a person could start from zero. We learned to respect her job and the demands it made on her body. We quickly developed the attitude that if you are using your body at work, you are an occupational athlete, and you deserve the same attention in training as an Olympic gold medalist. Since then, we've trained dozens of occupational athletes, so we know this plan can work for you. Let's take a look at some specific situations where occupational athletes can apply physiological principles to their activities to heal current pain and prevent further injury.

PROTECTING YOUR BACK WHEN YOU SIT ALL DAY

Sitting is a way of life for many people. While many activities could just as easily be accomplished while

John is a columnist for the *New York Times*. His back was killing him from years of sitting at his desk, working on a keyboard, and talking on the phone. He made his appointment with some urgency because his upcoming assignment was to accompany an expedition to the North Pole and cover their story, and he was gravely worried about his ability to handle it. The trip would require a lot of cross-country skiing, and, because was he out of shape, he was concerned that his back would never withstand the exertion.

Sitting seems like a relaxing posture, but it's killer on the body, especially when it's done at length by a writer. Like in most professional "sitters," John's glutes, hip rotators, and hamstrings were in constant compression. In examining him, we discovered that his hamstrings were tight from sitting, and he had only about 25 degrees range of motion. He also had nerve pain down his leg from pressure, and his abdominals were weak. The problems originated in the zone from his knees to his pelvis, but his back is where he felt the pain. There was really nothing wrong with his back that a little balancing act couldn't correct.

How John Got Out of Pain: John's biggest relief came from flexibility. We started to work with stretch ropes, training him to increase range of motion joint by joint. We focused on his hamstrings, glutes, and hip extensors. He was out of pain nearly immediately.

When he was flexible enough, we added strengthening. Initially, he was unable to do one abdominal curl, so we had to modify the move. This was particularly important because the abdominals support the back. We needed all his muscles back on duty, but especially his lower abdominals. Even with the modified exercises, he progressed very quickly, because little efforts add up fast.

John is an athlete at heart and a tenacious adventurer. He felt better after being stretched out, and he improved quickly. Four weeks later, all of his back pain was gone, and in just a few more weeks, he was in shape and ready for the expedition.

John's trip to the North Pole was a success. He sent us a photo of their campsite with a dogsled and a stretch rope. He told us later that he had all the expedition team lined up and waiting their turns to use it.

standing, we simply don't. We could stand at the counter to eat, but we sit at the table. We could stand while we watch television, but we sit in the recliner. We could raise our desks and stand while we work, but we sit in chairs. We could stand, but we don't. So we sit. And sit. And sit.

Sitting at a desk all day can take a terrible toll on an unprepared body, putting more stress on your lower spine than standing. And, no matter how ergonomically designed and seemingly comfortable your chair is, your back, hips, legs, and buttocks are going to fatigue and tighten up if you don't give them a break.

The other problem with sitting is that all your work is contained within a small, specific space—usually right in front and just below your face on a desk. Your arms and hands are usually up on the desk, and your neck is flexed downward toward your work. This bad situation is made even worse by your locking into this position and moving very little and very infrequently. Your shoulders and the area between your shoulder blades fatigue and strain as you maintain and sustain this torturous posture.

As long as we sit so much, we might as well be good at it. So let's take a look at ergonomics, the science of applying engineering principles to environments, tools, furniture, and equipment so that people are safe and productive at work and at home. It's a booming industry. The Occupational Safety and Health Administration reports that 1.8 million workers suffer from injuries that result from mistakes in ergonomics—a seemingly harmless desk too high, a chair too low, a mouse the wrong size.

As workers become more efficient at simplifying and streamlining operations, requiring less physical effort to get a job done, they're getting hurt more. For example, a secretary 20 years ago had to type on a manual typewriter, run back and forth to the file cabinet, carry a schedule ledger into the boss's office to review appointments, and dash to the bank to transfer money. On her way home, she stopped by the office supply store to order notebooks for a meeting. Today, all that can be accomplished with one computer in a few minutes.

There's no question that we're getting more done, but there's a heavy price to pay for all this efficiency. That price is paid in human suffering. Experts in ergonomics are trying to help.

These experts have identified problems that affect circulation, muscles, bones, connective tissues, eyes, ears, and nerves. (Gee, that pretty much covers every major system in the body.) Most of the problems that occur from sitting at desks are caused by cumulative stress and fatigue. Most desk jockeys are riding computers, so ergonomics engineers have identified specific complaints. The most common are neck and shoulder pain, back pain, eyestrain, and repetitive stress injuries such as carpal tunnel syndrome. We'll discuss this bad boy in greater detail in the section "Protecting Your Back When You Use a Computer All Day" on page 294.

Don't let the litany of possible injuries scare you—fight back! Some simple changes to your work

environment will make big differences. Most of the ergonomic guidelines deal with helping you maintain good posture and keeping your back is safe.

Use a towel or pillow to create the right angle. Your back has three curves: cervical (neck), thoracic (chest), and lumbar (lower back). All three curves should be in an upright alignment from your tailbone. To support and balance your lower back, place a pillow or rolled-up towel at the back of your chair so that you can lean against it. Also, set the angle of your seat so that your knees are slightly lower than your hips and your feet are flat on the floor. This forward angle also tips your pelvis forward and takes a lot of strain off your lower back.

Choose your chair well. The best chairs have seats that don't tip when you recline the back, so you won't have pressure on the backs of your knees and thighs. If your chair has arms, make sure they are adjusted to proper height so that when you rest your arms on them, your shoulders are relaxed and comfortable with no pressure on your upper back. Try to avoid crossing your legs. Scoot your chair in as close to your desk as you can, so that you don't have to lean forward and reach out to handle your work.

Position your computer and other tools appropriately. Make sure your computer screen is straight in front of your face so you don't have to extend or flex your neck to get a good look at it. Place your keyboard at a height that allows your elbows to be flexed at 90-degree angles. If you must use the phone, don't wedge it between your shoulder and your ear. Either hold it in your hand or use a headset.

Keep moving. Equally important as designing the perfect workspace is moving around whenever possible. Use every excuse you can find to stand up and walk around. File things. Drop things and then get up to retrieve them. Stroll down the hall to answer a question rather than use the phone. If it is inappropriate for you to stand, wiggle and flex while seated. Roll your shoulders. Lift your arms over your head. Extend your legs, rotate your ankles and feet, crunch your toes up and then relax them . . . do anything that gets blood flowing. Use your breaks and lunchtime to walk and relax your shoulders and back. Take a few deep breaths.

Use the quick releases. If you want real tension busters that take only a few minutes, require minimal space, and draw only a little attention, go to page 252 in chapter 12. We've outlined a few quick-release moves that will work the kinks out in record time and get your blood circulating.

Treat your back gently. A word of caution: Ergonomic experts who specialize in preventing back injuries warn us that back fatigue is tricky. It can sneak up on you when you least expect it, so always try to avoid sudden, jerking movements after you've been sitting awhile. To pick up objects that have fallen on the floor (or were tossed there by you as an excuse to move), gently slide to the edge of your chair and place a hand on your knee or your desk to support your back. Keep one foot in front of the other for additional support.

Make up for your job's demands in your downtime. Working at your desk all day means that you are not getting enough exercise, so you will want to put together an after-work fitness program that combines strength, flexibility, and cardio work.

To get the kinks out of your back after sitting, try this stretch.

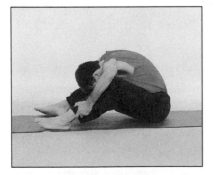

TRUNK EXTENSORS
See complete instructions on page 49.

PROTECTING YOUR BACK WHEN YOU STAND ALL DAY

Several years ago, we attended the summer graduation of a basic training group at a naval training center. The ceremony was held inside a large, stiflingly hot, unair-conditioned auditorium. Young men and women in crisp, white uniforms stood at attention for more than an hour through speeches and ceremonies. And in that hour, we watched them drop like flies. One here. One there. One in the far corner. If it hadn't been so disturbing, the people sitting around us probably would have started taking bets about which sailor would hit the deck next.

While you might not have to stand rigidly at attention without moving a muscle, we are going to assume that you are upright and on your feet throughout a work shift of some duration. So what happens now?

Your foot is literally a shock absorber, designed to take the vertical forces of your weight and gravity and translate them into horizontal force. When you walk, the arch of your foot sort of flattens out and then springs back up to give you a little lift with each step you take. It's a physical dynamic that is really quite remarkable. But when you stand all day and never lift those vertical forces off your feet, the arch flattens under your weight but never springs back into shape. As you move around, it might spring a little, but never fully. The arch and all the muscles that surround it become strained and exhausted.

Any imbalance in your foot, such as a slight roll of your ankle inward caused by a weak or flattened arch (inversion) or a slight roll outward (eversion), will be aggravated by standing for long periods of time. Those imbalances will travel up your ankle to your knee, which will eventually strain to try and keep you in balance. The strain in your knee will travel to your hip, and your hip could then throw your back out. This chain of unfortunate compensations sends the pain and strain straight up.

CASE STUDY: ED MATHEWS

Ed is a massage therapist and a musculoskeletal therapist. When he came to us for treatment of a painful back, he had already determined the causes. He spends many hours every day bending over some of the top dancers in the country, so he attributed his lower-back pain to constant flexion and exhaustion. He thought his upper back kept going into spasm from years of massage that tired his shoulders and arms. Ed was right about the stresses of massage. But we suspected that the real culprit was that he stood on hard surfaces every day.

The foot is far from the heart, so gravity and distance had caused some circulation problems as well as tired feet. As a skilled therapist in demand, he had worked hard, and the result was a punished body.

One day, he told us that he had dislocated his ankle several years earlier. The injury had been severe and had left him with a fallen arch in his foot that rotated his ankle toward the midpoint of his body. We looked at each other and smiled—we knew something that Ed was about to learn.

When the ankle is unstable and the arch falls and rolls the foot in, the knee gets strained. When the knee is strained, the hip compensates. When the hip compensates, the lower back is strained and weakened. And that will shoot right up to the neck.

Not only that, but when the arch isn't stable, it's not able to do its job at first point of impact in a foot strike. It's the shock absorber for the body. It's supposed to take the weight, dissipate the shock, and then spring back into shape to give lift to the step. Ed's couldn't do it. All that shock was traveling straight up the leg. The body finds the weakest link, and Ed's was in his shoe.

How Ed Got Out of Pain: Instead of throwing Ed on the table and working on his back, we used Active-Isolated Stretching to unlock his body. We needed to restore range of motion to his joints and get circulation going again. Then we taught him a couple of exercises specifically to strengthen the foot and lower leg.

Ed is highly attuned to his body and took the workouts seriously. Once we had him feeling better, we added the full strength routine with emphasis on glutes, adductors, abductors, and hamstrings. His back stopped hurting very quickly, but full recovery took 6 weeks, because Ed had so many levels of dysfunction from years of being hard on his body.

We're proud to say that Ed studied our systems and made them his own. In fact, he now works in our New York City clinic.

Your circulation is also affected. One law of physics states, "What goes up must come down," but no law states, "What goes down has to come up." The heart does a remarkable job of pumping blood down and usually does a remarkable job of pumping it back up, but gravity is a formidable foe. Being on your feet all day can cause your circulation to become sluggish. Metabolic wastes from firing muscles in your legs and feet may not be flushed sufficiently.

Fluids may pool in muscles and around joints, and you may find yourself swollen from the knees down, which is called edema. You can tell you have it if you lift your sock away from your leg, and the imprint of the weave and the elastic band are visible in your leg as though you've been embossed. Not good. When leg and feet tissues swell, nerves are compressed, and you may experience aching.

Additionally, the fainting sailors remind us that

when blood and fluids are accumulating in your lower half, they're not supplying your upper half. When blood can't make its way back to your brain in sufficient amounts, you faint. Getting your heart pumping and your blood circulating is a matter of moving once in a while. But if you wait too long and feel as if you're about to keel over, sit down and put your head between your knees or lie down and elevate your feet. ("Face pale, raise your tail.") Gravity will do the rest.

As soon as blood gets back to your brain, you'll feel better. Don't allow foolish pride to keep you from preventing a fall. When you faint, you have no control over how or where you will fall. It's better to have hurt pride than to have a hurt back . . . or worse.

Combating these problems is a matter of proper planning. Here are a few suggestions for keeping your back healthy on the job.

Wear suitable shoes. Good footwear that supports your feet in perfect balance with plenty of room for comfort will go a long way in preventing problems. Whether you are wearing shoes or boots, you need to make certain that they fit properly and provide support and cushioning appropriate to your job and the surface on which you must function.

Explore inserts. Beyond the shoes themselves, you can buy gel insoles and slip them into your shoes to help take some of the strain off your feet. Make sure they fit the shoes you'll be wearing and feel comfortable.

Cushion your standing area. Try a padded mat on the floor where you stand. Mats made of a soft gel diffuse vertical force and feel cushy (but not too cushy) beneath your feet. Available from commercial suppliers, these mats are slip-proof. They will not correct imbalances in your feet and ankles, but they can make you more comfortable, since your feet are protected from the hard floor.

Kick your feet up—but just temporarily. By the end of your shift, you'll be tired of standing and tempted to hurl yourself into a recliner to get your feet and legs up. Not a bad idea, as long as you don't stay there too long. Being tired is one of the most common excuses for skipping a workout. We urge you to push through fatigue if you can. Don't be tempted to eliminate all exercises that work you below the waist, thinking that you've had enough for one day. Becoming stronger, more flexible, and more balanced will help you withstand the rigors of standing all day.

To get the kinks out of your back after standing, try this stretch.

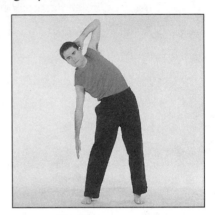

TRUNK LATERAL FLEXORS
See complete instructions on page 51.

PROTECTING YOUR BACK WHEN YOU LIFT AND HAUL ALL DAY

Recently, we had the opportunity to work with a highly trained male dancer from one of the most successful and longest-running musicals on Broadway. In every performance, one of his most spectacular moves was to catch a tiny, leaping female dancer and lift her over his head before she slid down from his upreached arms, to his chest and into his embrace for a showstopping moment of romance. He did it in rehearsal. He did it for eight performances a week. But one night came when the tiny, leaping female dancer leaped, he caught her in midair, but he couldn't lift her. She slid down his face, and he slid down right next to her for a showstopping moment of disaster.

His lower back had simply shut down in a

painful spasm, and he couldn't support her weight. How could an experienced professional dancer suddenly seem so weak? Easy.

Like most of us, he lifted all his weights in front of his body . . . including his partner. His back side, imbalanced and weaker than his front side, struggled to participate in the lifting. He had become so weak that to lift her, he arched his back to create a sort of fulcrum with his body to balance her weight. His lower back, buttocks, and hamstrings stayed continually contracted, impinging nerves and shorting out, getting weaker and even more imbalanced with every lift, until things started shutting down.

When the muscles in his lower back could no longer handle the load of the lifts or support the forces of impact and lift, muscles in the front had to work harder. But they weren't strong enough to carry the whole load by themselves. Plus, he started having difficulties with muscles in his arms and shoulders, and then his lower back was screaming as he arched and absorbed the forces of lifting another dancer. From that point forward, his lifting days were numbered. This was a man in need of balance.

We can't assume that a person who lifts and hauls for a living is totally fit, despite having a highly physically demanding job. Frequently, the opposite is true. Fitness is defined as health, strength, cardiovascular fitness (endurance), and flexibility. A person who lifts and hauls for a living may have only one of the components: strength. He might look great and still fall far short of being fit. If you want to do well in your profession and work injury-free, you must make sure that you have all the fitness pieces in place.

In lifting and hauling, injuries are both acute (like sprains) and overuse (like tendinitis). Most common are sprains, strains, and soft-tissue injuries of the lower back, shoulders, biceps, deltoids (behind the shoulders), elbows, forearms, wrists, hands, groin, thighs, and hamstrings. If it looks as if we just listed every body part as being in serious jeopardy, don't panic. Notice that we did not mention knees,

ankles, and feet. It's harder to get hurt in your lower extremities. Still, it's important to remember that although lower extremities are not the targets of injury, they can be the causes. Imbalances in your lower extremities translate right up through your hips and back as your muscles try to compensate and soft and connective tissues are strained.

Be advised that lifting and hauling can also cause one-sided muscle hypertrophy. This means that the muscle is highly developed in the lift (concentric contraction), but not nearly so in the opposite direction—say, when you lower whatever you've lifted (eccentric contraction). Because this muscle develops only half of its functional strength, it isn't flexible. And because it's inflexible and firing on only half of its pistons, other muscles are continually recruited to assist whatever task is at hand. Imbalances are common. A truly strong muscle can shorten to lift a weight and then lengthen to lower that same weight with the same speed and control as the lift, with both phases of movement through the full range of motion. All the way up, all the way down. Nice and easy.

Using common sense should help you avoid many of the injuries associated with lifting and hauling.

Stay well. Don't lift and haul if you are injured or feeling under the weather. When you're not well, your body diverts energy into healing. In this weakened state, you're out of balance and your muscles might not be able to fire at full capacity.

Don't rely on a back belt to give you support. These belts look spiffy and keep your waist and lower back warm, but they don't live up to their promises. They give the illusion of support, so you might feel invulnerable and try something that ultimately will hurt your back. Also, they restrict range of motion and cause muscles to get lazy and atrophy from disuse. Make no mistake: You *are* muscularly developed enough—especially your abdominal muscles—to support the weight you are lifting or hauling. The only back belts we endorse are those worn by competition weight lifters. These are specifically designed for well-trained athletes who use them for one purpose: to protect the lower back in a lift. You'll note they're not neoprene with suspenders.

Know your limits. If something is too heavy for you, use your brain, not your brawn. Either figure out another way to move it (like with a pulley) or ask for help.

Put your body against the object you're lifting. This tightens your center of gravity and removes some of the load from your lower back. Never stand away and reach out for something heavy. Instead, snug up tight, bend your knees, and lift with your legs. Focus your energy. Don't hold your breath. Lift slowly and smoothly.

Do a little dance. If you're carrying something and you have to change directions, don't twist or turn your torso. Keep the load of this weight distributed right where it is—directly in front of you and close to your body. Change directions with your feet.

Lower with your back straight. When you're ready to put the weight down, keep your back straight, hold the object as close to your torso as possible, bend your knees, and lower slowly and smoothly. (It's okay to make the "ughhh" sound!)

Use a stepladder. If you have to lift something from a level higher than your shoulders or place something higher than your shoulders, stand on something stable that will support your weight and get you where you need to be. No "heave-ho."

Don't forget your stretching. No matter how much you lift and haul during the day, you need *total* stretch work for balance, so include an Active-Isolated Stretching workout in your training. A tight muscle—especially one with one-sided hypertrophy—takes more effort to move and can't move as fast.

Also, don't forget: No matter how hard you work or how you huff and puff, lifting and hauling are not aerobic. You need to do cardio training.

To get the kinks out of your upper back after lifting and hauling all day, try this stretch.

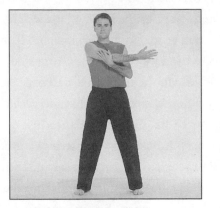

ROTATOR CUFF 1
See complete instructions on page 57.

PROTECTING YOUR BACK WHEN YOU DRIVE ALL DAY

To those who are stuck in an office job, driving commercially can seem like the ideal lifestyle. You just cruise around, listening to your CD player and watching the miles whiz by, right?

Wrong. The truth is that driving is one of the most mentally and physically demanding of all professions. You sit belted into one position for hours with your arms extended in front of you, your hands gripping the wheel, and your eyes glued hypnotically to the road ahead. All the controls for all the equipment are within inches of your hands or feet so you don't have to reach for them. Commercial vehicles—especially trucks—seem to be designed so that you *never* have to get out. The only problem is that efficiency and convenience leads to a sedentary driver whose only exercise is to rush to the restroom and back to the cab.

From the standpoint of physiology, driving makes several specific athletic demands upon the driver. Pressing on the clutch puts your left leg and foot to work, using ankle flexors (gastrocs in your calves) and knee extensors (quads in the fronts of your thighs). Braking engages hip rotators and adductors. Shifting also engages your arm: wrist flexors, arm extensors, triceps, and upper rear shoulder. Steering requires development in your chest (pectoralis) and shoulders (deltoids and rotator cuffs).

With arms out in front of you as your hands grip the steering wheel, you tend to relax arm muscles and rely on your grip to support their weight. Try this posture for a moment, and you'll notice a slight pull in your back between your shoulders. If you hold this posture for long periods of time, this slight pull becomes a big problem. Tension will set in. As the muscles in your upper back tense, blood supply is restricted. The muscle fatigues and starts shutting down, and metabolic waste from the effort is not easily flushed away, so pain sets in.

Your neck may be holding steady, rotating, and extending as necessary, but it's never enough. It will short out, guaranteed. The problem with neck fatigue is that you cannot relieve it as you drive by rolling your head or rotating it to get the kinks out. Doing this will not only take your eyes off the road (never a great idea), it will upset your equilibrium to the extent that you'll be a road hazard all on your own.

The sitting position puts more stress on your lower spine than standing. And, no matter how ergonomically designed and seemingly comfortable your seat is, your back, hips, legs, and buttocks will fatigue and tighten up if you don't give them breaks once in a while to stimulate circulation. Worse than that, with more work to do, one foot is dominant over the other, so you'll sit at an angle on one hip to get that foot ready to move. You'll stay that way throughout the drive—vigilant, ready, and prepared to move fast. With one hip hiked up, you've put your back into slight rotation. It fatigues from tension, even if the drive is under an hour. You've just created a serious imbalance, because the side opposite the dominant side is fatiguing while trying to hold you there.

When tension and fatigue set in, the piriformis muscle, which runs from your sacrum to your femur bone in your thigh, constricts in a spasm and clamps down on the sciatic nerve, which runs from your buttocks down the back of your leg. In piriformis syndrome, as it's called, your back aches, your butt and the back of your thigh hurt, and you'll slowly notice that you're losing function. This can cause a potentially dangerous lag between the moment when your brain tells you to move that foot and when that leg can transmit that urgent signal through a nerve that's no longer communicating well. It disrupts the message between the back and the foot; somewhere in there, the message gets retranslated to "This hurts so badly, I think I'm going to throw up!" Hitting the brake or clutch becomes difficult.

Piriformis syndrome doesn't automatically go away when you leave the vehicle and straighten up. You'll need to work a little to relieve it, which is your body's way of telling you that it needs flexibility, balance, strength, and a break once in a while. Luckily, prevention is simple.

Don't forget to *move*. Whether you drive a police cruiser, fire truck, passenger cab, utility van, or an 18-wheel rig, remember to move occasionally. From time to time, shift and wiggle in your seat. Crank up your music and do a little seated dance. Rock your weight from one side of your butt to the other and back again several times. Roll your pelvis forward until your back actually arches, hold for a second, and then roll it back as far as you can until it draws your chest slightly down. Clench and release the cheeks of your buttocks several times. This pumping action looks insane, but it recruits blood flow to the area. And get out of the vehicle a *minimum* of every 2 hours or so and walk around.

Smooth out the transitions. Many professional drivers also load and unload cargo. We can't stress enough how important it is to intelligently make those transitions from sitting to standing to walking to lifting. Think of yourself as a triathlete who has several physical activities to master: Each activity is different, and the transitions between them make the difference between success and failure. In fact, triathletes train for transitions as thoroughly as for their individual sports. You'll have to do the same.

Remember how fatigued your back can get from sitting. You may have weaknesses and imbalances that will make it difficult for you to make sudden demands on your back and upper body. After you roll out of your driver's seat, use the walk back past the trailer to sneak in a little stretch or two. At the very least, "shake it out" to remove tension from your back and get blood flowing to your arms and legs. Remember, when you lift, keep your back straight, keep your abdominals tight, and lift from your knees to keep as much pressure as possible off your back.

Boys in blue, beware. We have worked with police for several years and have spent a great deal of time evaluating and solving the physical problems of an officer who has been patrolling for hours in a seated position behind the wheel, but then has to throw on the brakes, leap out of the cruiser, and pursue a suspect on foot. The demands placed on muscles, joints, and heart are horrific when an officer goes from "sedentary" to "warp drive" in 2 seconds. Worse, at the end of this chase, there might be hand-to-hand combat. All systems have to be *go* immediately. If you expect to function at all, we suggest that you stay loose in the cruiser. Move as much as possible.

To get the kinks out of your back after driving all day, try this stretch.

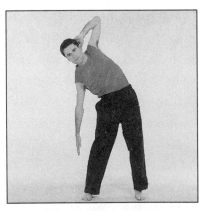

TRUNK LATERAL FLEXORS
See complete instructions on page 51.

PROTECTING YOUR BACK WHEN YOU USE A COMPUTER ALL DAY

Using a computer, or doing other kinds of keyboarding, can be a double whammy. Not only will you be sitting at a desk with all the perils that we listed above, you also add that notorious weapon—the keyboard.

Oh, sure, keyboards look innocent enough. Some even have designations like "featherlight touch" and "ergonomically friendly." But they can wreak insidious damage, better known as carpal tunnel syndrome.

Carpal tunnel syndrome is one of a group of injuries called repetitive stress injuries (RSI). The syndrome develops as fingers repeatedly strike keys over a long period of time. The hands and wrists fatigue; tendons, ligaments, and soft tissues swell. Just as stepping on a garden hose slows the flow of water, so the swelling compresses the median nerve fibers and slows down the transmission of nerve signals through the carpal tunnel, the passageway that runs from the forearm through the wrist. The result is excruciating pain and paralyzing numbness in the wrist, hand, and fingers.

Why are we including this in our discussion of backs? Because an alarming number of cases are directly related to the back. Either the pain of carpal tunnel syndrome sets off a series of compensations that travel directly up the arm to the shoulder to the back, or the back shorts out and sets off a series of fatigued muscles throughout the shoulder and down the arm to the wrist and hand.

We know that the body is an integrated system, with each part linked to every other part. When a wrist isn't operating properly, the lower arm kicks in to move the hands. But the lower arm fatigues. When the muscles start to fail, the arm above the elbow moves in to take up the slack. But that's not what the upper arm is for. It shorts out. When it falters, the shoulder kicks in. But the shoulder isn't good at managing movement in the wrist and hand, so it

Our favorite restaurant in New York City is Mana. It's owned and run by a pixie of a lady named Songee Lee. We eat at her place very often.

One day we noticed that apple crunch was missing from the menu. As guys of habit, this was deeply disturbing to our routine, not to mention disappointing. We asked Lee what happened to the apple crunch. She quietly and politely said that she hadn't been able to prepare it that day because of an excruciating pain in her arm.

How Lee Got Out of Pain: It was near closing time, so we cleared a couple of tables and hoisted her up so that we could get a look at her. Her rotator cuff and upper back were fatigued and shorted out. We unlocked her with Active-Isolated Stretching. (After all, apple crunch was at stake!)

We quickly learned that the source of her injury was not from chopping. It had started lower, with a hard, tiled floor in the kitchen, where she stood. Her back and hips had become fatigued, and that stress translated up her back to her shoulder, where the pain radiated down her arm. We have since trained her in the techniques of Active-Isolated Stretching and Strengthening, and she's feeling great. We haven't missed apple crunch since.

eventually strains. When the shoulder is strained, the back tightens. See how it works?

These links also work the other way. When the back spasms between the shoulder blades, the body strains to hold the torso up against gravity—particularly in the posture that we assume as we sit and type on a keyboard. As the upper back locks up, the shoulders lose their range of motion. When they fatigue, the upper arms work overtime to move the lower arms. When the upper arms tire out, the wrists and hands are strained. Spasm and swelling of tissue impinge the nerves in the wrist. Bingo: carpal tunnel syndrome. Cause and effect, directly linked both to and from the back.

While keyboards have been around for a long time, carpal tunnel syndrome has been epidemic for a mere 15 years. But the reason isn't a mystery. The old-style typewriter keys were harder to strike, so the hands got a better workout. And the carriage return made it necessary for the typist to reach up and whack it at the end of every sentence. In contrast, the computer keyboard has a soft, light touch, so the hands must work more subtly. Without a carriage return, there's no reason to move a muscle.

Computer keyboards are common at work *and* at home. Many people go from being mesmerized by one computer screen to another with only dinner in between. We can sit for hours without noticing that we're numb from the waist down, so we don't realize that our hands and backs are fatigued until it's way too late.

From your perspective as an athlete, you must view carpal tunnel syndrome as a classic overuse injury. "Overuse" means just that—used too much, overdone. But the good news is that we can prevent it or, if it's already setting in, we can turn it around.

Don't ignore the signals. People aren't suddenly struck down in the prime of their typing without warning. Indeed, carpal tunnel syndrome develops over a long period of time, settling in while a person ignores clear signals that something's not right.

The first signal is fatigue in hands and arms. You could feel it as "slowing down" or a slight lack of co-ordination. Eventually, fatigue will feel like a small ache. The solution is simple: Take a short break every hour to get things moving and keep them moving to improve circulation and restore range of motion.

Watch your form. Besides taking frequent breaks, you can also prevent carpal tunnel by taking a few simple precautions.

- Don't rest on the wrist pad or mouse pad when you're working.
- Keep your mouse as close to the keyboard as possible and at the same level so that you don't have to reach and strain your back.
- When you are not using the mouse, take your hand off and relax it.
- Keep your monitor screen at eye level and straight in front of you.
- Keep your document holder as close to the monitor screen as possible. Switch sides occasionally.
- Try to keep your wrists as straight as possible so that your hands will relax.

Don't forget your program. Prevention is a matter of training. Like any athlete, a keyboarder must be physically fit with specific training to withstand the demands of the job. Keyboarding requires strong arms, shoulders, and back, and flexible wrists, hands, and fingers.

Keep your eye on the bigger picture. As we've mentioned, carpal tunnel syndrome isn't the only treachery of keyboarding. Sitting at a keyboard all day can take a terrible toll on an imbalanced, untrained, unprepared body, putting more stress on your lower spine than standing. And, no matter how ergonomically engineered and seemingly comfortable your chair is, your back, hips, legs, and buttocks will fatigue and tighten up if you don't give them a break periodically. Your neck, shoulders, and the area between your shoulder blades fatigue and strain as you maintain and sustain an upright posture with your arms in front of you and your hands on the keyboard. You have to move.

Find and use every excuse you can to stand up and move around. Set a timer if you must. No more than 2 hours of sitting and typing at a stretch without a 5- or 10-minute break during which you work out the kinks. Take a look at the tension relievers in chapter 12.

If you work at a keyboard and are sitting all day, we guarantee that you are not getting enough exercise, so you will want to engage in a fitness program that combines strength, flexibility, and cardio work.

To get the kinks out of your back after keyboarding all day, try this stretch.

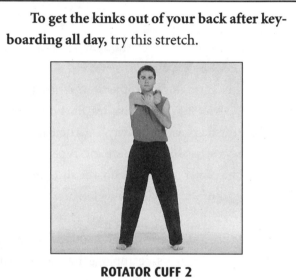

ROTATOR CUFF 2
See complete instructions on page 58.

Chapter 15

YOUR HEALTHY BACK AT HOME

We were called to the home of a high-profile client whose back was in spasm. We had been working with her to unlock painful back spasms that had gripped her since a high-speed horseback ride in a scene of a movie she was shooting. After this inexperienced rider had one too many takes, the pounding from the saddle of a galloping horse had strained and traumatized her back.

Although we usually worked on her in town, we were glad to make a house call. When we arrived, we found her on her hands and knees in the bathroom, cleaning the toilet. We got down on the floor beside her and raised the all-important question: Why would a famous actress be cleaning a toilet?

Her answer was simple. She liked cleaning toilets, and, besides, her back hurt too badly to get off the floor, so she was tending to chores that were low to the ground. We worked on America's Sweetheart right on the bathroom floor with a wet toilet brush propped neatly in the corner.

Home should be where the heart is, not where the hurt is. Preventing back problems is a matter of both learning how to go about your daily chores with the physical precision and skill of a trained athlete *and* taking measures to make sure your home is safe and efficient.

DON'T SLIP AND TRIP ON THE HOME FRONT

While most people will tell you that they feel most safe at home, recent studies tell us that every year people make more than 20 million medical visits on account of accidents in the home. Next to traffic accidents, the home is the second most common place for fatal injuries. Yikes!

Fatalities aside, the most common injury in a fall is the back, but almost all of these injuries are preventable. So why are they so common?

Researchers tell us that most people do not see the hidden dangers within their homes. They may not be in denial, but, on average, people really can't imagine how they could get hurt in *their* places, where they feel most secure.

Part of the problem might be that we own a lot of "stuff." In fact, most of us own more stuff than we have room to store neatly, so we pile things up. We get so used to the chaos, because we are so familiar with it, that we cease to "see" it. In the past, possessions were few, distractions were even fewer, and the pace of life was slower. In addition, women didn't work outside the home, so more attention was paid to simple tidying and maintenance. Not today.

Another part of the problem is that we are, by

Are You Fall-Proof?

Although no one can truly be safe all the time, you can *personally* do many things to assure that you won't take a tumble at home.

1. Wear shoes that fit well and are skid-proof. Flat shoes with cleated, soft-rubber soles and heels are best. High heels with minimal heel-to-surface contact, shoes with cleats only on the heels, and shoes with soles made of leather are the most likely to slip.

2. Walk purposefully, but not fast. When you walk fast or run, you land hard on the heel of your front foot and push harder off the sole of the rear foot. With those forces at work, it takes more work for you to pull out of a potential fall—you simply won't have

time. Changing direction quickly is the same problem. You're not balanced and ready to react.

3. Watch where you're going. One of the most-often-heard explanations for tripping over or slipping in something is "I didn't see it." Pay attention.

4. Don't carry things so bulky that they obstruct your vision. If you can't see over it, if you can't see around it, if you can't see under it, put it down.

5. Take your sunglasses off in low light. You might look cool, but your vision is as impaired as if you were standing in dusk. You can't judge surfaces well.

6. Don't wear skirts or robes that are too long, trousers that drag on the floor, or socks that don't fit. Aside from the fashion faux pas, you just may trip.

---

nature, optimists and procrastinators. Few of us are prone to sit around and think about the ways our homes could kill us; if we do think about the dangers, we're likely to wait until a situation becomes critical before we act to remedy it.

Homes are private and, therefore, not subject to inspections by experts who could tell us how to injury-proof our homes. Too bad, because we could all learn a lot from these professionals. Why not act as your own inspector? Try this checklist of common risks found in the home.

☐ **Are your telephone and electrical cords out of traffic patterns so that no one will trip on them?** Cords strung out across people's paths are traps set for falls. Move them or have an expert rewire the outlet to be closer to the place you need it. If you must string out a cord, make sure it's taped securely to the floor, centering wide tape along the length of the cord from wall to appliance. Also, don't run them under carpets or rugs, where they can create an invisible hump to trip someone.

☐ **Are all your area rugs and runners secured to the floor with either skid-proof rubber matting or carpet tape? Are all the edges flat to the floor so that no one will trip?** Carpet suppliers sell a lightweight webbed rubber that can be cut to the same size as your rug. Simply place it between the rug and the floor for grip you won't believe. Or run wide carpet tape along each edge of the rug.

☐ **Are your walkways free of clutter?** We aren't suggesting that your home be pristine and sanitized, but you will be safer if you can move freely about without tripping over things. Keep the floor and stairs clear all the time. Consider rearranging furniture so that people can circulate through rooms freely without having to wedge between or step over things. Think about creating clear passage from every major area in your home to every door.

☐ **Are all the legs of your tables, chairs, and stools tightly secured and level?** A chair with a broken leg can tip, throwing you off balance and wrenching your back. Or it can break completely and drop you to the floor. Nothing you own is worth the risk. Fix them or give them away.

☐ **Are you using maximum-wattage bulbs in all fixtures both inside and outside your home?** Impaired vision is a major contributor to falls. We recommend turning on every light and then deciding if it's bright enough. If you notice dark spots or areas where detail is so obscured that you would not be able to sidestep a fall, consider installing additional lighting.

☐ **Are the switches for all your lights easily accessible and logically located?** Never let there be a moment when you or anyone in your home gropes for a light switch. In emergencies, you have to be able to turn on lights quickly. At other times, you don't want to be feeling along a wall for a switch when you're unable to see things in your way.

☐ **Are you using a sufficient number of night-lights?** Night-lights are not just for children. They should be everywhere you might need to go at night.

☐ **Is each bathtub and shower outfitted with a skid-proof tub mat or textured strips or appliqués so that you won't slip when you're wet?** Wet porcelain is slick. And you'll always be on one foot as you step in or out. One false move and you're on the floor. If your tub or shower is not already skid-proof, make sure you do it yourself.

☐ **Do you have bath mats outside each tub and shower so that you won't slide across the bath-room floor when you step out?** Bathroom floors are notoriously slippery when they get wet. A bath mat will give you some traction. If you don't have a mat, throw a towel on the floor to prevent a fall.

☐ **Do you have grab bars to help you get in and out of the tub or shower? Are they affixed to structural support so that if you have to depend on one, it won't pull out of the wall?** Towel racks weren't designed to support the weight of an adult human who is doing a triple half-gainer. Grab bars are, but even they will fail if they're not installed properly. Make sure your bars are bolted into structural support, such as wall studs behind the tile.

☐ **Is the area around your bed clear of clutter, discarded slippers, or sleeping dogs?** Many nasty falls occur when a person stumbles out of bed and gets tangled up in something unexpected on the floor. Scoot your slippers under the bed when you take them off. Keep the clutter off the floor around your bed, particularly between you and the door to the bathroom and the door to the rest of your home. If your dog is a frequent visitor to your bedside, but you're never sure where he is, put a glow collar on him.

☐ **Do you have a telephone next to your bed?** If something happens, the ability to call for help is essential.

Teaching Yourself How to Fall

Of course, our primary hope is that you never slip or trip and fall. But if you do, you may as well know that there's a right way to do it.

Please don't misunderstand us: We don't want you to go out and literally practice. Instead, just rehearse this method in your mind a few times. When you fall, you don't think. You react. If these instructions exist somewhere in your subconscious, then you might fall correctly and suffer minimal injury. Here's how.

- Tuck your chin in, turn your head, and throw an arm up. It's safer to land on your arm than on your head.
- In mid-fall, twist or roll your body to the side. It's safer to land on your butt and side than to land on your back.
- Keep your wrists, elbows, and knees bent. Avoid attempting to break the fall with your hands or elbows. Try instead to spread out the forces of the impact by landing with as much of your body as you can. This absorbs the shock and distributes it more evenly. It's not exactly a cushion, but it might help.

☐ **Is your workshop tidy?** Even in an immaculate home, sometimes the workshop is a disaster area because it has become the dumping ground for all stuff that had nowhere else to go. Keep it as neat as your home. Mop up oil, grease, or water that's spilled on the floor. Keep all drawers and doors closed. Falling in a workshop is especially dangerous. You're in close quarters with sharp tools and solid cabinetry, and, because it's not in the normal traffic pattern of your home, chances are slim that someone will happen by if you can't get up. Not good.

☐ **Are the light switches for your workshop located near the entrance?** Because workshops are sometimes roughly designed or are areas that were originally designed for some other purpose, light switches can be helter-skelter. Make sure that you can turn on the light from the doorway. You must not try to feel your way through a darkened workshop to get to a switch.

☐ **Do you have flashlights located strategically around your home, so that if you have a power failure, you can find your way around?** Darkness greatly increases your chance for a fall. When a power failure occurs, you'll be plunged into darkness. Even night-lights will go out. Keep many flashlights handy. You also might want to buy one of those emergency lights that you plug into an outlet. It operates on battery and comes on only when the power is off.

☐ **Are the stairs in your home in good shape? All level? No loose boards? Free from clutter?** If you want to avoid a fall, give yourself a fighting chance. Stairs are dangerous. Level them. Repair any problems. And clear them off entirely. In addition, don't run up and down the stairs in your socks. If your stairs are wooden, you'll slip. If your stairs are carpeted, you'll trip. And don't put an area rug at either the top or the bottom.

☐ **Are the stairs in your home well-lit with switches at both the top and the bottom?** Under no circumstances should you be forced to walk up or down stairs in the dark. If you have a switch at only one end, get an electrician to install a second one.

☐ **Are the handrails on your stairs in good shape? Not wobbly?** If you start to slip, you need a handrail that will support your entire weight and stabilize you until you can get back in balance. If your handrails aren't sturdy, repair them.

☐ **Is the carpet on your stairs in good shape? No fraying or unraveling that might trip you? Is it firmly attached?** Imagine the thud you would make if you tripped and fell on the floor. Now imagine thud thud thud thud thud thud thud . . . splat. Stairs can multiply the injury of a simple spill many times over. Inspect every inch of the carpet on your stairs and make sure no hidden traps exist.

☐ **Are your steps outside constructed of rough texture or covered with abrasive strips?** Steps outside are particularly problematic because they are frequently wet and in the dark most of the night. Tiles and pavers that are designed for exterior use are skid-proof. If your steps are wooden, paint them with skid-proof paint. Or mix sand with paint to give it some "tooth." If your steps are concrete, affix abrasive strips. Do whatever it takes to make sure no one will take a tumble.

☐ **Are the stairs in your home and the steps outside your home even and of the same size and height?** Walking up and down steps requires a certain rhythm. In fact, building code standards dictate the height of each riser. Under no circumstances should your steps be uneven or randomly spaced; otherwise, the rhythm of the walking person will be completely cut off.

☐ **On any flooring, are there worn places? Uneven places? Nails or screws that are sticking up?** Inspect every square inch of flooring in your home. If you find anything uneven or anything sticking up or out of place, fix it immediately before someone stumbles. A variance of as little as $3/8$ inch can stub a toe and cause a fall.

☐ **Do you have any places, inside or out, on which standing water collects where people**

walk? Water on the floor can be as slick as ice. And worse, it's usually invisible and unexpected. The net effect is a jarring, shocking fall. If you've just spilled water, clean it up immediately. If you have a standing-water problem, remedy it. Water that's always there can develop a sort of microbial slime that makes it even more slippery. And although you and your family might remember that little puddle and manage to avoid it, your unwary guests will not.

Now that you've answered all the questions, you'll know where you have to concentrate your efforts to save your back from a nasty tumble.

DON'T LET YOUR BACK DO THE HEAVY LIFTING

When tackling a big load, you may be tempted just to heft it in a surge of effort. Later, your back pays mightily. Use your brain, instead of your brawn. Once again, protecting your back has everything to do with planning.

Before you lift, consider the following:

1. First, the obvious: Avoid lifting heavy objects whenever possible. Try to figure out ways to shove or roll or slide or drag it. Recruit a helper—two lifters are always better than one. Think about dividing the load into smaller, more easily managed pieces.
2. If you must lift the object, ask yourself these questions.
   - Am I in shape enough to lift this particular object?
   - Am I properly warmed up?
   - Is the object awkwardly shaped?
   - Is it sharp or does it have things on it that might harm me?
   - Is the weight evenly distributed throughout the object?
3. Give it a shove or tip it to test the weight. If you think you can handle it, plan what you'll do with the object once you've lifted it. Look for the shortest path from here to there and make sure it's clear and safe for you to walk there.
4. Decide where you're going to put the object down and make sure that the receiving end of this project is prepared. You don't want to stagger out to your car with a hefty crate, only to discover that you forgot to open the trunk.

Once you've done your planning, it's time to lift. Here's how the pros do it every day and live to tell the tale.

1. Stand close to the object with your feet spread shoulder-width apart and your knees relaxed.
2. Keep your back straight, bend your knees, and lower yourself until you can get a grip.
3. Wrap your arms around the object. Keep your hands wide open with fingers spread for maximum grip. Put your torso as close to the object as possible. Get against it if you can. This keeps your lower back from having to deal with cantilevered forces of gravity.
4. Contract your abdominal muscles and slowly rise by straightening your knees. Keep your back straight. Do not hold your breath.
5. Keep your elbows tucked in close.
6. Make every movement a slow, smooth one. If things aren't working out, bend your knees and lower the object back to the floor, then move on to Plan B—whatever that might be. Do *not* risk a back injury just to move something heavy. There's almost always another way.
7. If you have to change direction, move your feet first and follow with your shoulders and torso. Under no circumstances are you to twist or rotate from the waist and shift the forces of that load to the side.
8. When you're ready to put the object down, just do everything in reverse. Keep your back straight and bend your knees. Slowly lower your torso and the object until it's down. Make sure your fingers are out from under the bottom of the object as it hits the surface.

9. Stand up slowly, stretch your back, and shake out your arms and hands.

10. Do an inventory of your whole body to make sure you feel all right.

And here's one final tip from the experts: Never try to catch a falling heavy object. Just get out of the way!

How to Lift Something Light

If you think it's ludicrous to be concerned about lifting something light, think again. If you simply bend over from the waist and reach to the floor with your hand, you run the risk of straining your lower back. Sometimes the smallest, most simple movements are the ones that trigger spasm or aggravate an imbalance or injury. To lift something light from the floor, such as a magazine, lean over it, slightly bend one knee, and extend the other leg behind you. You'll look sort of like a sprinter on the starting line. Hold on to something or brace yourself against something as you continue to bend your knee and dip toward the object. Once you have it, simply straighten your knee, bring your back leg up, and stand tall.

PROTECTING YOUR BACK WHEN YOU WORK AROUND THE HOUSE

Susan Fielding came into our clinic 2 years ago with severe upper-back spasms and cervical pain. The stress and tension of running her home and managing two young children had shorted her out. She had a classic overuse injury. Her muscles had become so weak that they were restricting range of motion in her back, neck, shoulders, and, well, everywhere.

We decided to approach her treatment as if she were an athlete who had run onto the playing field without preparation or training. First, we unlocked her back with Active-Isolated Stretching and Strengthening, and then we taught her to do it herself. We were delighted when Susan told us that she always thought she was too busy to work out but that our program didn't take much time at all. In fact, because she was so much more flexible, strong, and energetic, she seemed to have more time in each day.

Individual tasks of housework can be real back breakers, so it makes sense to approach them as if they were athletic events. Do what you can to make sure you're flexible and strong. Pace yourself so that you don't tire out too much. And remember to drink plenty of water. We also taught Susan a couple of ways that she could keep her back safe when she works around the house.

Cooking: Preparing meals is generally not hard on the back—but it can be if you stand too long. Be certain that your counters are the right height for you. If you're going to be standing at the counter for a long time, put a box about 6 inches tall under one foot, or open a cabinet and prop your foot up on the bottom shelf. This takes the pressure off your lower back. And don't forget to straighten up and shake out the tension once in a while.

Standing to clean floors: Vacuuming, mopping, buffing, and sweeping can put a lot of pressure on the lower back because, as you stand, you also push and pull from your upper body, bending from the waist. Keep your back straight and bend from the hips as much as possible. Make sure that the handles and wands are long enough to allow you to maintain an upright posture with as little flexion from the waist as possible. As with kitchen work, give your back a break at frequent intervals by standing fully erect. Do a few of the quick-release tension relievers you'll find in chapter 12 on page 252.

To get the kinks out of your back when you've been vacuuming, mopping, buffing, and sweeping, try this stretch.

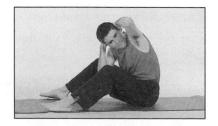

THORACIC-LUMBAR ROTATORS
See complete instructions on page 50.

Kneeling to clean floors: Getting down on your hands and knees to scrub requires that your back curves forward to allow you to reach the floor. But your back also has to support your weight because your hands are occupied and are not helping to keep you in position. Fatigue sets in very quickly, so be sure to take frequent breaks. Stand up fully and get the pressure off your back. Besides, from a standing position, you're better able to look down and admire your work!

To work the kinks out of your back when you've been scrubbing, try these three stretches.

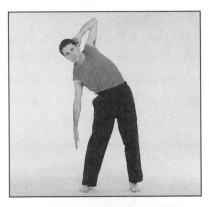

1. TRUNK LATERAL FLEXORS
See complete instructions on page 51.

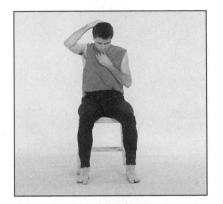

2. NECK EXTENSORS
See complete instructions on page 61.

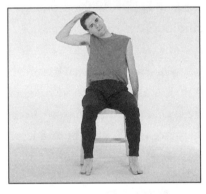

3. NECK LATERAL FLEXORS
See complete instructions on page 62.

Making a bed: Try kneeling rather than bending forward to tuck in a corner on the bed. Don't reach across the bed to smooth covers or tuck in a corner on the opposite side. Take the time to walk around. If the bed is against the wall and you can't get to the other side, consider putting the legs of the bed on casters so that you can roll or easily pull it away from the wall.

Doing laundry: Squatting is better than bending over at the waist for unloading a front-loading washer or dryer. If yours are top-loading, try to keep your back as straight as possible, by extending one leg and leaning forward from the hip on the other one. (If you know

To get the kinks out of your back when you've been making beds, try this stretch.

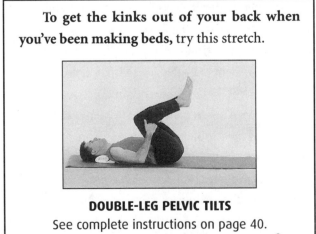

DOUBLE-LEG PELVIC TILTS
See complete instructions on page 40.

ballet, it's sort of an arabesque posture.) Keep the toe of your extending foot on the floor as you lean back. Lift it as you lean forward for counterbalance. These same techniques are good for loading dishwashers.

To get the kinks out of your back when you've been doing laundry, try this stretch.

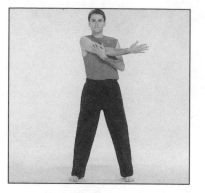

ROTATOR CUFF 1
See complete instructions on page 57.

PROTECTING YOUR BACK WHEN YOU'RE GARDENING AND DOING YARD WORK

When discussing matters of the home, gardening distinguishes itself and deserves a bit of extra attention. One friend is a master gardener who finds herself in our clinic with back problems from time to time. She often quips, "Green thumb. Bad back." As witty as we think she is, we're also deeply concerned that she's at the "root" of the problem. (Sorry, couldn't resist the pun.)

Serious gardeners are athletes, but many of them don't realize it. Their need for training and conditioning doesn't become obvious until something goes wrong. More than 400,000 gardeners seek medical or therapeutic attention every year. The physical problems they present to professionals are identical to those of athletes, but that's where the similarities end. Their training doesn't even come close to being comparable.

One of the problems is that gardening is seasonal. Spring and summer tend to be far more demanding than autumn and winter. Unlike an athlete who spends the off-season in training camps to prepare, a gardener might retire to the den to thumb through seed catalogs and dream of warmer days. When it's

time to come out of hibernation and get to work, the gardener is deconditioned from months of layoff, yet the work of early spring is especially hard: lifting, hauling, digging, weeding, tilling, planting, and pulling out and moving plants. But spring is in the air, so the out-of-shape gardener will leap right back into rigorous labor. Even when the work is not hard, you'll find a gardener on his knees, bending over little plants for hours at a time. Little wonder the back shorts out.

If you want to stay healthy so that you can enjoy gardening and stop referring to it as back-breaking work, you have to train for it during the off-season and then maintain complete fitness when your garden demands your attention. Before your day in the dirt begins, do your workout so that your body is strong, flexible, and warmed up, ready for work. If you have time for nothing else, do the stretch routine. And once you begin, use the right tools for the right jobs. We recommend lightweight equipment.

Specific jobs have specific remedies. Here are just a few.

Pushing a wheelbarrow: If you're pushing a wheelbarrow, make sure you've balanced the load within the bed so that one side isn't heavier than the other. Keep your back straight and let your legs do all the work as you lift the handles and maneuver it.

To work the kinks out of your back when you've been pushing a wheelbarrow, try these three stretches.

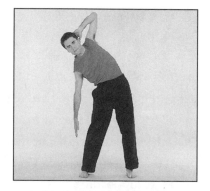

1. TRUNK LATERAL FLEXORS
See complete instructions on page 51.

(continued)

Know Ladder Safety

Experts in home safety have singled out the ladder as being particularly hazardous to your health. Anytime a ladder is used, it goes without saying that you're getting ready to leave the ground. Whenever you fall from height, there's farther to go before you land. Experts call these elevated falls, and injury is very often more severe than those that result from falls closer to earth. Here are a few pointers that will make ladder use safe.

1. Inspect your ladder for damage before you start. It should be dry and free from oil, grease, or mud.

2. Ladders should be set at a 4-to-1 angle, meaning that for every 4 feet up you go, the feet of your ladder should be planted 1 foot out. Make sure that the feet are firmly planted and that both of the side rails at the top are against the surface you're climbing.

3. Your ladder should be long enough so that when it rests against the upper support, you can work without your waist being higher than the top rung of the ladder or above the rung at which the side rails are resting at support. Good rules of thumb: Stop short by three rungs from the top of a straight ladder, and stop short by two rungs from the top of a stepladder. Tying the top of the ladder to the surface against which you're resting it will give you an added measure of safety.

4. The feet of your ladder should be slip-resistant. Be especially careful if you're planting the feet on a hard surface, like a driveway or a tiled floor. Sometimes you can compensate for a less-than-perfect slip-resistant base by planting the feet of the ladder on soft ground. But beware. In soft ground, one foot might sink lower than the other and pitch the ladder to one side under your weight.

5. Wear shoes with heels on them so that if you slip forward on a rung, your foot won't continue through. You can catch yourself by hooking your heel on the outer edge. Don't climb a ladder on tiptoe. Firmly place your feet on the rungs just ahead of the heel, resting on the midfoot or arch. Always climb facing the ladder, centered and balanced with both hands on the side rails at all times. Never turn around and never reach too far to either the right or the left.

6. Keep your hands free as you climb. If you need tools or equipment at the top, tie them onto a rope and pull them up after you're securely in position.

7. Never put more than one person on the ladder at the same time. If you have an extra person to help you, have him stand at the base of the ladder to stabilize it for you and make sure you're safe.

8. As a final note, never use a metal ladder in an environment where electrical wires might come into contact with it.

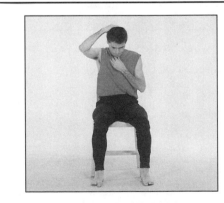

2. NECK EXTENSORS
See complete instructions on page 61.

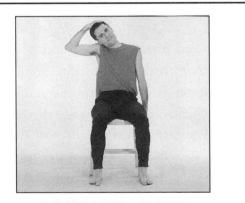

3. NECK LATERAL FLEXORS
See complete instructions on page 62.

Bending over your plants: Weeding and planting involve gripping, pulling, and twisting that can irritate muscles and tendons in your lower arms and hands. Work a little while, and then give them a rest. Stretch them a little to get the kinks out. Remember that gripping, pulling, and twisting can also irritate the back, so make sure that you're stabilized and that you don't strain. Also be aware of bending over, even at slight angles, for extended periods. Small irritations to the lower back over long periods of time will short it out.

Bending over while kneeling is very hard on your lower back. Take frequent breaks to straighten out your legs and back. If your back is really bothering you, consider using a long-handled tool from a standing position. Or sit on the ground and work. We even have one client who lies down on her abdomen and rests her chin on one folded elbow while she works with the other hand on something right in front of her face. If you're going to be on your knees, put a pad under them to cushion the pressure. (If you lift something, please refer to the section in this chapter that describes proper technique for lifting both heavy and light loads.)

When you're pulling out shrubs, wear gloves. Loosen the soil around the base of the plant. Stand close to the shrub with your feet shoulder-width apart. Keep your back straight and your face forward. Bend your knees and lower yourself until you can get a firm grip. Take a firm hold. Straighten your knees and lean *slightly* back as you rise slowly. Stay alert to that subtle moment right before the shrub lets go, and relax some of your pull. You don't want to keel over backward with a shrub and a ball of dirt on top of you. When you have successfully pulled the shrub, stand fully upright, relax your back and shoulders, and stretch.

To work the kinks out of your back when you've been bending over your plants, try these stretches.

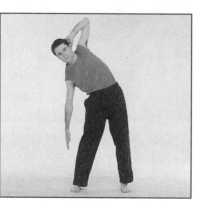

1. TRUNK LATERAL FLEXORS
See complete instructions on page 51.

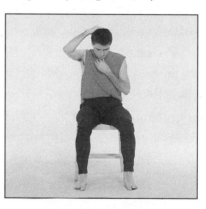

2. NECK EXTENSORS
See complete instructions on page 61.

Raking and hoeing: Raking and hoeing are deceptively hard on the back, because you reach forward and pull backward from a standing position. Additionally, these actions are rhythmic and repetitive. It's easy to get lulled into underestimating the demands they make on your lower back. Make sure you are sufficiently warmed up, change positions often, and take frequent breaks to stand fully upright, to take the tension off your lumbar spine.

To work the kinks out of your back when you've been raking and hoeing, try this stretch.

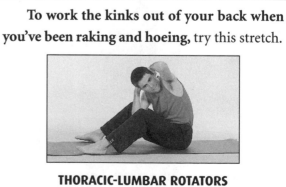

THORACIC-LUMBAR ROTATORS
See complete instructions on page 50.

Digging and shoveling: Stand with your feet shoulder-width apart when you're digging and shoveling. Be sure to use long-handled tools. Work close to your feet, resisting the urge to bend at the waist and reach out to work. Lift only small amounts of soil with your shovel so that the weight will not strain your back. And always remember to take frequent breaks.

To work the kinks out of your back when you've been digging and shoveling, try these stretches.

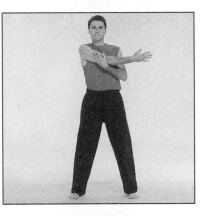

1. ROTATOR CUFF 1
See complete instructions on page 57.

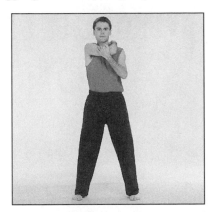

2. ROTATOR CUFF 2
See complete instructions on page 58.

Hauling: Hauling is about reaching and lifting, so it's important to protect your lower back from strain. Keep the load close to your body and let your legs do most of the work. Keep your spine straight at all times.

To work the kinks out of your back when you've been hauling, try this stretch.

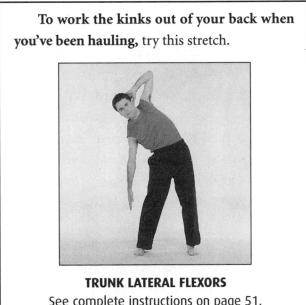

TRUNK LATERAL FLEXORS
See complete instructions on page 51.

A FINAL WORD ABOUT WATER

When you're gardening, it's easy to become so engrossed that you forget to drink. Hydration is as critical for you as it is for your precious plants. If you've waited to drink until you feel thirsty, it's too late. Thirst is a symptom of dehydration, and dehydration decreases plasma volume. With less blood getting to the skin, the systems that control heat dissipation fail. Once this happens, a gardener overheats even more quickly. Work suddenly seems to take superhuman effort.

Symptoms of dehydration include muscle cramping, excessive sweating, dark urine or infrequent urination, weakness, nausea, rapid heart rate, headache, light-headedness, increased body-core temperature, heat exhaustion, and heatstroke. If symptoms are too subtle for you, check your urine at the end of the day. If it's darker than the color of straw, you're not doing a good job of hydrating. Your goal should be urine that is clear or nearly so.

Plan to hydrate before, during, and after your work. Keep a bottle of water next to you or drink out of the hose. Every time you water a plant, join in.

Chapter 16

YOUR HEALTHY BACK ON THE ROAD

We have a client who always stops by our New York City clinic on his way home from La-Guardia Airport. In fact, we have a sneaking suspicion that his travel agent books his flights and then makes a reservation in our clinic for his arrival home.

This client always returns from traveling with a litany of tensions and imbalances that start in his back and don't quit until he's racked with pain. We can usually unlock him within the hour, but we're going to teach you how to avoid travel problems altogether.

The travel industry is often called a leisure industry, but the means of getting to your destination and home again can be anything but restful. Whether it's the cramped indignities of a tiny airline seat or the tense shoulders that come from driving to beat the weekend traffic, travel is rife with potential pains in the back. The best way to prevent, and repair, the damage comes down to foresight, planning, and some on-the-spot common sense.

We've culled these strategies from our hundreds of trips around the globe, tending to other peoples' pain while trying to avoid our own, and we're delighted to share them with you. Whether you travel by plane, bus, or train, most of these tips will help you keep your back limber, healthy, and flexible for the trip and beyond.

GETTING YOUR TRIP OFF TO A GOOD START

A good beginning can set the tone for your whole trip. Do your best to plan ahead and get things done in advance so you're not rushing around at the last minute. Tie up loose ends at home and at work so that you can completely relax about leaving. Make sure the details of your trip are well-planned and all your reservations and appointments are confirmed. Planning is the best thing you can do to make your trip a success.

If you're rushed, you're pushed. We've traveled often enough—and have clients who do as well—to know how rushing to catch a plane or train can really get the grip on your back. If you think that you can stress out while preparing for your trip until your back is in knots and then relax on the plane, think again. Releasing tension takes some space, which you probably won't have, and movement, which you probably can't have. Strapping into one of those upright seats (with the tray table in its upright position) is practically guaranteed to make everything worse. Upright seat. Upright tray table. Uptight you.

Be on time, if not a little early. Create a buffer between you and a meltdown at the curb.

Book the bulkhead. When traveling by plane, ask to be placed in the first row, also known as the bulkhead. Because there are no seats directly in front of you, you'll have extra leg room and be more comfortable.

We learned this trick from marathon runners who have to fly right after they've run 26.2 miles and while they're suffering the effects of the race. With the extra room, they can move and stretch their legs to get the kinks out. You can even lie down on the floor and do a few stretches, provided you are friends with the other passengers sharing your aisle. Still, when you whip out a stretch rope and throw yourself on the floor, you may have some tough explaining to do. Caution and courtesy are advised.

PACKING AND HANDLING BAGS TO PROTECT YOUR BACK

The process of hefting and hauling your stuff from point A to point B is also rife with threats to your back. Take these steps to treat your back gingerly.

Pack as little as you can. And if you can't do that, at least plan to carry as little as possible. Unless you're a professional sherpa, it's worth saving your back if you check your heavy bags and wait at the luggage claim for a few minutes at the end of the flight.

If you won't check your bags, at least roll them. We don't know how we managed before some brilliant person invented suitcases with handles and wheels. We highly endorse them. If your luggage has no wheels, rent some. Put a couple of dollars in the little machine and get yourself a cart. Or tip a baggage handler to help you. This minor investment will pay off in keeping the strain off your back.

Balance the load you carry. If you're going to haul your bags, always carry two of the same weight, so you can balance them. Weight on one shoulder will put tremendous strain on your back and your hip on the opposite side. If you're weighed down evenly, you might huff and puff, but your back will thank you.

Think before you lift. When you reach down to pick up your bags, keep your back straight and bend at the knees. Try to pick them both up at the same time, rather than recruit an assistant who drapes them on you one at a time. If the bags are heavy, your assistant will heave that first one slightly higher than your shoulder and, when it's in position, let go, dropping it onto you. It will hit you quickly and heavily, jarring your back. By the time you receive the second bag, the damage will already be done.

Try to avoid sudden jolts. Even when you put the bags down, be smart: Just follow the same advice as picking them up, only in reverse.

Wear your backpack correctly. If you carry a backpack, resist the urge to look very cool with it slung nonchalantly over one shoulder—wear both straps over your shoulders. Carrying all the weight on one shoulder will throw your back off balance and put too much strain on the opposite hip.

When you pack the backpack, try to get the heavier items as close to your hips or as low in the pack as possible. This puts the center of the load near your hips, where it's easier for your body to balance and carry. We encourage using fanny packs, which always distribute all their weight low on the back.

Send your luggage ahead. If your back is very fragile and any sort of load is problematic, consider shipping your belongings to the hotel by one of the courier services to arrive before you get there. Put your name on the box, the date of your arrival, and the word "Hold." Alert the manager that the hotel should expect it and allow plenty of time for the package to get there.

If you want to be really organized, take tape and a mailing label for shipping the package home. Most hotels ship and receive every day and will be glad to help you get this taken care of.

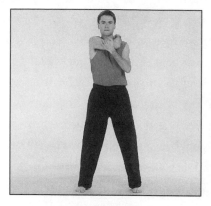
KEEPING FIT AND HEALTHY ON AN AIRPLANE

Andrew Weil, M.D., famous author and physician, heard of our work and invited us to his Center for Integrated Medicine at the University of Arizona in Tucson. It was a thrill to introduce our work to the first class of physicians coming through his program.

Dr. Weil is a wonderful man, an avid hiker and gardener. But he admitted to us that he was experiencing back pain from traveling on airplanes and lugging around bags. We were only too pleased to quickly unlock his back and train him in the techniques of Active-Isolated Stretching and Strengthening, so he could work out himself. He was so excited by the results that he sent his personal trainer to New York to study with us.

Dr. Weil stops into our clinic when he's in town. We're always gratified to note that he arrives at our door from a long flight and is still standing tall and pain-free. We're happy to see that the program fits his busy schedule. Here are a few ways to make sure you keep your program up while you're on the road. (By the way, we use the same methods whether we travel by plane, train, or bus.)

Use waiting time in the terminal to get some exercise. While you're waiting, walk back and forth in front of your gate. Swing your arms and be sure to stop 10 yards short of that place that sells cinnamon buns and chocolate croissants. In fact, you can use that place as a turnaround and quicken your pace as you walk away from it.

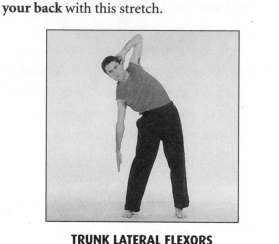
Get as much exercise as you can on the plane. We know for sure that those plane seats were designed by the best ergonomic engineers on the planet—but their one-size-fits-all definitely doesn't fit everyone. How delightful to have to sit with your belt tightened and seat flat, knees jammed, hips thrust forward, and midback arched to the back in a curve that resembles the letter C. Oh, let's not forget that your head is thrust forward and held there by a pillow that hits you anywhere but where you need it. Nice try, airline industry. Not comfortable or good for your back, especially for long flights.

For this reason, you need to get up and move. Walk up and down the aisle, stand for a while, and do some of the quick releases we show you on page 252. When we explain to the flight attendants that we're not out of our minds, we're merely suffering athletes, we are always welcomed into the space next to the galley. There's a little more floor space. On more than one flight, we've been joined by other passengers in the galley to do a small stretch class.

Drink plenty of fluids. The altitude and dry air in an airplane causes dehydration. When you are dehydrated, healthy cells that are usually plump and juicy shrivel up. They don't work as well when their composition and function are disrupted. They don't slide as easily against each other. In fact, they actually shred.

If your back is tight because you're tense, and you're also dehydrated, you'll exacerbate the damaging effects of the tension on your muscles. Take the flight attendants up on their offer to serve you drinks. Start with water. We carry our own 2-liter bottles of water with us. Not only do we stay hydrated even when the flight attendants are busy, we have an excuse to walk to the restrooms frequently and get more exercise.

If you are wild for variety, drink decaffeinated beverages and juices. The caffeine found in some carbonated drinks, coffee, and tea is a diuretic that will dehydrate you further. You may think that you need a stiff cup of coffee to perk you up, but please balance it with an equal amount of water.

Alcohol doesn't count at all. Sorry, but it doesn't hydrate you, and it has lots of empty calories. Experts tell us that it's far easier to get drunk at 30,000 feet than at sea level. If you are drunk and fall asleep, you're likely to droop into a posture that strains your back—and stay in that position too long without moving. You'll feel relaxed, but you're doing damage that will affect you once you're on solid ground. It's better if you are sober and conscious just enough to wiggle a little. Save the wine until you're on the ground.

Make sure you're warm enough. If you're cold, you'll shiver and tense up. Before you know it, your shoulders will be up around your ears. Your back, between your shoulders, will fatigue from tension and eventually begin to short out. When you arrive at your destination, you'll feel tired, but the exhaustion isn't the true exhaustion born of healthy effort—it's from weakness and impeded blood flow to your back.

Once you get to the hotel, you may be tempted to stand under a hot shower or climb into a hot bath, but wait. Stretch first. Then try a little ice, to recruit blood to the area and flush out the metabolic wastes that have accumulated while the muscles were constricted. Move a little. Then go ahead with that hot shower or bath.

Avoid salty foods the day before your flight and during the flight. Of course, this seems nearly impossible advice, considering that a little bag of salted peanuts is traditional, standard fare on an airplane. But the sodium makes your tissues retain fluids, which causes swelling of your extremities. You're going to have enough of that to worry about all on your own without the help of salt.

Instead of accepting the peanuts or other salty snacks, why not bring something of your own to enjoy during the flight? Food service has become limited on many flights, so brown bagging might be a great option. As long as you are tidy and courteous, and avoid anything flambé, there are no restrictions about what you may bring on board.

Take care of your legs and feet en route. Swelling of the lower extremities is caused by sitting still in one position with your feet on the floor. You're sitting so still that your circulation starts to slow. Your heart pumps blood all the way down to your toes, but you don't make it particularly easy to get it back up. If the plane is cold, the situation is even worse. Edema and wretched circulation are the results.

The consequent swelling can be uncomfortable and last more than 24 hours after you get onto the ground. We wear the most comfortable shoes we own and then take them off to wiggle our toes and move our feet around. We want blood flow—as much as we can get. Don't hesitate to lift up your feet and massage them vigorously with your hands.

Keep moving. Get up and wander around the cabin. Do everything you can to stay active in flight. Believe it or not, your life might be at stake.

Blood clots can form when blood pools, most often in the legs, during periods of inactivity. Called deep-vein thrombosis, or DVT, these clots can break off and travel throughout the bloodstream to the lungs, brain, or heart. Heart attack and stroke can result. Some people have died, although this is rare.

CASE STUDY: PAT DEVANEY

Pat Devaney is a footwear designer for DaDa and Deckers. For years, he has designed the shoes that put the elite-level athletes at the top of their games. He's a high-energy guy who travels the world constantly. We worked with him frequently and ran into him at trade shows and expos for sports equipment. We noticed, however, that his back was always in flexion. He was stooped with his shoulders caved in, and he was developing a dowager's hump. What a contradiction—Pat himself is a fine athlete, a competitive marathon runner.

How Pat Got Out of Pain: One day, when he was looking especially tired, we took Pat aside and said, "Look, you're not supposed to be like this. You don't need to be in this much pain. Let's work on it together." We examined his lifestyle and discovered that he sat hunched over a drafting board much of the time, but the real culprits were long flights compressing his back, followed by his carrying his own bags—heavy ones loaded with shoes and books. We gave him the Active-Isolated Stretching and Strengthening program, pointing out that a rope wasn't too heavy to carry. And we advised him to turn *all* his bags over to porters from now on. He's doing better.

Many of the victims of DVT developed the condition on long flights, such as those over 15 hours. But experts warn that shorter flights do not guarantee safety. If you have poor circulation and sit still for longer than 2 hours, you, too, are at risk. It's so common, in fact, that it's called economy class syndrome, referring to cramped seats and minimal leg room. The key to prevention is to increase circulation by moving around and keeping blood flowing. Additionally, researchers now know that eating and drinking during the flight increases blood volume and helps keep DVT at bay, but eating too much will divert blood from the legs into the digestive system and increase risk. Prevention is simple: Eat a little, drink a lot, and move.

Dress for success. We always travel in loosely fitting clothing that we wear in layers. If we're cold, we can keep all the warm garments on. If we're hot, we can start peeling. We wear the most comfortable shoes we have and make sure that we can wiggle out of them easily without having to make a production out of it.

Another key tip: Men, take your wallet out of your hip pocket and carry it somewhere else. Having a lump on one side of your butt lifts your pelvis to an angle you'll regret later when your back shorts out.

Work out in your seat. To get your blood circulating and keep it going, you need to get moving with the following four stretches: rotator cuff 2, ankle evertors, tibialis anteriors (on page 314), and trunk extensors. A measure of caution is in order if you're seated next to other passengers who might not enjoy your enthusiastic workout. But if you explain what you're doing, they might not assume you've lost your mind . . . and might even join you.

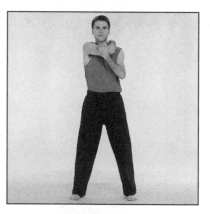

ROTATOR CUFF 2
See complete instructions on page 58. You can perform this stretch while seated.

ANKLE EVERTORS

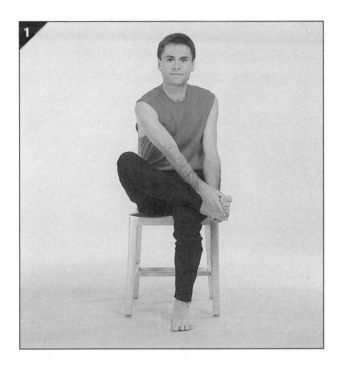

Active Muscles You Contract: Insides of your feet and ankles

Isolated Muscles You Stretch: Muscles on the outsides of your feet and lower legs

Hold Each Stretch: 2 seconds

Reps: 10 on the right, 10 on the left

This keeps circulation in your ankles and feet moving. You can avoid swelling, and you'll be able to sprint off the plane while others are hobbling.

1. While sitting in your seat, bring the foot of the exercising leg up and place it on top of the thigh, just above the knee, of the nonexercising leg. Reach straight down and grasp your forefoot with both hands.

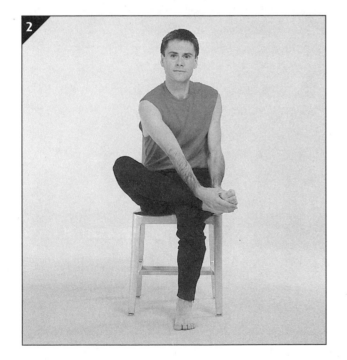

2. From the ankle, rotate your foot inward, pointing the sole of that foot up. You may use your hands for a gentle assist at the end of your stretch.

Note: You may want to use one of those little airline pillows on the top of your thigh, under the ankle of your exercising leg.

TIBIALIS ANTERIORS

Active Muscles You Contract: Muscles in the backs of your lower legs

Isolated Muscles You Stretch: Muscles in the fronts of your lower legs

Hold Each Stretch: 2 seconds

Reps: 10 on the left, 10 on the right

To keep your legs from cramping in the signature fetal position that makes flying such a special joy, let's work out your lower legs.

1. Bring the foot of the exercising leg up and place it on top of the thigh, just above the knee, of the nonexercising leg. Reach straight down and grasp your forefoot with the hand on the side of the nonexercising leg. Use the other hand to apply gentle pressure on the inside of the knee of the exercising leg to stabilize it.

2. Flex your exercising foot. You may use your hand for a gentle assist at the end of your stretch.

Note: You may want to use one of those little airline pillows on the top of your thigh, under the ankle of your exercising leg.

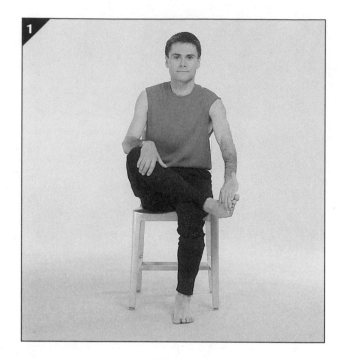

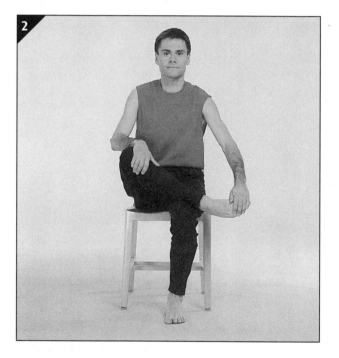

PAIN-FREE SOLUTIONS FOR EVERYDAY SITUATIONS

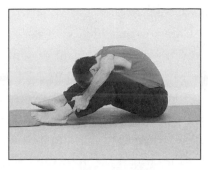

TRUNK EXTENSORS
See complete instructions on page 49.

Trunk extensors will keep your lower back from fatiguing after being locked in with a seat belt. Be really certain that your tray table is up for these. There's nothing worse than knocking yourself unconscious on the way down.

STAYING RESTED WHILE YOU TRAVEL

Doing without sleep for a few nights is enough to put a damper on your whole trip. Even among those who love to travel, losing out on shut-eye is a one-way ticket to fatigue, pain, and misery.

Store up rest. Get a good night's sleep the night before you travel. Being in "rest deficit" before you fly will cause your muscles to fatigue more quickly and easily. Also, if you're exhausted when you sit down, you'll fall asleep and your body will drape itself from a sitting position into relaxation that not only will be unattractive but also will likely strain your neck and back. Sleeping in a sitting position is hard on your hips, back, and neck. If you think you can justify it by pointing out that the seat tips back to cradle you, we assure you that those 10 degrees will make little difference.

If you must sleep on a plane, support your back and neck. There is no good way to sleep sitting up, from the perspective of your back and hips, but you can help a little. We recommend a cervical pillow that wraps around the back of your neck like a stuffed horseshoe and holds your head in an upright position if you're leaning slightly back. Some are inflatable, so carrying one is easy. And some are stuffed

but always light. Additionally, try taking one of the airline's little pillows and placing it at the small of your back for extra support. If you don't have a cervical support pillow, and if other passengers have beaten you to the airline pillow supply, simply reach into your bag and grab a T-shirt or a towel. Fashion anything you need by folding and rolling it until you're comfortable. We do it all the time.

Be aware of the effects of a sleep deficit. Experts tell us that if you arrive at your destination worn out, you will lack concentration and motivation. You'll have trouble following instructions and directions. You won't remember details; you'll be irritable; and your immune system can be compromised by fatigue, leaving you susceptible to illnesses. These misfortunes can't be good for either conducting a business meeting or enjoying a piña colada on the beach.

Crossing time zones is especially problematic. Every human has an inborn personal clock, called a circadian rhythm. That clock is set in your own time zone, so when you pass from one zone to another, your circadian rhythm is disturbed, resulting in what's known as jet lag.

NASA scientists say that you need one day for every time zone you crossed to reset your circadian rhythm and feel normal. If you traveled 6 hours out of sync with your own time zone, you'll need 6 days to equalize.

Flight attendants advise that if you're traveling east, don't rush to your hotel and go to sleep. Try to "push through" and stay awake and active. Eat on a local schedule. And tuck in for the night fashionably early. If you're traveling west, just go to bed at the time you normally do when you're in your own time zone.

Stick to your normal routine. If you're on vacation, going off your normal routine would seem precisely the point. A break does you worlds of good. But when you eat and sleep on a different schedule, your body will be confused. You'll have to cope with adjustments that might take a few days to work out.

We aren't suggesting that you should be rigid in adhering to a disciplined schedule, especially if you've changed time zones. We're suggesting that you try to keep within the broad range of basic functions, or adjust slowly to changes.

Make sure your hotel bed is a good one. Try it out. Like Goldilocks, you'll find some too hard, some too soft, and some just right. If the bed is too hard, call housekeeping and have the chambermaid put three or four blankets under the mattress pad for you. If the bed is too soft, pull the mattress onto the floor.

If the bed is just right, check out the pillow. Order extra pillows if you need them or take the cushions off the chairs and couch. Even a rolled-up towel from the bathroom will sometimes give you the support you need.

If you have back problems and always find hotel pillows unacceptable, consider traveling with your own. We have one friend who ships his favorite pillows to the hotel in advance of his arrival. They are too bulky for him to handle in luggage, so he packs them in a box and sends them ahead. He's never had a problem.

BE AN ATHLETE ON THE ROAD

David Nelson is recently retired as the president of Harcourt Brace, a publishing company. He's a wonderful guy who was looking forward to his retirement, but years of stress and flying and working on airplanes had taken their toll. He came to us with constant lower-back pain. He had tried everything, but nothing was working.

We unlocked him and taught him the techniques of Active-Isolated Stretching and Strengthening, and he swears that he has never felt better. And it's a good thing, because among his retirement plans is travel. We're training him to fly and travel like an athlete, so he'll never have another problem.

You don't have to wait until retirement—make your program part of your day, no matter where you wake up.

Pack workout clothes and your stretch rope. Because you are now an athlete with a deep commitment to working out, you'll want to continue that even while you're away. Don't forget to pack your workout clothes, walking shoes, and stretch rope. You might even be tempted to take your weights, but before you pack them, call ahead to the hotel. If they have a gym, they might also have the weights you'll need.

If you can, pack your rope in luggage going into the baggage hold. Because of heightened security, airport security personnel may interpret it as something more malicious than a tool to help you with Active-Isolated Stretching.

Look for workout facilities. Most hotels have a little spa with a treadmill. Sometimes if the hotel has no workout room, they have special discount pricing at a nearby health club that you can use. No matter what the facilities, it will have little impact on your program, because your workout routines are self-contained.

The only problem you may have is finding weights, and a little imagination goes a long way: Search your hotel room for something that weighs about the same as the weight you use, and then figure out how to lift it. We often use a tube sock into which we stuff something heavy enough to be useful. You can tie the open end of the sock around your arm or leg. Trust us—it works nicely. And we've used some fairly bizarre things.

If you walk around the hotel, make sure it's safe. Take a card from the front desk and print your name and room number on it with a ballpoint pen, so if you sweat, the ink won't run. Then pin it on the inside of the waistband of your shorts. If there's an emergency, you and everyone else will know who you are and where you're staying.

We once had a client who left a "big, gray hotel with glass doors" in the middle of a complex of hotels in Tampa and went for a long run. Not only did he get lost, he couldn't tell anyone where he had come from. Every hotel in the complex fit the description. It was both embarrassing and dangerous. Tell the desk clerk that you're leaving to walk, where you intend to walk, and approximately what time you'll be back. If you don't show up, the clerk can sound the alarm. If you don't want to go outside, consider walking the halls and stairwells of the hotel, or go down to their weight room and hop onto the treadmill.

STAYING FIT ON A CRUISE

Cruising is the fastest-growing industry in tourism, so there's a good chance that you will one day find yourself standing on the deck with the salty wind in your hair, toasting a glorious sunset with a drink containing a little umbrella. Cruise ships today are floating palaces. Every consideration has been given to your pleasure, safety, and comfort. In addition, cruise lines are set up to handle your bags . . . and just about anything else you don't want to mess with. In other words, they're there to spoil you rotten.

Take advantage of the luxuries. This effort to spoil you extends to the spa. Most liners have an on-board massage therapist who will be glad to keep you relaxed and loose. Also, you'll find a full-service gym and a variety of exercise classes. Just join right in, but don't overdo it. It's very easy to get carried away when you're having this much fun.

Look for the measured running route on the deck of your ship. Ask the purser which deck is designated and how far the loop is. Be courteous to other runners and walkers. And be sure the deck is dry—you don't want to slip.

See the experts. If you have any problems with your back or with anything else, the ship has an on-board physician to take care of you. You'll be surprised at how well-equipped the clinic is. Don't hesitate to seek assistance if you need it.

Don't fear the motion of the ocean. If you've hesitated to take a cruise because your back is unstable and you're concerned about keeping your balance as the deck pitches, you've been watching too many pirate movies. Today's ships are huge and have special motion-control engineering that keeps the world on an even keel, literally and figuratively. You'll probably never notice any movement other than forward.

Practice temperance. Be a little careful of being too festive. Getting caught up in the party atmosphere of a ship is all too easy—there's plenty to do, and it's all packaged to delight you and be fun. Practice moderation and use good judgment. The midnight limbo to the rhythms of steel drums on a beach lit by torches might seem like a good idea at the time, but if you haven't limboed lately (and, frankly, who has?) and aren't trained for it, you might pay for it later. Doing a few modest things is better than doing one spectacular limbo and spending the rest of the cruise in traction.

If you don't have it, ask. If you wish to have extra pillows in your stateroom so that you can modify your bed to support your back, inform the cabin steward. Stewards live to serve your every whim. You'll never encounter a person more willing to bring you extra pillows, blankets, and towels.

DRIVING WITH A HEALTHY BACK

Steve Frankfurt is a television and film producer and a public relations executive with an incredibly heavy work schedule. He came to us with back pain so severe that even we winced. The culprit? His commute: He drives an hour into New York City every morning and an hour home every night. For those 2 hours a day, his back muscles were in constant contraction to the extent that he was stooped over, putting even more pressure on his back. With Active-Isolated Stretching and Strengthening, we were able to reduce his pain and straighten him up a little, but we're still working on it. Commuters have a long road they travel every day, but if they take the proper precautions, the road to recovery need not be as long.

Whether you're riding in an airplane or driving your car, most travel today is a matter of sitting still for long periods of time, so all the rules that govern smart travel on an airplane apply to drivers and their passengers. Automotive engineers have made sure that you can do everything without moving from a seated position. You can honk your horn, roll down your windows, lock your door, get into gear, put on the headlights, release the emergency brake, signal, see behind you, and adjust the speakers on your CD player with almost imperceptible movements. This efficiency is nothing if not hard on your body.

While driving, you're also susceptible to all the physical difficulties of an airplane passenger: dehydration, swelling in your feet and legs, fatigue in your back and shoulders, and deep-vein thrombosis. But when you drive, you can add a couple more hazards.

You learned in driver's education to hold the steering wheel at 10 o'clock and 2 o'clock and to grip it firmly so that you are in full control at all times, especially in case you need to steer quickly. Because your arms are out in front of you as your hands hold the steering wheel, you tend to relax your arm muscles and rely on your grip to support their weight. While this works very well, you'll notice a slight pull in your back between your shoulders. If you hold this posture for long periods of time, this slight pull becomes a big problem. Tension will set in. As the muscles in your upper back tense, blood supply is restricted. The muscle starts shutting down and gets fatigued, and the metabolic waste from the effort is not easily flushed away, so pain sets in.

When you drive, you extend your legs so that your feet can reach the accelerator, clutch, brake, and anything else mounted there. Whether your car is manual or automatic, one foot is far more active than the other, so you'll hike up on one hip to get that foot ready to do its job. The bad news is that you'll hold that position, with your back in slight ro-

tation and your hip hiked up, for the duration of your drive.

When your back is held in this odd position, even if the drive is under an hour, it fatigues from tension and creates an imbalance. If, like most people, you hike up on the right, the left is working hard to hold you there. Then the piriformis muscle, which runs from your back to your hip and buttocks, constricts and impinges a nerve that runs from your buttocks down the back of your leg. In this painful and debilitating condition, called piriformis syndrome, your back aches, your butt and the back of your leg are in pain, and you start to lose function. Suddenly, hitting the brake or clutch with your left foot is difficult. Most disturbingly, there's a lag between the moment your brain tells you to move that foot and when that leg can transmit that urgent signal through a nerve that's no longer communicating well. You won't be paralyzed, but you'll be slowed down. Dangerously so.

Prevention is simple. Here are a few suggestions of how to do so without disrupting your trip too much.

Just move. From time to time, shift and wiggle in your seat. Consciously shift your weight from one side of your buttocks to the other and back again several times.

Do a pelvic tilt. Roll your pelvis forward until your back actually arches, holding for a second, and then rolling it back as far as you can until it draws your chest slightly down. It might also help to clench and release your buttocks several times. (If you do it right, it will actually elevate your body. Don't worry that you'll look like you're bobbing up and down—just focus on the fact that it recruits blood flow to the area.)

Take a pit stop. Get out of the car and walk around at frequent intervals, no longer than 2 hours in between breaks. It's important to get out of the car, because you cannot relax your neck,

Choosing the Back-Friendly Car

Ensuring your back against travel-related back pain can begin before you even set foot in your car. Next time you're in the market for a new vehicle, keep these tips in mind—they could help you prevent pain well into the future.

1. Make sure you can get in and out easily. If the car is too low to the ground, you might have trouble.
2. A tilt steering wheel can make getting in and out easier on your back. Consider this feature.
3. The driver's seat should feel firm, contoured, and comfortable. Look for several features: easy forward and backward adjustment, adjustable lumbar support, lateral bolstering to "cuddle" your buttocks and thighs, tilting seats, and headrests that can be adjusted to make contact with the middle of your head.
4. Electronic adjustments for the seats will save wear and tear on your back and keep you from having to wrench and work to get things right. Consider automatic buttons and toggles.
5. Take a test drive to make sure the suspension is firm to assure you of a smooth ride that will not vibrate or jar your back on long-distance trips. You want the car to absorb shock, not your back.
6. Try to find a car with a shallow trunk. Deep trunks force you to bend over and reach for items you are lifting in and out. This strains your back.
7. Take your favorite passenger along and make sure he or she is as comfortable as you are in the car.

---

back, and shoulders while driving. Rolling, rotating, and nodding your head will throw off your equilibrium—and you'll get pulled over for weaving all over the road.

Hit the self-serve lane. If you stop for refueling, get out and pump your gas. Walk around and check your tires. Vigorously wash your windows. Clear the interior of the car of trash. And walk into the building to use the restroom. Work hard to be as active as you can while you have the chance.

Bring a healthy picnic. We all have a natural human tendency to mistake fatigue for hunger. But if you're truly hungry, avoid drive-thru windows. You might gain a burger, but you'll lose an opportunity to move.

Remove that wallet. We mentioned this earlier when we talked about planes, but, please, men, take your wallet out of your hip pocket and carry it somewhere else. Having a lump on one side of your behind lifts your pelvis to an angle you'll regret later when your back shorts out.

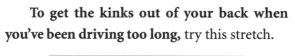

To get the kinks out of your back when you've been driving too long, try this stretch.

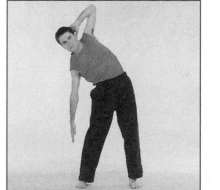

TRUNK LATERAL FLEXORS
See complete instructions on page 51.

Travel, whether for business or pleasure, is one of the great adventures of the human experience. Enjoy yourself. Get the most out of every minute that you're gone by taking care of yourself. And when your trip is over, we'll welcome you *back*!

Chapter 17

YOUR HEALTHY BACK AT PLAY

Although our practice began with coaching and rehabilitating collegiate and Olympic swimmers and runners, word of our work spread fast. Before we knew it, our appointment books were overflowing with a wide range of athletes representing a mind-boggling variety of sports. We even once treated a champion show dog that was faltering in international competition due to a hip problem. We flew to Iseo, Italy, to meet with our new client, a Great Dane who was suddenly, maddeningly, inexplicably limping on one of his back legs. With an unbalanced pelvis and a ragged gait, this athlete couldn't impress the judges and bring home the biscuits.

Following a few short sessions, we had that big guy back out in the ring. (It was the only time we ever had a client lick us.) The point is that after so many years of working all over the world with athletes from a wide range of disciplines, we know that while the biomechanics of activities will differ, *fun* remains the constant.

Once you're in good shape and your back feels great, it's time to return to play. Maybe you'll even find a new sport. Maybe you'll return to a long-forgotten pleasure. The better you feel, the more you can play. The more you can play, the better you'll feel. It's a wonderful cycle of fitness synergy.

We've selected a few activities that are common among our clients and from which you might choose. To get you off on the right foot, we've included brief discussions with sound advice very similar to what we deliver to our new athletes. As a bonus, we've given you a secret-weapon stretch or two, which you can do right before your games begin, that will make all the difference in your performance. Get out there and have fun!

BASKETBALL

We have worked with a number of basketball players in our career, including the New York Knicks, and we can tell you one thing: Flexibility is critical—for us! We are relatively short guys, so when we're talking to a 7-foot-tall basketball player, our necks and backs are in serious flexion from looking up. Good thing we're strong and flexible, or we would be in traction simply from talking to these big guys.

The bigger they are, the harder they fall. Although regulations are aimed at keeping body contact to a minimum, collisions send these players to the floor or somersaulting over sportscasters on a regular basis. Because players don't wear protective gear, a moving body meeting an immovable object can provide some fairly spectacular falls—most are pretty minor, but some result in serious injuries.

Basketball is a rigorous, fast-moving, highly ballistic sport that keeps the players in perpetual motion.

As a result, most players are in good shape. Repetitive movements, like running, jumping, pivoting, rapidly changing direction, rotating, and shooting—some of which is airborne!—characterize the sport. These skills, sharpened by drills and honed by long games, put an athlete's body at risk of physical injury, particularly to tendons, ligaments, and muscles that stabilize joints. Landing from a layup, for example, produces forces seven times your body weight; a jump shot produces forces five times your body weight.

The good news is that back injuries are rare and most commonly the result of trauma, particularly among young or inexperienced players. In kids under the age of 15, basketball is the fourth leading cause of injury in both unorganized and organized team sports. Girls and women are injured more frequently than their male counterparts, and their injuries tend to be more serious. Here are a couple of ways you can help prevent injuries on the court.

Know your weak spots. Most injuries take place in practice, and most often in the feet and ankles, where supersized feet can become stress-fractured by supersized workouts on a hard floor, or fractured by collision or stomping. In addition, strains and sprains are common. Trainers keep vast stores of tape in the locker room for just such occasions. In order of physiological demand, from most to least, your body's most vulnerable points are the knee, ankle, lower back, shin, hip, shoulder, neck, wrist, foot, groin, and fingers.

Proper stretching and conditioning, using the Active-Isolated method, can help prevent most of the overuse or traumatic injuries in these areas.

Shop for smart shoes. Perhaps the best precaution you can take is to be very selective about your shoes. Basketball shoes are specifically designed to provide a little cushion between your foot and the floor, give a little support to the ankle, and to pivot by virtue of special engineering on the sole, particularly at the ball of your foot, where you'll bear the weight of that move.

Get a clean surface. If you're playing on an outside court, inspect the court first to make sure it's free from debris and the surface is smooth without holes or buckles in the paving.

Kids, take precautions. Experts advise that children wear knee and elbow pads, mouth guards, and eye protection. (Frankly, adults could take a cue.)

Hydrate—carefully. Remember to drink frequently, so you're always hydrated, but be sure to keep your water off the court. A wet, slick spot can send one of your teammates skidding.

Know your secret-weapon stretch: tibialis anteriors. The floor of a basketball court is hard and the cushioning in basketball shoes is minimal. Because you'll be running, stopping, turning, pivoting, jumping (and winning), you need to make sure that your heels can strike the floor without damaging the fronts of your shins. When the heel is down and the forefoot is up, your shin strains. It's exacerbated by the lightning-fast hammering your feet take as you thunder up and down the court. Don't hide this stretch from your teammates, because you'll want them all to benefit from it, but don't ever do it in front of your opponents and give away one of the best-kept secrets in injury prevention and flexibility in movement.

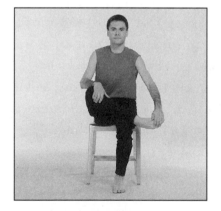

TIBIALIS ANTERIORS
See complete instructions on page 314.

BIATHLON: SKIING AND SHOOTING

We'll talk about skiing in its own sections (see pages 324 and 328), but let's talk for a moment about shooting. Shooting puts a unique set of contradictory demands on an athlete. On the one hand, you have to be strong so you can extend, support, and stabilize the weight of a weapon at lightning speed when your adrenaline is pumping you into overdrive. On the other hand, you must create a stillness around you so you can focus like a laser, take accurate aim, and squeeze off the shot with a tiny, almost imperceptible contraction of one finger. Shooters claim that in that split second, nothing else in the world exists except the marksman and the target. Your whole body goes to work while your mind locks in.

Shooting is really easy—shooting accurately is tough. Since the dawn of guns, accuracy has required practice, and practice in any physical activity almost always leads to the evolution of that activity into sport. Shooting has been a part of the Olympic Games since 1896, and today the sport boasts several different specialties: free pistol, rapid-fire pistol, small-bore pistol, prone, skeet, and moving target for men; and sport pistol, air rifle, small-bore standard rifle, trapshooting, and skeet for women.

In shooting, your body must be relaxed but balanced in perfect equilibrium. This requires tightening your entire muscular system to give you a backward slant and simultaneously rotating your trunk. After you have rotated and leaned, you lock into position with your abdominal muscles (in the front), the muscles in your back along your spine (the erector spinae), groin (psoas), and the middle and lower back (quadratus lumborum). Your pelvis is braced by the hip abductors and adductors along with the hip flexors and extensors. Your upper ankle joint, the front of your leg (tibialis anterior), and your lower leg (a couple of muscles that form the triceps surae) must be both strong and flexible to provide the endurance required in holding the stance and maintaining balance.

Stability of your weapon is provided by the arm holding it and the shoulder on that same side. Your elbow and hip on the opposite side are also part of the stabilizing muscles, helping take some of the burden off the muscle behind your shoulder, the pos-terior deltoid. You might *look* like you're standing stock-still, but your back is working like a dog, as long as you're twisted and supporting weight on only one side.

One year we worked at the World Track and Field Games in Göteborg, Sweden. We were working as therapists for the Mizuno athletes. One of the Swedish coaches approached us to take a look at an athlete, but he wasn't a runner—he was a biathlete suffering from upper-back pain, a full two seasons after his last competition.

The athlete was a tall, friendly guy, but his height might have been part of the problem. His back was working against gravity in a challenging stance—holding the rifle cantilevered out in front of his body and contracting all his muscles to hold still to pull the trigger. These muscles had been cold and exhausted from skiing before he even began. We found minor imbalances and weaknesses that were easily remedied with the stretching and strengthening program. Two years later, he made the team and did very well. He taught us a few things about successful shooting.

Treat it like any other sport. Shooting, like any sport, is more successful and enjoyable if you are fit. A full supplemental stretching and strengthening program is in order, as well as a cardio workout.

Focus for safety. In the heat of competition, you may be rushing to get to the next target, but take good care of your weapon and practice safety at all times. You know this is one sport where a mistake can take a life.

Take precautions for the weather. Be careful about working out when you're cold. It's a good idea to start gently and work your way up into enthusiasm.

Know your secret-weapon stretch: hip abductors. In addition to your regular Active-Isolated Stretching and Strengthening and cardio workout, we have one stretch just for you. Do it right before you shoot to enhance your performance by helping to steady your stance.

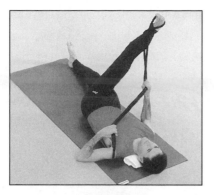

HIP ABDUCTORS
See complete instructions on page 44.

CRICKET

For the past couple of years, we've helped runners prepare for the Barbados Independence Day marathon, which starts at 4:30 in the morning to beat the heat of the Caribbean sun. In the week before, we conduct workshops to give runners tips on preparing and recovering. But it seems that the marathon pales in comparison to the intense cricket matches that go on in the field next to our hotel, all day and well into the night. One year we noticed that, among the runners we were coaching, were men and women dressed not in nylon running shorts but in pressed white uniforms. Cricket players had sneaked into our stretch classes. We loved it.

Cricket appears to be an innocuous, highly civilized game played by well-mannered gentlemen and gentlewomen who follow polite rules that have governed the game since antiquity. They are, after all, wearing white. So if it's so civilized and well-manner and polite, why is it necessary for a cricket player to wear a helmet fitted with a shatter-proof face visor, a high-impact-resistant chest protector, forearm guard, gloves, genital protector, thigh pads, and shin pads? What could eclipse a thousand years of gentility? A little 5.5-ounce ball rocketing toward you at a scorching 90 miles per hour—so much for manners.

Of course, getting beaned by a ball that moves faster than you can duck is not your only concern. Protective gear and a dead-eye bowler will assure you

a bean-free day. Injuries in cricket are specific to the aspects of the game.

Bowling—propelling the ball—is less like overhand pitching or underhand tossing in American baseball and more like throwing the javelin. Injuries to the bowler are nearly identical: lower-spine strain is common as the bowler runs into position, arches his back, rotates his hips, and then swings into and through the bowl, javelin-style. The mandatory straight elbow that distinguishes the "bowl" from a "throw" strains the shoulder, specifically the rotator cuff. Nerve impingement and overuse injuries of the shoulder are the most common problems in the sport.

In fielding, injuries occur when a quietly waiting player springs into action. From standing, alert and waiting, muscles are not prepared to move. When the ball rockets into the field, the player reacts quickly and dynamically. It's not uncommon for something to strain or tear.

Most batting injuries are caused because the back foot must remain on the ground when a player bats, so the Achilles tendon can suffer irritation and run the risk of rupture.

The wicket keeper's knees may strain and fatigue from squatting for long periods of time. And we'll tell you something else. An extensive Australian study of injury in cricket suggests that fatigue is as great a contributor to injury as anything else. Playing twice, as in a day–night game, increases risk.

Although cricket is generally considered to be a low-injury sport, it has its risks. You'll prevent injury and play better if you are strong and flexible and in shape. Preventing injuries, maximizing performance, and winning are matters of training and preparation.

Focus on your back and shoulders. The back, when bowling or batting, needs to be strong and flexible in order to avoid straining. The shoulder requires particular attention because it's the most commonly injured joint in cricket, most often damaged in throwing. Strengthening the primary muscles such as your shoulders (deltoids), the top of your upper back (trapezius), and your chest (pectoralis) is necessary.

Don't forget to stretch. Equally critical are flexibility and generous ranges of motion in all joints. When you're loose and warmed up, you can move more quickly without irritation. Also, the greater your ranges of motion, the greater your reach, the longer your stride, and the more torque and power you can put into rotation and windup.

Train hard. Being fit goes a long way in championship play. The good news is that cricket players are in better shape today than at any other time in history, because training methods have improved along with our understanding of the complexity of the game's demands. Also contributing to high-level athletics is the popularity of one-day play, which has put increasing demands on the players to survive the rigors of the accelerated game.

Know your secret-weapon stretch: rotator cuff 2. With ballistic throwing and catching, your shoulders need all the help they can get. The shoulder is the most mobile of all our joints. And yet, it's the most delicate, held together not by interlocking bone, but by muscles and connective tissue. It's highly susceptible to injury. To stay in the game and win, you have to keep your shoulders in great shape.

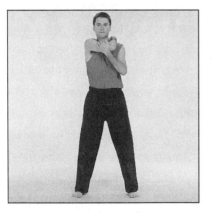

ROTATOR CUFF 2
See complete instructions on page 58.

CROSS-COUNTRY (NORDIC) SKIING

Rodoy, Norway, boasts a rock with a crude line drawing of a hunter on skis, the first evidence of cross-country skiing, dated as early as 2500 B.C. The first skis were basic transportation—a way to travel across deep snow—but around 1000 A.D., some Icelanders figured out that skiing was fun and turned it into a sport (along with betting). Although it has changed much since its early days, some things remain: Cross-country skiing is good transportation, good sport, and good fun.

As the snowmobile has eclipsed the cross-country ski as deep-snow transportation, cross-country skiing has been elevated to high art in the world of sports. Technology makes new advances in design and materials every season. Gone are the heavy wooden skis that dragged. Today's Fiberglas and graphite skis are smoother, lighter, and slicker on the surface of snow. But all this means that the skier has to be stronger to control direction and speed. Moving might be easier, but it's harder to control in many ways.

We are avid cross-country skiers ourselves, relying on it in the winter to keep up our cardiovascular fitness when running would sink us in a snowdrift up to our eyeballs. We recommend it highly—this unparalleled workout puts all major muscle groups to work and really gets your heart rate up. Not only is it spectacular exercise, it's really easy on your joints. Besides, we are big fans of fresh air and sunshine.

We also have a cross-country ski machine in our clinic for those times when the snow has melted but the call of the mountain backcountry beckons us with its pleasures. Many of our clients own them, too. They are inexpensive and easy to assemble, take up little space, require no electricity, and can be outfitted with all sorts of bells and whistles to monitor your workout and make it more entertaining.

It's impossible to single out muscles when describing the physiology of cross-country skiing, but that's precisely our point. It works everything from your buttocks and legs that power you forward, to your hip flexors (muscles along the fronts of your hips) and thighs that drive the momentum. In perfect concert, your arms are swinging, pushing, pulling, and poling from your shoulders and back. Your abdominals and back provide stability and balance. Everything works together in perfect rhythm. And everything requires strength and flexibility,

CASE STUDY: JASON ALLEN

Jason is a runner who also coaches cross-country skiing in Vermont. He was in constant pain on the left side of his lower back that wrapped around his hip. He had tried everything. Some things gave temporary relief, but nothing held up under normal activity. Pain returned with a vengeance. He was fearfully concerned that there would be no more fun in the snow. His life as an athlete looked bleak.

We sometimes travel to Vermont, so we met with him there. When we evaluated Jason, we discovered that he was simply imbalanced. His outer thigh was weak, so his hip was compensating and fatiguing. The hip was transmitting that compensation to the glute, which was shorting out. And the glute was passing the misery right up to his lower back. There was no flexibility in his pelvis, and it wasn't stable.

How Jason Got Out of Pain: All we did was calm everything down and restore range of motion through a plain, old Active-Isolated Stretching routine. Jason experienced immediate relief. When he was flexible, we added strengthening with special emphasis on the adductors and abductors in his thighs. Once they were strong and balanced, his pelvis stabilized, and his back no longer had to overwork.

In 3 weeks, we had stabilized that pelvis and relaxed his back. Usually, a program takes 6 weeks before a muscle is fully reprogrammed, but when a muscle is really weakened, little things make a big difference. A weakened muscle loses its neural drive—its ability to read and respond to signals from the brain. As a consequence, it actually loses the ability to fire properly. In small moves, Jason not only strengthened his muscles but also restored their ability to respond to the brain's command.

Jason's problem is solved. He's now working out with Active-Isolated Stretching and Strengthening . . . and waiting for snow.

---

and endurance that comes from cardio training.

Pinpointing injuries in cross-country skiing is tricky, because unlike injured downhill skiers or snowboarders, who present themselves to the ski patrol and are transported to the hospital where statistical data is compiled, cross-country skiers are elusive. What we do know is that because the skis are narrow, they tend to be unstable. And the boots are little more than fancy sneakers attached to the skis with lightweight bindings. It's easy to get off balance, particularly in turns. Fortunately, injuries appear to be uncommon. Here are a few ways to prevent those that can happen.

Warm up adequately. Your back is at risk because of all the poling you'll be doing—a cold muscle going into a cold environment tends to contract

Before you begin, remember to get your muscles warmed up. A few quick stretches before you step out onto the snow will get your circulation flowing and begin the warmup. Another tip is to start your course slowly and gently. When you feel warmed up and ready, you can increase speed and effort. As you ski, you'll feel warmer and more comfortable, and your back will be all right.

Loosen up. Of the few injuries that do occur, most are of the thumb, caused when the skier falls onto an outstretched hand still holding the pole. These injuries are easily prevented by remembering to loosen your grip as you fall.

Watch your edges. Injuries of note are the boot-top fractures and ankle sprains from catching a ski edge and falling—the ski stops, but the skier doesn't. Be mindful of the grooves in which you run your skis, so you can keep in perfect balance.

Rehydrate regularly. Remember that cross-country skiing is hard work and you'll be sweating, so drink plenty of fluids. Take a bottle of water with you.

Protect yourself from the sun. The protective atmospheric levels are diminished at altitude. Compound that with glare off the snow, and you have eyestrain and sunburn. Wear eye protection and slather sunscreen on all exposed body parts.

Leave word behind. Like a pilot "filing a flight plan," it's good to have backup . . . just in case. We suggest that you tell someone where you're going and when you'll be back. And if you're within range, carrying a cell phone is a good safety measure.

Know your secret-weapon stretch: psoas. Cross-country skiing is easier when you rely less on hip flexors and recruit deep muscles in your groin and upper thighs to power the glides. Get on your hands and knees. Make sure that the snow is soft enough to cushion your knees and the tops of your feet, but not so soft that you sink in up to your face. With the knee bent, extend your left leg until your foot is off the snow.

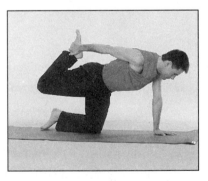

PSOAS
See complete instructions on page 45.

CYCLING

Cycling started out as basic transportation and remains so for many people around the world, but the complex partnership between an athlete and a bicycle can be thrilling. For some, it's a reverent way of life; for others, it's a joyful ride with the wind in their hair and a passing countryside. For everyone, cycling can be a great workout.

Many years ago, we started our practice in Gainesville, Florida, one of the best-kept secrets in training meccas. This wonderland of fantastic weather, landscape loaded with good trails, and plenty of sports medicine professionals overflows with sports teams who come to train in privacy. When we worked with one of the major cycling teams, we noticed that their hamstrings were tight, their quads had blown up, and their backs were trashed from hundreds of miles of training a week.

Their hamstrings and quads were easy to recover, but their backs were not. In a rider, the back is always in flexion, bent over and stabilizing to hold the cyclist in perfect aerodynamic position. This position does not promote circulation, relaxation, or recovery at all. Also, some of the younger, less-experienced riders tightened their hands around the handlebar grips and translated that tension up through their arms and shoulders and straight into their backs. Even short periods of time holding the grips too tightly would do it. We had to teach everyone to relax. And almost all the work we did with them was to unlock tortured backs.

Because cycling is primarily pedaling, the legs are the drivers in rotation. When pressing down and out on the pedal, you use hip and knee extensors (quads) and ankle flexors (tibialis anterior). In assisting to bring the pedal up in rotation, you use your hip and knee flexors (hamstrings) and ankle extensors (gastrocnemius muscles). These rotations and the forces that drive them are consistent side to side, particularly with the use of toe clips that lock the feet into position on the pedals. Arm extensors help you turn the bike and support some of the weight of your body as you lean into the grips in that signature aerodynamic position. But the weight isn't fully supported by your hands on the grips; your flexed back and contracted abdominals stabilize your torso—transmitting the support work of your arms to your legs. Your upper back and neck are holding your head up, face forward and made heavier by a helmet. As you pedal, you are getting a no-impact aerobic workout.

But cycling is not a perfect exercise. Pedaling around and around in a tight concentric circle shortens the muscles when they work, particularly the hamstrings. In order to be healthy and balanced, a muscle needs to be elongated as well as contracted and shortened, but cycling can produce imbalanced, inflexible muscles. Sports medicine experts also rank cycling high in injury statistics. In fact, injury is an inherent part of cycling. Most common injuries are traumatic and the direct result of impact and skidding on pavement. Common are road rash, cuts, bruises, and broken bones. We also see repetitive stress injuries and overuse injuries that we can help you avoid with these tips.

Take steps to combat nerve compression. Among the most common overuse injuries we see are nerve compressions of the hand (ulnar nerve) and forearm (radial distal nerve) from pressure on the handlebar grip—holding on too tightly for too long or resting one's weight too completely on the palm of the hand. Contracted muscles tighten up and put the nerves into compression, causing pain, numbness, fatigue, weakness, and irritation. Wear padded gloves and remove your hands from the grips one at a time, shake them out, and wiggle your fingers to get blood flowing.

We also see some nerve compression in the foot from wearing tight shoes, keeping too short a distance between the seat and the pedals, putting too much force down on the pedal for extended periods of time, and having weak muscles of the lower leg. Flexibility training will probably get you out of nerve compression, but it may take some time before you are 100 percent.

Stretch and strengthen to avoid inflammation. We see inflammation of the tendons at their attachments at the hip, knee, and ankle; overly tight quadriceps compressing the kneecap against the joint (major discomfort); pressure on the nerves of the cervical spine at the back of the neck from hyperextending and fatiguing the neck in holding the head up; lower-back pain as we explained earlier; and pain deep in the buttocks (sciatica, or piriformis syndrome). Flexibility and strength will prevent all of these problems.

Select your seat carefully. Another injury we see is nerve compression between a rider's legs from sitting too long on a seat so hard that circulation is cut off. Avoiding nerve compression between the legs is a matter of lifting your booty once in a while—just stand up on the pedals and get the pressure off your butt. Another option is to get a better seat, one that is cushioned by padding or diffuses pressure with gel. Try as many as you can until you get a perfect fit for your physiology and comfort level. There are even seats that support your "cheeks" but have a gap where more-sensitive body parts can be free. Unfortunately, this is one area where a stretch rope just won't do.

Vary your posture. Sit straight upright from time to time and take the pressure off your back and neck. Move your head from side to side, but carefully. You don't want to throw off your equilibrium.

Be prepared for problems. Keep a repair kit and a spare inner tube with you in the event of a flat, and always cycle with a cell phone.

Don't forget the water. Remember to drink plenty of fluids. When you're flying along, it's so easy to get fooled into thinking that you're not really sweating, because at high speeds, sweat quickly dries to cool you.

Safety first. And *always* remember to wear your helmet. We want you to survive a spill.

Know your secret-weapon stretch: quadriceps. The correct rotation of the pedal limits range of motion in your joints and builds muscles that can easily become out of balance. Strong and flexible quads are essential for powering the cycle.

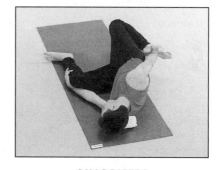

QUADRICEPS
See complete instructions on page 46.

DOWNHILL SKIING

In skiing, control is a matter of simple physics—a breathless lift into weightlessness followed by digging in or side-slipping that causes a change in direction or speed.

Skiing is also a matter of shock absorption. And we're not talking about bouncing off a pine tree. We're talking about taking a pounding in moguls. All these dynamics in combination really put the body to work. Your hip extensors, knee extensors, and plantar flexors carry your lead leg forward. Your rear leg is held forward by your hip flexors. Your abdominals and back support your torso, providing stability for your leg extensors. The metatarsal arch in your foot bears your weight when you plant your foot, providing stability during any balance of weight shifts from side to side.

Speaking of shock absorption, the design of today's ski closely mirrors the shock-absorbing properties of the human foot: There's a slight arch in the center of the ski, which takes a hammering but then quickly dissipates those forces outward. You swing, lift, plant, and maneuver around your poles using your back, shoulders, arms, hands, and wrists. With exercise like this, it's easy to fatigue everything, especially your back.

According to the National Sporting Goods Association, more than 10 million people ski each year. Skiing can be wonderful fun and great exercise, but it can also be risky. The good news is that injuries are down from the early days, because of better equipment, better slope development and maintenance, and better training. Lower-limb fractures used to top the list of maladies, but the high-tech, impact-resistant boots have provided a measure of protection that has lowered the statistic significantly.

Unfortunately, although ankles and shins are safer, the knees are still taking a wallop—particularly the anterior cruciate ligaments. This is the most common of all injuries. The boots allow limited movement of your ankles, so when you decide to change the angles of your feet and skis, you must effect that change from your knees and hips, exerting force on the front and sides of your shin to translate your decision down through the boot to the ski to the snow. The tibialis anterior and the triceps surae in your lower legs are also involved.

When you first begin skiing, you'll notice that the smallest moves make big differences, especially at high speeds. Good skiers make it look easy with very subtle, controlled adjustments in position. A beginner who is not quite as strong has to throw the whole body into a maneuver, which can be awkward and exhausting. As a skier improves, all movements are stronger, more subtle, and more quickly performed—all of which is helped incredibly by overall fitness.

As we researched back injuries among skiers, we discovered that although back injuries don't top the list, no body part is immune from getting hurt when you're hurtling down a mountain at top speed and something goes wrong. The best defense is experience and training. In fact, inexperienced skiers hold the record for all accidents: four to one over the experts. Here are a few ways you can better those odds.

Stay in shape throughout the year. Strength and flexibility will give you some of the skills you need. You need good reflexes, coordination, and balance. And all of these qualities can come from working out.

Don't forget your cardio. At some less-advanced levels, skiing is not a complete exercise, so you'll want to supplement your training with some cardio workouts. Running, cycling, or inline skating at altitude yields superior cardiovascular benefits. At altitude, the air isn't as dense in oxygen, so your body adjusts to it by increasing red blood cells to carry the little oxygen they can get as you cycle air through your lungs. This increase in red blood cells—and that little extra boost—is amazing when you return to sea level.

Eat and drink for fuel and warmth. Remember that being cold causes your body to shiver to keep you warm, which will burn extra calories. Eat small amounts often so that you can keep your blood sugar levels up for maximum, consistent energy.

Additionally, we encourage you to drink water. Dehydration can creep up on you without warning.

Beware the weather. The blinding sun reflecting off the snow can be beautiful—but very dangerous to your eyes and skin. Wear goggles to protect you from glare and use high-SPF sunscreen. Also, dress in layers that will keep you warm and wick sweat away from your body.

Don't take unnecessary risks. Stay on marked slopes and trails. Please stay on slopes that are at your level. (Here's a hint: Black Diamond to a beginner means, "Ski here and die.") Mistakes in skiing can be dangerous—for you and others. Be smart.

Know your secret-weapon stretch: hip abductors. Everyone will think you're making a snow angel, but this stretch will keep you loose on the slopes and make maneuvering and shock absorption easier on your legs. Lie down on your back on hard-packed flat snow with both legs extended straight out.

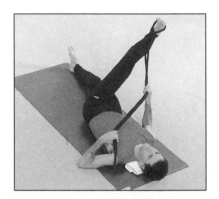

HIP ABDUCTORS
See complete instructions on page 44.

DUATHLON (OR BIATHLON)

We like duathlons (known commonly as biathlons), because they are an eloquent testimony to the power of cross-training. Competitors are challenged to keep performance levels high in more than one discipline, which generally produces a more well-rounded athlete.

Duathlons are sporting events in which you bike and run, or bike/run/bike, or run/bike/run, or run/swim, or ski/shoot. Which sports are included usually depends on where the event is held and who is organizing the competition.

Duathletes are usually in great shape, not only because of the high levels of performance that demand top conditioning but also because of the transition between the two sports. In order to arrange a physical and mental transition between the two, you have to have skill and focus, but being able to do it is half the fun of competing.

In order to explore the stretches for your duathlon, you'll have to look up each individual sport. We would, however, like to discuss your transitions, the principles for which are the same, no matter what the sports are.

Have a transition strategy. Because of the buildup of metabolic waste in the initial activity, the transition to a different activity requiring different movement puts a greater stress on your body than if you just continued on with the initial event. Your muscles may tighten and lock up because they are "shocked." They have no opportunity to recover and stretch out. They may be in a pattern of contraction or fatigued to the point that they will be signaling difficulty—which you'll be forced to ignore in order to move into the next stage of competition. Practice your transition as often as if it were a third sport in the competition.

Know your secret-weapon stretch: standing gluteals (on page 330). In duathlons, the risk of injury increases twofold: double the sport, double the opportunity for pain. You might be a great runner, for example, but running potentially could be irritating if you do it right after you cycle. Staying flexible will help.

STANDING GLUTEALS

Active Muscles You Contract: Abdominals and muscles from the fronts of your hips down the fronts of your thighs

Isolated Muscles You Stretch: Muscles in your lower back that rotate your torso, the muscles that rotate your hips, and buttocks

Hold Each Stretch: 2 seconds

Reps: 10 on the right, 10 on the left

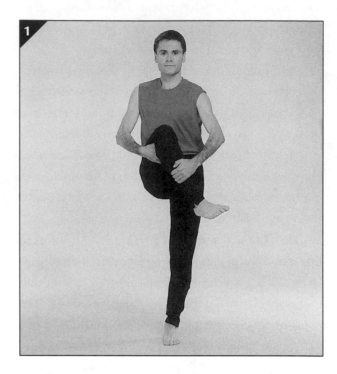

1. Stand with your feet shoulder-width apart and your knees relaxed. Start with your right side. Place the palm of your right hand on your outer right thigh. Using your abdominal muscles, inner thigh, quadriceps, and hip flexors (muscles along the fronts of your hips), bend your knee and lift your right thigh up and toward your left side until you can feel the stretch in your hip. Gently guide the stretch with pressure from your hand on the outer thigh.

   If you want a deeper stretch, you can grasp the outside of your shin with your left hand and assist the stretch toward the midline of your body. Don't force it. Add the slightest pressure, extending the range of the stretch just a little more. Hold for 2 seconds and then relax in preparation for the next stretch. Repeat on the left side. For efficiency, do 10 stretches on the right and then 10 on the left.

GOLF

A few years ago, Roger Fredericks, the director of instruction at the Kaanapali Golf College in Maui, Hawaii, noticed some significant changes in performance of one of his players from the previous year. This player's swing had been limited by his stiff back, but when the golfer returned to Maui from a trip to New York, his game improved like magic.

The golfer confessed that, aside from standard tourist fare, his trip to New York had also included a visit with us. We had unlocked his back and hips with Active-Isolated Stretching and Strengthening, taught him all the techniques, put a stretch rope around his neck, kissed him on both cheeks, shouted "Aloha!," and sent him back to Maui. Roger Fredericks was impressed and curious, so he hopped on a plane to New York to study with us for a week. Now he starts every golf lesson with Active-Isolated work. "I can't improve a golfer's game or swing until we unlock his or her pelvis," he says. "It's the *only* way I've found to get the pressure off the back and turn that golfer loose."

A golf swing is one of the most complex of all athletic endeavors. The swing demands a full range of motion from nearly every joint in the body, so full flexibility is essential. The areas of your body that most affect a swing are your abdominals for stabilization and rotation; your hip, trunk, arm, and shoulder for the golf swing; and your wrist for grip, control, and stability.

The forces that propel the swing start low, in your ankles and feet, travel up your legs as you begin your torque, go through your knees up your thighs to your hips, accelerate through your trunk, and drive up through your chest and shoulder as you tightly coil to draw back and lift into position your arms, wrists, and hands. From this position, you're in full rotation with your eye on the ball. At this moment, you're gauging forces, speed, direction, finesse, and power necessary to strike that ball perfectly to put it where you want it. You experience a moment of complete stillness, and then—pow!—you unwind explosively, sweeping your arms, wrists, and hands down in that controlled, graceful arc that forms your swing.

Power and momentum drive your follow-through into a reverse "C" finish. And here is a simple lesson in physics for you. The more flexible you are, the farther you can bring the club away from the ball as you wind up. Increasing this range creates more swing speed, which gives you more distance and accuracy on your drive. And being able to sweep into your follow-through means that you have smoother control of your shot. Flexibility means more power, control, distance, accuracy, and fewer overuse injuries.

In professional golfers, the most common injuries are to the wrist, back, hand, shoulder, and knee.

In amateur golfers, the situation is different. Amateur injuries line up as the lower back, elbow, wrist, shoulder, and knee.

We want you out there on the links, so do your best to avoid injury by trying some of these strategies.

Work on that swing. In both professionals and amateurs, most injuries are caused by ineffective swing mechanics and inefficient warmup. The difference between amateur and professional lower-back pain is that amateurs, less trained, load the spine more. And they lack the organized muscle-firing patterns that develop only with time and experience.

Emphasize flexibility. Professional golfers have the highest incidence of back injury of any professional athlete. The culprit is usually torsional stress on a back that is too inflexible to absorb the rotation in the hips, knees, and shoulders, and is unable to spread the stresses over the entire spine, which is where they should be. Lower-back pain can be caused by a poor swing. And a poor swing can be caused by lower-back pain. Get strong and flexible, and your swing will improve.

Prepare your body. Although you may be itching to get out there, take the time to warm up and cool down. Preparing your body for exercise is always important, but Mark McLaughlin, M.D., from the department of neurosurgery at Tufts University School of Medicine in Springfield, Massachusetts, says it's especially important when your back is hurting or weak.

Don't be proud. If your back is in pain, move your ball out of angled lies, thick rough, and pot bunkers rather than take the shot. If you're not up to playing, take some time off. A little rest now can preserve your game for the long term.

Take along your water bottle. You're going to be out in the sun, so stay hydrated.

Get in some of your cardio. If you can, leave the golf cart and walk. If you can carry or pull your own clubs, all the better. Still, remember that golf will not give you a well-rounded workout. You'll need to augment your fitness program with other cardio, strength, and flexibility training. Now go out there and have a great time!

Know your secret-weapon stretch: lateral trunk flexors. In addition to your regular workout, here's a stretch that you can use in the locker room right before you step out onto the course. It gets your circulation going and loosens up the muscles in your back and along the sides of your trunk. The result? More dynamic torque in the windup and release of your swing.

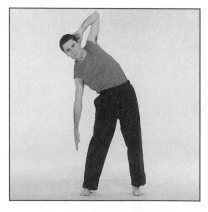

TRUNK LATERAL FLEXORS
See complete instructions on page 51.

HIKING AND BACKPACKING

We define the difference between hiking and walking this way: Hiking *is* walking, but it usually involves covering distance and is usually done in a rural or wilderness setting. Hiking is often combined with other activities such as backpacking, high-country fishing, mountaineering, and bird-watching.

Hiking not only gets you out the door and into the great beyond, it's also a great workout for your hips, back, legs, and feet. Hiking can be a decent cardiovascular workout if you intensify the pace or add hills that cause you to work a little. At sea level, on flat paths, at strolling pace, and while carrying nothing, hiking can be an easy saunter; at altitude, clawing your way up a graded trail at a searing pace with a 35-pound pack strapped to your back, hiking can be an amazing workout. One sport, variable levels. Your choice.

With hiking, injuries are few unless you stumble and fall or are subject to some unfortunate accident like a landslide or an encounter with some unfriendly wildlife. But now, let's talk about backpacking. Physiologically speaking, backpacking is hiking after you strap on a considerable amount of weight, which probably includes the gear needed for setting up a camp, preparing food, and sleeping. How heavy or light your pack is makes no difference—your body is not used to having your center of gravity moved behind you and bearing the extra weight. Moreover, we are willing to bet that you are planning to carry that weight for a considerable distance over uneven terrain.

When you put a pack on your back—even a light one—it tends to pull you over backward. To compensate, you'll automatically lean forward at the waist and tighten your lower abdominals. Muscles in your lower back contract to keep you upright, causing your pelvis to rock slightly forward and arch your back to take the pressure off. On short hikes, this is no problem. For longer hikes, if you're not conditioned, you might fatigue. Take some precautions to help keep your hikes pain-free.

Train in advance. The problem is that unless you're a forest ranger, hikes are intermittent. The workouts can be spectacular, but they're infrequent and inconsistent. You lose fitness levels in between treks, so you can't really rely on hiking to be your entire workout program. You have to do some extra work in flexibility, strength, and cardiovascular conditioning on a frequent basis to be fit enough to enjoy a good hike. (And it wouldn't hurt you to do some walking in your hiking boots on local pathways and hills, just to stay in practice for managing uneven surfaces.)

Buy the best boots you can afford. Footwear is the most important aspect of guaranteeing a good hike. Invest in shoes or boots that are manufactured specifically for hiking. Today, these are lightweight and comfortable, designed to support your ankles on uneven surfaces and help keep you from fatiguing over long distances.

Have your boots professionally fit. If your boots are too big, you'll slide in them. Downhill hiking will jam your toes to the front. Uphill hiking will jam your heels to the rear. And you'll never be steady and stable on uneven surfaces if your foot moves but your boot doesn't.

Keep your feet dry. Another miraculous hallmark of good hiking boots is their ability to keep your feet dry by creating an ingenious one-way moisture barrier that keeps outside dampness from seeping in, yet allows sweat to wick out. When you have a dry foot, you're less likely to develop pressure "hot spots" or blisters.

Choose the right socks. You'll also want to wear sports socks designed to wick sweat and prevent blisters. They are soft and tightly woven, and they don't have seams on the inside to rub. Make sure they fit you tightly enough to prevent bunching, and be sure to try them on with the boot you've selected.

Break out the petroleum jelly. A blister-prevention secret from marathon runners who put 26.2 miles of pounding on their feet at one time: Put a thin film of petroleum jelly on the soles of your feet and your toes before putting on your socks. It will reduce friction.

Hike prepared. If you're going to be out for more than an hour, you'll want to carry a few supplies. For short trips, you'll need only the basics: water, a snack, a little first-aid kit, a compass, a cell phone, binoculars, a camera, and a whistle.

Keep the load light. Carrying anything, no matter how small, does two things to your workout: It adds weight that increases your load (good for increasing stamina!), and it adds that weight to your back, unbalancing your natural gait (bad for increasing pressure on your back!). Trim down to the essentials and carry extras in a fanny pack or a little ruck sack.

Invest in a good pack. Today's pack, although it's carried on your back, is actually supported by your hips, cinched with a padded belt to your pelvis below your waist. This takes the pressure off your spine. The shoulder straps, often a suspension system, merely stabilize the bulk of the pack and keep it from falling backward.

You can make it even better if you pack most of your heavy items in the bottom of the pack near your pelvis, or against your back, where they are closer in to your center of gravity. If you know what you're taking on your trip, practice carrying that much weight before you get out on the trail. You'll have more fun if you're in shape.

Don't forget to drink. Backpacking is demanding. You need water. Outdoor suppliers have figured out how to make powdered food, but they have yet to figure out how to make powdered water, so you'll have to carry it.

If you can't carry enough water for the entire trip, make certain that you are hiking near potable water sources, carry a filtration system, or bring along some tablets that you can drop into almost any slime and make it drinkable.

Know your secret-weapon stretch: trunk extensors. The only competitor you'll find on the trail is your own lack of flexibility and strength. Hiking on uneven surfaces and covering the ups and downs of the trail are hard on your lower back, especially if you hike with a pack. This is a two-in-one stretch. It not only stretches your back nicely but also allows you to contract your abdominals, the muscles that support your back. Sit on flat ground or a flat rock with your back straight, your knees bent, your toes pointed slightly up, and your feet resting on your heels.

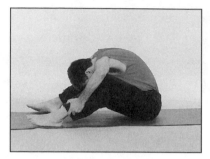

TRUNK EXTENSORS
See complete instructions on page 49.

INLINE SKATING

Inline skating was developed by Scott and Brennan Olson of Minnesota as an off-season training tool for skiers and ice hockey players. Done downhill, this skating closely approximates the physics of skiing, complete with weight transfer, edging, and turns. Some ski resorts even have inline skating trails for training in the summer. On the flats—the way most of us will do it—inline skating closely approximates the physics of ice hockey. In fact, we've seen many a summer hockey game here in Central Park.

Skating provides low-impact (mostly!) aerobic exercise and can be done right out your front door. The skates and protective gear are inexpensive, and it can be great fun. Although it is enjoyed by people of all ages and persuasions in life, it's now officially designated as an "extreme" sport, a reputation earned by daring young skaters who defy gravity (and sometimes mortal injury) with impressive acrobatics.

For most of us, inline skating is uncomplicated. All you need is one inexpensive pair of skates, as much protective equipment as you can

put on, and a vast expanse of pavement. Although the first thing you must learn to do is brake, skating begins with balance and coordination. (Adding speed and learning fancy moves come later.) You learn to roll forward, then add pushing off, with each foot in a stabilizing diagonal from which pressure can be exerted to move the other foot forward. You shift your weight over the advancing skate and repeat the process, which propels you forward.

To stabilize, you use the abductors in your hips, buttocks (gluteals), thighs (quads), and calves (soleus). Your trunk flexes forward from your hips with your back straight, engaging and contracting your abdominals, lower back, and hip flexors and extensors to create that signature forward thrust. For turns and changing direction, you use hip abductors and adductors. For spins and rotations, you fire your hip and trunk rotators. For jumps, you lift off with your gluteals and abdominals and absorb shock with your hips. For backward movement, you turn your head with your neck rotators, hyperextend your hip for direction changes and abduct and adduct your hips for propulsion. Arm and torso swinging (rhythmic side-to-side motion) is controlled by your hip rotators, abductors, and adductors, with your back and abdominals providing stabilization. In other words, you get nearly a full-body workout.

Most injuries from inline skating are the results of trauma. Skaters fall down, crash into or fall off things, or slam into each other. But skaters have a high incidence of lower-back pain related to the repetitive movement and the extreme forward flexed position of the skater's trunk. This pain can be easily bypassed with stretching and adequate warmup. Also, it's a good idea to stand up straight and take some of the tension out of your back with a few quick releases. Here are a few tips to make your inline skating injuries a little less "extreme."

Spare no precaution. We weren't kidding: Wear

every bit of protection you can. Padding and bracing are critical for protecting knees, elbows, and wrists. Also, we insist that you wear a helmet. Head injuries are very serious and totally unnecessary.

Compensate the upper body. Inline skating, when you're really pumping, is a wonderful aerobic workout that lets you work your lower extremities, but your upper body is sort of neglected. You'll want to supplement your training with general strength and flexibility and with attention to upper body work.

Don't forget your lower half. Even though you're working your lower body pretty hard, don't forget that the skate boot restricts your foot and ankle movement and prevents your legs from getting a complete, well-balanced workout. Also make sure that you work legs, ankles, and feet in your stretching and strengthening program.

Boost your cardio. Again, it's a great cardio workout—but you can make it even better by buying yourself a set of ski poles with rubber tips and using the poles as you skate. Or join in a hockey game and swing a stick.

Know your secret-weapon stretch: ankle evertors. Because your ankles are going to be strapped into your boot and held rigidly, you have to introduce some flexibility for quick turning and shock absorption when you jump. Your skating will be smoother, and you'll feel better when you change from skates to street shoes.

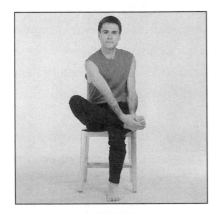

ANKLE EVERTORS
See complete instructions on page 313.

MARATHON

Ever since 490 B.C., when the Greek messenger Phidippides ran from Marathon to Athens to spread the word about a military victory, runners have been measuring their grit by this race of 26.2 miles. We both are marathon runners who work with and train marathon runners all over the world, so this is by far our favorite sport.

Grete Waitz, the undisputed Queen of the New York Marathon, has won it more times than any woman. When she was competing, she trained at the highest levels and was plagued by back pain. We worked with her and taught her to do our work on her own. She's said publicly that she never leaves home without her stretch rope—so now you know a secret of one of the marathon's greatest champions!

Running is running, but what makes the marathon such a challenge is the distance and the consequent fatigue of pounding 26.2 miles, often up and down hills. In fact, the fatigue can be so severe that an unconditioned runner or one who isn't properly fueled will "hit the wall" or "bonk"—he can literally slow down to a stop. This usually happens around miles 18 to 22—the body runs out of the glycogen that the muscles use as fuel to fire and switches instead to metabolize other things—like muscle tissue—as fuel sources. Take it from us, it's painful.

Whether a marathon runner bonks or just gets fatigued, the body mechanics can become sluggish and sloppy, and a series of compensations ensue. Typically, one of these adaptations will be the "marathon shuffle"—shortened stride, deterioration of the gait, and flexion of the trunk (tightness in the lower back) from stooping forward. Or the head will fall forward, seriously fatiguing the cervical spine and upper back. Or the arms will drop, caving in the chest and bringing the shoulders forward, further straining the back, constricting the chest, and impeding breathing.

Khalid currently holds the world's record in the marathon and is as fine an athlete and nice a man as one will ever meet. He first came into our New York City clinic in autumn 2000—5 short weeks before the Chicago Marathon in October. He had pulled a hamstring and needed to recover fast.

As we spoke of injury, he revealed that 2 years earlier he had pulled his Achilles tendon and had stress-fractured his lower leg, which had led to a series of compensations that had severely weakened his adductors and hamstrings. Instead of concentrating on the pulled hamstring, we followed the weak links down his leg to the source—his Achilles tendon, ankle, and arch—and started to work on many things all at once.

Khalid came in two or three times a week and did Active-Isolated Stretching at home every day. The results were remarkable. Five weeks after we met him, in his first marathon as an American citizen, Khalid broke the American record, winning the marathon in 2:07:01.

But the story doesn't stop there. And neither did the friendship. In summer 2001, Khalid was training to represent the United States in the World Championships marathon in Edmonton, Canada. As part of his training, he ran two very competitive shorter races within several days of each other. In the second one, he pulled a muscle in his lower back. He was in full spasm, in great pain, and unable to move. The pain radiated up and down his back. The next day, his brother literally carried Khalid into our clinic. It was the hamstring injury again. It had tightened from running up and down hills in the Utica race. Muscles had locked down, as nature designed them, to protect the hams from further injury. We started right away with gentle, small movement, restoring range of motion to his hips and legs. Ice. Lots of it. Light strengthening. More ice. And more little movements. The spasms released. Three weeks later, he ran in Edmonton.

In spring 2002, months of hard training in

Most injuries are overuse injuries—shocking, huh? Most common are strains, tendinitis, inflammation, and stress fractures. Lower extremities, starting with the pelvis, are at great risk. When you multiply the miles of training and competing—and add the pounding—injury rates rise exponentially.

You probably won't be surprised to discover that in order to prepare your body for the intense demands of the marathon, your training should include—in addition to running—strength training of your upper body and lower body, and flexibility to maximize range of motion. If you want to stay out of

pain—or, let's be honest, minimize it—try a few of these suggestions.

Lengthen your gait. In evaluating two runners competing in the 1992 New York City Marathon, researchers analyzed their gait patterns and counted their steps. They discovered that, although the gaits of the two were very similar, the runner with the longer stride took fewer steps to cover the 26.2-mile course, ran more comfortably, finished first, and recovered more quickly.

We have confirmed these observations time and time again by taking a good runner, increasing his flexibility and lengthening his stride, and dra-

New Mexico and the mountains of Mexico had left Khalid's body exhausted, with highly contracted muscles. He took all that training and raced in Japan. But he knew he was in deep trouble, or about to be. He flew directly to New York and came straight to our clinic, because the London Marathon was 8 weeks away, and he was concerned about his ability to withstand the pounding. He asked our opinion. We said, "Let's get to work and see how you feel, buddy. Wait and see."

That searing back was again the result of that problematic hamstring, so we went to work to release the muscle and then to strengthen it. It had been stuck, sort of welding the muscles together. There was no blood flow. It was contracted. In an intensive effort with Active-Isolated Stretching and Strengthening, he was able to lengthen his stride and—wonder of wonders—his back stopped hurting. Khalid decided to take on London. He broke his own world record again with 2:05:38.

Not bad for a guy who couldn't stride out 2 months before.

How Khalid Got Out of Pain: With Khalid, periodic rehabilitation always begins with arches and ankles. Running 26.2 miles in record time pounds the foot. It's always a challenge to balance the demands of the sport against the balance of the body, and herein lies the champion's secret. We have to keep his arches strong and strengthen his adductors so they won't lock up his hamstrings and destabilize the pelvis. When we do all that, we can take the strain off his back.

In addition to the routines in this book, modified with pillows, that we suggest to relieve strain during the workout, Khalid also uses the ankle-weight-in-the-sock and the towel-bunching routines. And we make sure he doesn't skip abdominals and back stretches and lifts. Khalid is the most fit athlete in the world, and he takes care of little problems before they get big. He does the work every day.

matically improving his time. Even at an elite level, we've seen enhanced athletic performance *without* increasing mileage, logging more time on the road, losing more weight, or spending a month on top of a mountain to altitude train. Plus, injury rates drop.

Ease into your long-run schedule. Long runs in your training schedule, gently increased in distance incrementally over a period of time, will slowly train your body to adapt to the demands of distance. They'll also give you a chance to fine-tune your clothing, bathroom breaks, and shoes—all of which can be problematic on the course.

Don't forget: water, water, water. Hydrate before, during, and after every run—in training or during the real deal. When a distance runner is low on fluids, efficiency is compromised, blood volumes drop, oxygen-carrying capability is diminished, core temperature rises with the inability to sweat and dissipate heat, thinking becomes confused, and some serious problems can set in.

Know your secret-weapon stretch: standing gastrocnemius (on page 338). This is a great stretch, because it releases your calves but requires very little energy. And you need all the energy you can get for those 26.2 miles that loom before you.

STANDING GASTROCNEMIUS

Active Muscles You Contract: Muscles in the fronts of your lower legs

Isolated Muscles You Stretch: Calf muscles

Hold Each Stretch: 2 seconds

Reps: 10 on the left, 10 on the right

1. Stand with your feet shoulder-width apart and your knees slightly bent. Put your left foot slightly in front of you and lock your knee. Keep your heel flat on the floor.

2. From your heel, flex your foot back toward your ankle, aiming your toes toward your nose. For an advanced stretch, use your stretch rope for a gentle assist at the end of this movement. Remember to keep your knee locked and upper body still. For efficiency, do all the left side stretches first, and then move to the right.

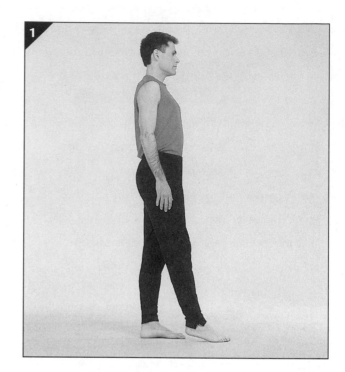

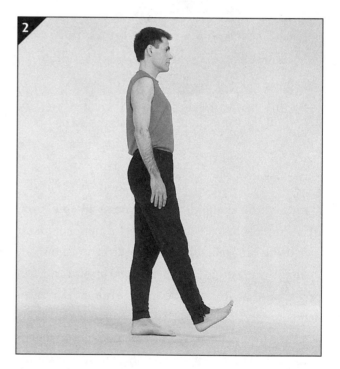

RUGBY

Rugby, to an American, is like stripping a football team down to its shorts, tightening up the field, removing about half the rules, sending the referees out for pizza, pumping everyone up into a frenzy, and turning them loose for a free-for-all. The professional level of this game is most common in Australia, northern England, France, New Zealand, and New Guinea, but amateur and college teams are common in the United States.

Rugby has been described as "controlled violence," but it's not as controlled as it looks. Fifteen percent of all injuries are from *illegal* moves, so somebody's not playing nice, and few seem to mind. Like many of the Olympic sports (like wrestling or modern pentathlon), rugby, too, has its roots in battle, mano a mano. So it's easy to get carried away in the passion of the moment.

The game begins with a scrum: players from both teams wadding up in the center of the field with their arms around each other. Welcoming their opponents and wishing them well? Forget it. The scrum is the first opportunity to intimidate the opposing team and show them who's boss. From the opening whistle, the scrum is a tangle of pushing, pulling, and kicking. It's not uncommon for a scrum to collapse and afford even more opportunity for physical contact, only this time everyone's off balance and on the ground head first. Stompings are common. Considering the spikes on the bottom of everyone's shoes, it can get pretty ugly.

Now we're going to shock you. Although study of rugby is not as comprehensive as for other sports, incidence of injury appears to be fairly low. The most common injuries are cuts, half of which will require stitches and most of which are in the head and face. Second most common are joint injuries, usually incurred as one player defends the ball against another player—or the entire opposing team. After joint injuries are the following: neck strain, cervical spine injury, shoulder and arm injuries, and trunk trauma.

Drop the beer, pick up the stretch rope. As with all sports, strength, flexibility, and cardio fitness will help you stay alert and give you an advantage in defeating the opposing team. Warming up before a game is critical to get all muscles ready for contact. We don't want to see you in rehab. We want to see you in PREhab.

Know your secret-weapon stretches: neck extensors and neck lateral flexors. Rugby is one sport where the back and neck are at risk, and there's little to be done about that, except to be highly conditioned and to stay out of the way of the thundering herd. Because tackling and scrummaging can get out of hand, the neck, in particular, is at risk. Make sure you're strong. Your mouth guard will do little to keep you from an injury in the cervical spine.

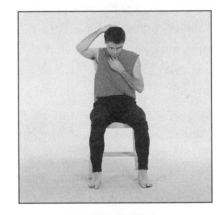

NECK EXTENSORS
See complete instructions on page 61.

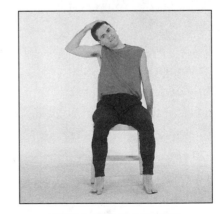

NECK LATERAL FLEXORS
See complete instructions on page 62.

RUNNING

Perhaps the most beautiful thing about running is the basic biomechanics. Your running gait is in three phases: the foot plant (when one foot is planted on the ground and your body literally rides over the top of it); the push-off (when that foot leaves the ground behind you in a thrust from your glutes and swings forward to receive your weight in front of you, literally when the back leg becomes the front leg); and airborne (when both feet are off the ground before the front foot plants again and right after the back foot pushes off).

The third phase, airborne, is what distinguishes running from walking or racewalking. In the foot-plant phase, your ankle is the power generator, out-working your knee by 150 percent and your hip by 300 percent. (In fact, the ankle is responsible for 60 percent of the total power, followed by 40 percent from the knee, and 20 percent from the hip). Power for your push-off phase comes primarily from your gluteus maximus. Literally, you thrust, rather than lift, your knee and reach out with your leg for the next step. Your arms pump, amplifying forward momentum and counterbalancing your body.

As you run, your arms are pumping to help you stay in balance and rhythm and to amplify the energy of forward momentum. Your abs and back are holding you in an erect position. Your hands are relaxed. Your head is up. Your chest is open. And you are breathing.

Running is a superior cardiovascular workout, but because runners hold a specific form, the body gets very little variety. Weakness and imbalance can set in. Because of this, runners hold the record for overuse injuries among all athletes in all fields—a whopping 70 percent. Thirty-seven to 56 percent of all runners get hurt every year, although the injuries might be only minor. Injuries of the knee are most common, followed, in order of frequency, by feet, hips, upper legs and thighs, and lower back.

Get strong and flexible. While running is great for your cardiovascular system and gives a good workout to many muscles, it's not a perfect exercise. You need to supplement it with Active-Isolated Stretching and Strengthening. Not only is variety good for complete fitness, it will improve your running.

General Active-Isolated Strengthening will help you hold your form and maintain efficiency, and it also will give your muscles some variety so that you can avoid imbalance and weakness. Flexibility training will allow you to lengthen your stride.

Don't forget to drink. Running is strenuous, sweating work. Hydrate before, during, and after you run. Staying hydrated can help keep your blood volumes up, which helps your heart more efficiently pump blood and oxygen to the muscles that need them to fire then carry metabolic waste away.

Invest in good running shoes. With every footstrike in running, you hammer 1.5 to 5 times your body weight down through your legs to your feet at more than 110 footstrikes per mile or 5,000 footstrikes per hour. If you weigh 125 pounds, this can be as much as 625 pounds of force 5,000 times an hour. Whoa! Running places great demand on your body, but your foot is remarkable in its shock-absorbing ability, made even more amazing by the addition of a good running shoe. Go to a running store and have them fit you for the best shoes you can afford. You'll feel the difference immediately. Once you have a decent pair, you'll never go back.

Rest. And remember to get some rest once in a while. One of the greatest secrets to top-level training is that a day off between hard workouts allows the body to recover and rebuild. You'll get stronger and faster if you integrate easy workouts or complete rest between sessions of tough training.

Know your secret-weapon stretch: standing quadriceps. This stretch is the best, but unless you have been blessed with superhuman balance and coordination, you might want to stand facing something against which you can steady yourself. There's nothing more heartening to your opponents than to see you topple over on the starting line.

PAIN-FREE SOLUTIONS FOR EVERYDAY SITUATIONS

STANDING QUADRICEPS

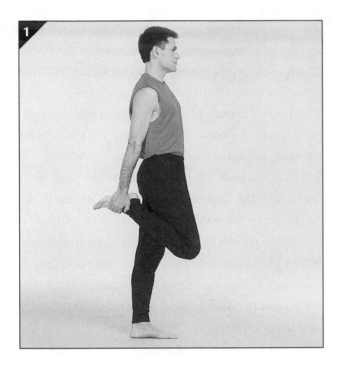

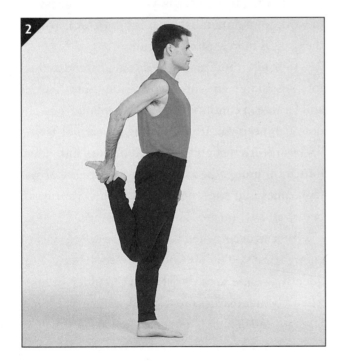

Active Muscles You Contract: Muscles in your buttocks and backs of your thighs

Isolated Muscles You Stretch: Muscles in the fronts of your thighs

Hold Each Stretch: 2 seconds

Reps: 10 on the right, 10 on the left

1. Brace if you must. Stand with your feet shoulder-width apart and your knees slightly bent. Be careful to keep your back straight. No arching or bending forward. Start with your right leg. Bend your right knee and lift your heel toward your buttocks. Use your hamstrings in the backs of your thighs and your gluteals in your buttocks to swing your leg back and bring your heel up. Reach down and back with your right hand and grasp your shin (or ankle or forefoot).

2. Gently assist at the end of the stretch. Return to neutral position, and then stretch your left quad. One right and one left constitutes one rep. For efficiency, do all 10 stretches on your left leg, and then move to stretch your right leg.

SCUBA DIVING AND SNORKELING

A friend phoned us from the Florida Keys in a panic. She had injured her back on a diving trip. Her neck was frozen into a painful spasm, and there weren't enough rum drinks in Key West to kill the pain or relax the spasm. (She had already tried that.)

Seems funny that just snorkeling languidly on the surface above a reef could cause an injury, but by floating facedown and keeping her head and snorkel above water, her neck had been in hyperextension all day. Plus, she was dehydrated. The fatigued neck and dehydrated muscles in the upper back had simply shorted out.

As gentle as diving and snorkeling seem, they also boast an impressive list of hidden risks. For example, you start the day on the pitching deck of a dive boat. It is 120 degrees of sweltering heat made more intolerable by your zipping yourself into a form-fitting, head-to-toe neoprene wet suit. You waddle to the dive platform, taking giant duck-steps over 15-inch hard-rubber rocket fins you have strapped onto your unsteady feet. Your dive buddy helps you into your backpack: two compressed air tanks that effectively double your body weight and put your center of gravity way behind you.

You struggle as you sway back and forth in relentless rhythm with the angry swells that toss your boat. But soon, in one breathtaking moment, after you have rolled into the water and before your bubbles clear, the bulky equipment seems to melt away, and you're free as a bird in flight. Truthfully, we think diving is a magnificent sport, providing you with unparalleled opportunities for adventures in the beautiful and mysterious realm below the surface of water. And diving gives you a chance to explore your body and its ability to move without regard for gravity. You can roll and tumble in all directions, stand on your head, and balance on one finger. You can be a gymnast, a ballet dancer, and a dolphin. You can glide back and forth and up and down with the flip of a fin.

As a diver or a snorkeler, you need strong, flexible hips and trunk in order to support equipment and transfer pressure to the surfaces of your fins to maneuver. For the most part, you'll free-float from a facedown position and roll your head up to look around or reorient yourself, starting with a flex from the waist and lower back and continuing through your neck. You need your arms, wrists, and hands for stabilizing your posture in the water, as rudders for changing direction, and for holding and lifting.

Now, let's talk about standing on the boat. They don't call it the "bounding main" for nothing. When you're out on the water in a boat, your whole body is engaged in constant compensation. In rapid response to the gyroscope-like sensor mechanisms in your inner ear, your body continually must adjust to the pitching of the deck to keep you upright and to keep you from catapulting over the sides and into the briny. Gentle bobbing on still water or being tossed around by raging whitecaps, your body is still having to work to maintain balance. If the water is rough, the work is merely more difficult.

Your hip stabilizers—the adductors and abductors—assist in maintaining your equilibrium. Ankles and feet are in continuous motion. Obliques and abdominals keep you from pitching forward or falling backward. It's difficult for us to discuss individual muscles or groups, because your whole muscular system comes into play automatically when your brain perceives that you are losing your balance.

Injuries occur when you cannot compensate fast enough and you fall or knock into something. Frequently, we see arm, wrist, and shoulder injuries when a boater reaches out to break the inevitable fall. Strength and flexibility go a long way in allowing you to compensate for a pitching deck and for preventing an untimely zig when you should have zagged.

Injuries in divers and snorkelers are few, but when they do occur, they are usually preventable, generally serious, and potentially deadly: running out of air, getting trapped or snagged, cardiovascular and medical problems triggered by the stress of increased pressure at depth, and unexpected, unfamiliar reactions to drugs and medications. Divers and snorkelers are wise to remember that water is a beautiful, yet hostile environment—and humans are merely tourists, who need strategies to survive.

Learn all about it. Don't forget that underwater flora and fauna can injure a diver in a myriad of ways—running the gamut from being stung by deceptively innocuous slime to being eaten by a shark. Even the diver's own body changes at depth. Education and caution go a long way.

Give your whole body a workout. As a complete-body workout, diving and snorkeling fall short. Your shoulders, arms, wrists, and hands need extra work. Additionally, you'll need to supplement your training with some aerobic workouts for a fit cardiovascular system. Maintain maximum flexibility so that you can enjoy your amazing, new range-of-motion opportunities.

Don't get addicted to fins. The minute you strapped on your first pair of fins, you discovered the miracle of propulsion with very little effort. But, you also became a lazy swimmer. Do yourself a big favor and take those fins off occasionally so you can maintain your skill as a swimmer.

Wear sunscreen. The sun's rays are intensified by the water. Wear waterproof sunscreen with a high SPF while diving and snorkeling. Sunburn is a problem for people who are busy and distracted.

Bring your own water. Don't forget to hydrate properly. This sounds odd, considering there's water, water everywhere, but it's easy to forget to drink.

Don't skimp. Be smart and insist on the best for yourself: the best teachers, the best books, the best equipment, and the best dive buddies.

Know your secret-weapon stretch: trunk extensors. Before you put on your wet suit and strap on your fins, sit on the dive platform of the boat with your back straight, your knees bent, your toes pointed slightly up, and your feet resting on your heels. Put a towel under your fanny and your heels so that you don't slip. If the water is rough, make sure

you're in a stable position and won't pitch overboard with one well-placed wave.

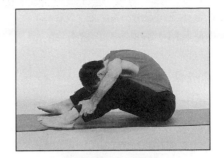

TRUNK EXTENSORS
See complete instructions on page 49.

SNOWBOARDING

Snowboarding actually made its debut in the 1920s, but today, it is not only the fastest-growing winter sport in the world but also the fastest, period. It has graduated from the exclusive domain of hotdoggers with their hell-bent downhill runs to choreographed, aerobatic, balletic international competitions. Snowboarding has been designated as an "extreme" sport.

When you snowboard, you use your legs for stabilizing and your ankle flexors and extensors, knee flexors and extensors, and hip abductors and adductors for balancing and turning. Your trunk is generally flexed forward. Your abdominals provide support.

Your arms and wrists are extended for balance and counterbalance or for gripping the board to guide it. You are loose and relaxed, guiding the board by shifting your center of gravity and putting pressure on one edge of the board. The physics are nearly identical to surfing, in which digging in on one side propels you in the opposite direction.

The most common snowboarding injuries are strains, sprains, fractures, and bruises—and most of those, especially those above the waist, are caused by wiping out. Interestingly, since both feet are strapped to the board with the left foot in front, most leg and foot injuries occur on the left side. No mystery that beginners are more at risk than veterans, but prevention is very logical. Use common sense!

Stretch and strengthen before you hit the trails. Strength and flexibility are crucial for maneuvering your board quickly and accurately. Because snowboarding is not a complete exercise, you'll want to supplement your training with some lifting and stretching.

Being fit means having more fun. Running, cycling, or inline skating at altitude yields superior cardiovascular benefits. In fact, athletes in other endurance sports often retreat to high-altitude areas before major competitions. When they work out at altitude, their bodies adjust to the thin air by increasing oxygen-carrying capabilities. When they return to sea level, their performance levels improve measurably. We encourage you to take advantage of your location. Increased cardiovascular health translates to stamina: more fun for longer periods of time.

Respect the weather. Being out in the elements demands that you pay attention to them. Make an effort to stay warm, wear eye protection (from sun, glare, and impact), and use sunscreen on your face and lips. Hydrate adequately.

Know your secret-weapon stretch: thoracic-lumbar rotators. Here's one stretch that you can do before you hit the slopes. It will warm up your back for maximum maneuvering and control.

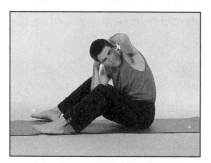

THORACIC-LUMBAR ROTATORS
See complete instructions on page 50.

SOCCER

In 2001, for more than a month, we worked in Napoli, Italy, to prepare their teams for the World Cup. Division One soccer in Italy is as competitive as it gets. The players are recruited worldwide and are elevated to celebrity status previously afforded only to Roman gods, especially when they're performing at the top of their game. Although we worked with the whole team, we were especially touched by Francesco Baldini. He had lost some of his speed because of constant back pain, and his "Roman god" status was in danger of fading from fickle Italian fans. Baldini was more concerned about his team than the fans. When we worked with him, his injury responded so well that he brought in his whole team. Seventeen of the 30 teammates were injured. Their title was on the line. We got 16 of the 17 back on the field. (The one holdout had a broken collarbone. We're good, but we're not that good.) It was incredible. They beat Rome, ranked number one, and Florence, ranked number four. It was a testament to solid training and preparation combined with strength and flexibility.

We love soccer. It's the world's most popular game, played in nearly every country in the world. Estimates place the number of amateur players worldwide at 40 million. When we work on marathon runners in Kenya, we see young boys and men travel by foot for 5 hours from a neighboring village to play soccer on a Saturday in Eldoret, where the marathon camp is located. At the end of a joyful day, they spend another 5 hours going home. You have to admit that there's something pretty compelling about a game for which people will go to that much effort. We heartily endorse soccer as a sport for nearly everyone without regard for age or gender. There are teams to suit everyone, regardless of ability.

Soccer is a great workout. The demands of play put most players into excellent physical condition with unusually refined coordination, power, speed, and control. Repetitive, explosive movements define the sport: running, jumping, changing of direction, rotating, pivoting, leaping, diving, heading, and throwing. Unfortunately, they're also the explosive movements that cause injury, particularly to the connective tissues: tendons, ligaments, and muscles that stabilize and mobilize joints.

While you're going to be running the equivalent of a 10-K during every game, you'll also be developing the skills of a sprinter: ballistic and high-speed. On the field, you're constantly on the move (aerobic exercise), then, frequently, you kick into warp drive (anaerobic). In fact, the workout provided by soccer is so intense that studies of top professional players reveal that, similar to what marathoners experience, soccer players can completely deplete their glycogen stores during the course of a game. (Glycogen is the energy fuel source your body stores and uses to fire muscles.)

At the same time you're running hard enough to exhaust glycogen, your arms and shoulders are pumping to help you stay in balance and rhythm, to amplify the force of your running, and to balance and counterbalance you as you quickly change direction and change the distribution of your weight. Your back and chest are holding you in an erect position. Your hands are relaxed. Your head is up. All your senses are on alert.

In soccer, most injuries occur in the lower extremities. Bruises, ligament sprains (particularly of the ankle), and muscle strains of the ankles and legs account for 75 percent of all injuries. Other injuries we see are iliotibial band (ITB) syndrome, an irritation of the outside of the knee; tendinitis; and other similar overuse problems caused by ballistic changes in direction. The constant hard charging sometimes leads to stress fractures of the tibia (shin). Collisions can fracture. Chronic groin pain seems to be an occupational hazard and is caused by forceful kicking when a player isn't flexible and strains connective tissue—tendons and ligaments. Goalies get injured by impacting with the ball, the ground, or a player diving to make a goal. In fact, goalies suffer 18 percent of all injuries in soccer but comprise only 6 percent of the total players. Statistically, that's a significantly increased risk. Here are a few ways to make soccer safer.

Watch your head. Soccer also claims an unusual injury found only in one other sport, boxing: A cyst forms in the center of the forehead just over the bridge of the nose, caused by repeated blows to the head. Boxers get it from being struck with a fist in a boxing glove. Soccer players cause it themselves by heading the ball with their foreheads. Studies of players who said they headed the ball more than 10 times per game also scored lower than average on tests for attention, concentration, and overall mental functioning, compared to other players. But that's not the only risk: When you get whacked on the head, your neck suffers a horrific jolt. There is no support or padding worn around the neck to protect it from serious injury, so it's up to you to protect your cervical spine by being careful.

Do extra work on your upper body. Because soccer is strictly a "hands-off" sport, relying mainly on your legs, you are deficient in work on your shoulders, upper back, arms, wrists, and hands. We would like to see you work overtime on developing a strong back and neck if you want to excel at twisting, turning, and heading. Being strong, flexible, and well-trained through practice will help you.

Guard against the elements. Because soccer is almost always played outside, you need to protect yourself from the effects of the sun and the heat. Stay hydrated with plenty of fluids before, during, and after the match. And don't forget the sunscreen.

Use protection. Also, if you are offered safety equipment, such as shin pads, seize the opportunity. Remember that soccer is a contact sport played at top speed. A lot can go wrong very quickly. Give yourself every advantage.

Know your secret-weapon stretch: hip adductors. In addition to your regular workout, here's a stretch you can do in the locker room to warm up your hips for a longer, more controlled gait—great for running and kicking.

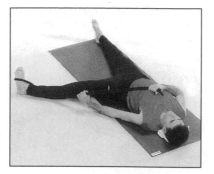

HIP ADDUCTORS
See complete instructions on page 43.

SOFTBALL

Softball is the kinder, gentler version of baseball and is said to have been originated by the Farragut Boat Club in Chicago in the 1880s, where members played with a boxing glove for a ball and a broom for a bat. The first games were called "mush ball" or "kitten ball" or "playground baseball." It all sounds so safe, so wimpy. Well, maybe it was then, but do not be deceived. There is very little "soft" about softball anymore.

Pitching is a complex set of precise movements, requiring a delicate balance between mobility and stability, coordination and depth perception. It may look like an action of your arm and shoulder, but your whole body winds up to power the throw, starting with your legs and through your rotating trunk. Throwing is hard enough to get right when you're standing on the mound or behind the plate—it gets even trickier if you are running, diving, or leaping into the air. If you ever want to convince yourself that your lower body is more than heavily involved in throwing or pitching, sit in a chair and try it—a pitch by even the strongest pitcher will only go one-tenth the distance he's used to throwing. What a good lesson in total-body mechanics and dynamics!

Even though we call it "running the bases," softball players aren't runners—they're sprinters. You'll go from a standing or crouched position and explode into a sprint down the baseline or to make a play. Like other sprinting, sprinting in softball requires thrust from the hip and trunk, agility from the foot and ankle, and power from shoulders and pumping arms to amplify the dynamics of your gait for greater balance and speed. Not only do you sprint, you have to stop quickly, often to initiate another move such as throwing, catching, tagging, or sliding. All of this takes great skill and precision.

In hitting, the primary stress point is your knee. We see dislocated kneecaps from sudden twisting and pivoting around a stationary and planted foot that doesn't yield, thanks to some spikes that hold the shoe in place—the knee twists one way, the foot doesn't.

Sliding is responsible for more than 70 percent of softball injuries. Diving for the base either face first or foot first is always a risk. Players can get hurt on impact with the ground, or they can slam into someone—or both. Most incidents are the results of bad judgment, inability to gauge distance, exuberance, bad technique, poor timing, lack of coordination, or alcohol. Whether you prefer the head-first approach or a foot-first slide, dirt diving converts a vertical force into a horizontal force against surface. Breakaway bases help reduce injuries from impact but are not 100 percent effective because there are too many other ways to get tangled up, too many other things to snag, too many other people to knock over. Sliding requires flexibility, strength, and plenty of great skill to avoid damaging ankles, feet, hips, trunk, wrists, fingers, face, and head.

The catcher just might play the most physically demanding position: squatting and standing, catching and throwing, chasing balls, and avoiding collisions with balls, bats, base runners, and misplaced umpires. Overall fitness levels should be exceptional with emphasis on knees (squatting), shoulder (throwing), and hands (impact from ball).

In fielding, we see explosive bursts of activity

PAIN-FREE SOLUTIONS FOR EVERYDAY SITUATIONS

from a still and tense posture. Success requires coordination, flexibility, strength, agility, and the ability to sprint. Injury prevention is a matter of strength and flexibility and practice in drills. Try to emphasize the work on your hip and trunk, shoulder, forearm, and wrist and finger flexors.

According to the National Electronic Injury Surveillance System of the USA Consumer Product Safety Commission, softball and baseball are two of the top contributors to emergency room visits. In order from most to least, injuries are related to sliding, collisions, falls, and overuse.

While many of these injuries can't be foreseen, you can do your best to prepare your body for impact and overuse.

Don't just stand there. When we consider the overuse injuries, we know that many of them are caused by holding still and then exploding into action. These are complicated and difficult transitions. Any time you're on the field, anticipate that this is going to happen and keep moving. (Notice that the pros skitter and fidget constantly. Use every minute to stay warmed up and alert.)

Consider it a hobby, not a workout. If you're like most players, you play too infrequently and are on the field for too short a time for this sport to qualify as a good workout. This is one sport for which you must train to get fit. You need to add running (sprinting) to your training, so you're ready for that dash to home plate. And, of course, you need flexibility and strengthening.

Protect yourself. Even if you're playing a casual weekend game, wear a batting helmet—it just makes sense. And if you're the catcher, make sure your team invests in the full getup before you get behind the plate.

Know your secret-weapon stretches: shoulder internal rotators and shoulder external rotators. To get your back and shoulders ready to bat, pitch, catch, and wave to the fans, you need to warm up the rotators of your shoulders.

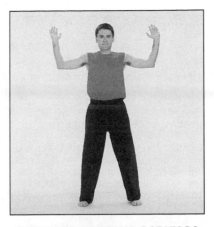

SHOULDER INTERNAL ROTATORS
See complete instructions on page 55.

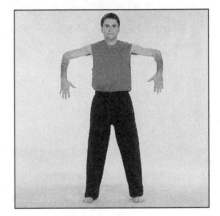

SHOULDER EXTERNAL ROTATORS
See complete instructions on page 56.

SPRINTING

Sprinting differs from basic running in two ways: It is explosive—much faster—and the sprinter strikes the track on the ball of the foot as opposed to the heel or midsole. You start from two positions: from crouching in the starting blocks and bursting off or from running upright, when you have to pour it on at the finish line of a race. Both require a push-off from the forefront of your initiating foot, a drive upward of the opposite thigh, and tight amplification of your arms. You position your weight in front of your legs, in a "reaching" posture. As in normal running, the basic gait is in three phases. (See "Running" on page 340 for a full discussion.)

One of the real challenges in sprinting is running

CASE STUDY: ROCK WILK

Rock lives here in New York City. He's a musician and a producer for Toni Braxton and Patti LaBelle. He's also a former sprinter and former football player for Colorado State University. He had seriously torn a hamstring when he was a sprinter, and the injury nagged him into adulthood. But his back was the problem in his focus.

He came to us after an inexperienced therapist, who was treating his painful back and hips, had overstretched him and said, "Whoops! I've really screwed you up. You need to see the Whartons!" The well-intentioned therapist had gone so deeply into his muscles that Rock was experiencing severe nerve pain.

When he hobbled in, he had a bad back and was unable to move his upper thigh. He was locked at the hip. His head and neck were damaged, and the ligaments in his back were lax. We were dealing with chronic injury from injuries that had happened years before, accumulated and compounded until they nearly shut down a dynamo of a man.

How Rock Got Out of Pain: Rock was one of our most difficult clients to treat, because as we restored tiny ranges of motion, got a little circulation going, and opened up some of the muscle adhe-sions, his entire body would spasm. Ice wasn't enough to reduce swelling and inflammation. We had to submerge him in a cold tank—a full-body ice pack of sorts.

We called Rock our "Science Project." We put him in the cold tank every day and worked to release the hamstring and strengthen the muscles in his hip and back that had been compensating and shorting out. As with all our clients, we started out with stretching and worked our way up to strengthening. We worked on the foot and ankle, abductors and adductors, hip flexors, glutes, and abdominals to support his back. Once we were able to stabilize his pelvis, things got better more quickly. It took a lot of work and patience on his part. Eventually, we were able to undo 20 years of biomechanical mistakes caused by a single hamstring tear.

Although it took only a few sessions to help him feel better, it took 3 months to get him balanced and pain-free. He worked with the diligence and focus he had honed as an athlete. His back is strong, balanced, and pain-free.

Today, Rock runs. And he says, "When I do stretching and strengthening, everything is fine. Just have to do it."

---

anaerobically—over the aerobic threshold, where conversation is impossible and you're sucking wind. Metabolites and waste products build quickly in the fast-twitch muscles of a sprinter at a faster pace. Lactic acid builds, and extreme fatigue sets in with excruciating pain. The reason sprinters pant is that rapid inhalation brings in oxygen and rapid exhala-tion expels wastes. It's difficult. And recovery at the finish line is a matter of getting respiration, heart rate, and pain under control before a sprinter can talk.

The most common injury in sprinters is a hamstring pull or strain, which is usually the case if the muscle is tight or if warmup is not efficient.

We also see injuries that are caused by running on the toes: stress fractures, calf strains, lower leg problems, and Achilles tendinitis.

Fortunately, the Active-Isolated Stretching and Strengthening program can help you as it's helped hundreds of elite-level runners. Here are a few more strategies.

Turn around. Banked tracks can cause a litany of imbalances throughout the legs and feet. For this reason, sprinters and all track athletes should run in the opposite direction once in a while.

Take your stretch rope to the track. Competition causes tension. A good stretch can warm up your body and relax you before you get to the starting block.

Drink as much as you can. Experiment with drinking in training, so you'll know how to hydrate and stay that way during competition. Waiting until you are thirsty will be too late. Also, drink cold fluids—they leave the stomach and are absorbed more quickly than warm fluids.

Train intelligently. Sprinting is brutal on the body. Work with a good coach who can help you make sure that your form is good and that you advance in time and intensity only when your body is ready.

Be kind to your feet. Racing flats have very little cushion, and with so little between the track and your foot, the pounding can be punishing. Wear racing flats only in training and competition, and take them off when you leave the track. For quick recovery, soak burning, aching feet in ice water for 10 minutes.

Know your secret-weapon stretch: standing straight-knee hamstrings. Shown on page 350, this stretch requires balancing on one foot, so find something or someone stable on which you can lean if you need to. You'll probably want to use a teammate or a coach of your own—it's bad form to shamelessly use an opponent right before you leave them in the dust.

SQUASH AND RACQUETBALL

Squash has been called the fastest of all racquet sports. That's a good thing. Generally, the faster the sport, the better the workout. On the downside, however, being the fastest also means there's greater opportunity for getting hurt. In fact, it has the highest rate of injury in all racquet sports—59 percent. (Sometimes we wonder if the origin of the word *squash* was the sound of a human body splatting against a cinder block wall after shouting, "I've got it!")

There's no way to identify individual muscles involved with the biomechanics of a squash player, because when you play, you work nearly everything, combining gymnastics, acrobatics, aerobatics, and racquet skills. When you're on the court, you're a blur of motion nearly 70 percent of the time.

Racquetball is so similar to squash in terms of physiology and injury, sports medicine experts tend to consider them in terms of being identical to one another. The games both require enormous control, endurance, strength, finesse, eye–hand coordination, and visual acuity. It all sounds wonderful, except that a falter in any one of these talents and skills can result in an injury to yourself or your opponent. Compared with all sports, injuries are few, but the majority of them are traumatic: slamming into the wall, getting whacked with a racket, tripping, and falling.

Very few injuries are from overuse, and those that are often occur when the player is competing over his skill level or is on the court too long and is tired. Overhead strokes can cause shoulder problems such as rotator cuff strains and nerve impingement, leading to pain and numbness. Because the racquet is lightweight and the player snaps or slaps a stroke, the elbow and wrist may fatigue and strain. Ballistically changing directions from side to side or from front to back and pivoting to catch a shot can result in sprains and strains of the ankles and feet. But, by far the most dangerous documented injuries in racquet sports involve the eye and the head. It's easy to

STANDING STRAIGHT-KNEE HAMSTRINGS

Active Muscles You Contract: Fronts of your thighs (quadriceps), muscles along the front of your hips

Isolated Muscles You Stretch: Large muscle in the backs of your thighs (hamstrings), just behind your knees

Hold Each Stretch: 2 seconds

Reps: 10 on the right, 10 on the left

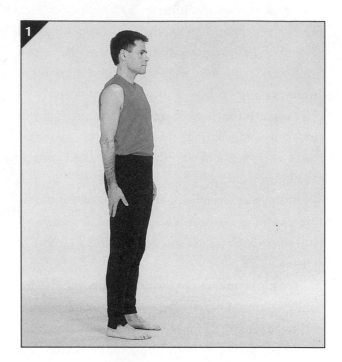

1. Stand with your knees shoulder-width apart. Start with your right leg. Keep your knee straight.

2. Leading with your right foot, lift your leg up. Don't swing it. Lift it with your quadriceps in the fronts of your thighs, and your hip flexors (muscles along the fronts of your hips). Put your hands under your right thigh for support and to assist the end of the stretch. Don't strain your back. Return to neutral position and move to your left side. One right and one left constitutes one rep. For efficiency, do all 10 stretches on your right leg, and then move on to your left leg.

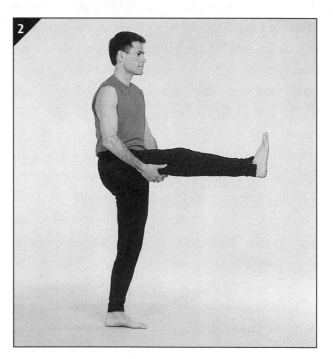

get into the line of fire of a rocketing ball or a racquet badly swung.

Do what you can to stay *out* of that line of fire, and stay healthy with these tips.

Focus on balance. Squash is decidedly one-sided—unless you're ambidextrous and you switch the racquet from side to side, only one arm, shoulder, and side of your back are going to be worked out during the course of a game. The other side will end up being weaker unless you plan your training to make certain that both sides of your body are strong, flexible, and balanced all the way up and down the line.

Get fit first. Squash is a wonderful way to work off the tensions of the day and get a good workout, but it's not recommended as a way to get fit. Instead, think of it as a game to play *after* you're conditioned. We hate to tell you this, but sports medicine experts cite squash as having the potential for heart attack in players who play too hard without proper conditioning. Stamina and endurance will not only give you the edge over your exhausted competitors, it might save your life. Put a high-level cardiovascular workout into your program.

Wear eye protection. Choose shatterproof glasses made especially for racquet sports. Make sure they fit properly and are secure on your face.

Don't skimp on stretching. Warm up properly so that the sudden, ballistic movements required in squash will not damage unprepared, cold muscles.

Choose court shoes. Leave your running shoes in your workout bag; they're made for moving forward only. Wear shoes that will support your feet as you pivot and move side to side. Make sure they fit properly and are tightly fastened.

Safety first. Never enter a court while a game is in play. Make sure your door is closed so that someone will not haplessly wander onto your court. And stay alert on the court. We don't want to hear the sickening sound of "squash" coming from your court, deal?

Know your secret-weapon stretch: hip abduc-

tors. This quick stretch is perfect for the locker room, right before the match. It will prepare your back, hips, and upper legs for the demands of lunging, pivoting, and jumping.

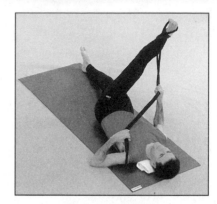

HIP ABDUCTORS
See complete instructions on page 44.

SWIMMING

Swimming is the ultimate repetitive-movement sport, from kicking with legs to stroking with arms. Each movement takes place over and over and over and over . . . until something in the body becomes fatigued and strains.

In our work with Olympic swimmers, we've seen repetitive stress manifest itself most often in the shoulder. Tendinitis of the supraspinatus or biceps tendon—a syndrome known as swimmer's shoulder—is found in about half of all competitive swimmers at some time in their careers.

No wonder the shoulder is so susceptible to overuse injury. As the most mobile of all the joints in the body, it is the most fragile with very little skeletal support. Strokes that are powered by the shoulder have to rely on complicated stabilizing and mobilizing relationships among the rotator cuff muscles, the shoulder capsule, tendons, bones, ligaments, and muscles of the chest and back. It doesn't take much to upset those balances and set off a cascade of injuries—many of which manifest in the upper back. Other overuse injuries in the swimmer's body include strains, sprains, irritation, and tendinitis in the feet, ankles, knees, elbows, and back.

CASE STUDY:
BRIAN VALENZA

We met Brian at a workshop we were conducting at his swim club on Long Island. He was a champion Junior Olympian, specializing in butterfly. He was a junior in high school at the time. He was also out of the water.

Brian had a frozen shoulder and severe upper-back pain. An examination showed that the infraspinatus muscle in his rotator cuff had become shortened in the butterfly. He had only about 5 degrees range of motion in the joint, radiating pain into his forearm and hand. Back muscles that cross over the cuff spasmed to protect it. It wasn't long before they were overloaded from compensation and shorting out. Because his forearm and hand were screaming and losing function, his shoulder was frozen, and his back was aching, he did his workouts in the pool with legs only. He was miserable. And he hated being left off the team.

How Brian Got Out of Pain: His injuries were serious, so we started his therapy with very minimal movements so that we could get things moving and get neural control back for him. We started by unlocking his body with Active-Isolated Stretching. When we tell you that the movements were minimal,

we mean it. We measured a stretch in millimeters. Every move was gentle. But he kept at it.

Eventually, we were able to unlock Brian's cervical spine, but there was a lot of scar tissue within his muscles that had to be broken up. Swimming powerfully and rotating his neck and lifting his head against water resistance had taken a mighty toll. We had to repattern his muscles and restore neural drive so they would react to commands from his brain.

Once we released his cervical spine, his frozen shoulder started to give. When we could get him through a stretch routine, we moved into strengthening. Again, we had to go very slowly and recognize that little improvements were adding up fast. Even though he was a big kid, we started with 1-pound weights. Eventually, we got him up to 25-pounders. It took time, but Brian learned the work and did it. He was back in the pool at competition levels—and without pain—within a couple of months.

By the end of his senior year, he earned a swimming scholarship to the Naval Academy. He's now a Navy Seal. And he gets other Seals to work out with stretch ropes.

Although back injuries in swimming are few, the cervical spine and lumbar spine are at risk when you dive, with rapid extension and flexion changes and severe arching of the back after entering the water. The butterfly kick is also distinguished as being hard on the lumbar spine, because of the extension and flexion of the back and legs against the resistance of the water. Especially at risk are younger swimmers.

The good news is that swimming is great for treating back injuries. The pool provides a spectacular workout without any jarring or pounding. The weightlessness of a body in water tends to take a lot

of pressure off the back, so that some measure of fitness can be maintained or even enhanced without irritating the back further. Make your swimming even safer with these tips.

Don't forget your bones. Although swimming is a wonderful exercise, it doesn't provide a full workout, so you'll want to supplement your training with strength and flexibility. Remember that swimming isn't a load-bearing exercise—that is, swimming does not put any impact on the bones. Women who rely on exercise for osteoporosis prevention need load-bearing work and should consider adding some more appropriate fitness components to their training, such as strength training and walking.

Keep that whistle wet. When you swim, it's easy to forget that you need to hydrate adequately. When you're already wet, you might forget that swimming is hard work and you're sweating. Drink plenty of fluids. Keep a bottle of water by the side of the pool and stop by for a drink at regular intervals.

Know your secret-weapon stretch: shoulder external rotators. Swimming is extra tough on your shoulders because you have to move powerfully—but you have to do it against the resistance of the water. To be sure, it's a superior workout, but it's also hard on your shoulders and upper back. Let's warm you up with a stretch that will give you an advantage.

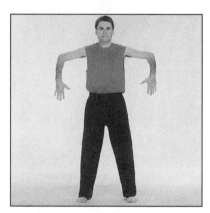

SHOULDER EXTERNAL ROTATORS
See complete instructions on page 56.

TABLE TENNIS

Challenging, fun, safe, and risk-free, table tennis (or "ping-pong," a much more melodic name) scores big points on the Wharton index. This wonderful sport is enjoyed the world over by people of all shapes and sizes. Few people we know have not, at one time or another, grabbed a little paddle and bellied up to a green table bisected by a tiny net.

Now, before you decide that table tennis is an easy game, think again. Few sports are played at higher speed. The ball is rocketed back to you practically before it has cleared your paddle headed the other way. You must have speed-of-light reflexes, a mastery of geometry to be able to anticipate where the ball will return, superhuman eye–hand coordination, an acrobat's sense of balance, a lighter-than-air touch in a powerhouse arm, and a supple body to get into position before the ball does. This combination of strength and finesse is highly unusual.

As you position yourself at the end of the table to serve or return, your legs and feet—quads, hip flexors, calves, and foot extensors—are all put into action to stabilize you and yet allow you to move. Your knees are bent and relaxed, and you are forward on the balls of your feet. You are ready to change positions quickly: pivoting, darting left and right, moving forward, or backing up. The trunk of your body bends forward as you volley. Your racquet arm hyperextends with the help of your shoulder, triceps in the back of your upper arm, and biceps in the front. Your wrist flexes and extends as you make decisions and adjust the direction and speed of your paddle. The opposite arm counterbalances you.

Injuries (and they are mercifully few) result from overuse of the shoulder, arm, wrist, hand, and back. In severe situations, we would expect to see fatigue, strains, and nerve impingement (where the muscles contract and trap nerves). Table tennis places slight stress on one side of the body, and when this happens, a player runs the risk of physical imbalance, with one side becoming stronger than the other. Please arrange your training program to include strength and flexibility for both sides, and work hard to stay in balance.

Give your hands a stretch break. Your hands must remain flexible for the entire match. Putting your paddle down from time to time during your game, and stretching and wiggling your wrist, hand, and fingers will get blood flowing again and take some of the strain off fatigued areas.

Stake out your playing surface. Another risk factor in table tennis is that it is played in facilities that may have different surfaces: hardwood floors, carpet, poured concrete, porches, ship decks, backyards . . . almost anything. Explore the surface of the entire area in which you will be playing so you can discover uneven surfaces without having to trip or fall during competition. Test the surface by "dancing" on it before the game starts.

Choose your shoes wisely. Your shoes can do much to compensate for the differences. Choose shoes that will keep you from slipping but will allow you to move quickly. Stay away from running shoes. Their soles are specifically designed to let you move forward and backward but not pivot.

Know your secret-weapon stretches: wrist flexors and wrist extensors. In addition to your regular Active-Isolated workouts, these are two stretches that will warm up your back and shoulders and put speed and power into your serves and returns. (See pages 355 and 356.)

TENNIS

We have worked with tennis players for many years and find them to be among the most fit of all our athletes, from which we draw one conclusion: Tennis is a spectacular workout, which also seems to be a lot of fun. After all, the equipment is fairly inexpensive (unless you lob a *lot* of balls out of the court), there are indoor courts and outdoor courts almost everywhere, and partners and coaches are plentiful.

Tennis is a game that keeps you on high alert at all times. You have to be ready for anything, from diving to the ground to leaping into the air. These high-speed maneuvers are both the blessing and the bane of the sport. Although they help develop a powerful athlete, they also put a great deal of stress on the body.

The most common injuries of tennis players, in order of frequency, are the shoulder, back, elbow, knee, and ankle.

Notice that we start at the top and move south? Most injuries are the result of overuse—repetitive movements that simply fatigue and then damage. In tennis, repetitive movements are also traumatic. Players hit hard, and even the smallest little injuries can become problematic after the 100th time they're irritated. Eventually, these small traumas will result in tendinitis, strain, and stress fractures. A good example of a tennis injury made worse by repetition is tennis elbow—lateral epicondylitis.

Not all injuries result from repetition and hammering. A little over a third of all tennis injuries are simply accidents: turning an ankle, wrenching a knee, or fracturing a bone in the foot.

As for the back, it's involved 110 percent. Tennis is second only to squash in back injuries, and nearly 40 percent of professional players have missed tournaments because of back pain. The back takes massive force to haul back at the shoulder, go into rotation, and then unwind in an explosion that gets the ball over the net. Small imbalances can create big problems. Follow this advice to make sure you play only when you're strong and flexible and have the endurance to beat your opponent.

Look for a mentor. Your form is very important, so you'll need time to perfect it. One great way to avoid injury is to study with an experienced coach who will make sure your moves are perfect.

Go at your own pace. Also, be sure to advance slowly from one level to the next. Too much, too soon guarantees fatigue, discouragement, and injury. Build a solid foundation every step of the way, and your game will be much stronger.

Cross-train. To play tennis well, you have to be light on your feet. Active-Isolated Stretching and Strengthening are the perfect programs because you need flexibility for quick moves and strength, not bulk, for driving the ball.

You also need a good cardio workout to supplement your training and playing. Tennis is far too much "stop and start" for you to get your heart rate up and keep it there long enough for a good cardio program, but you must have stamina and endurance. We recommend running, cycling, swimming, cross-country skiing, or inline skating.

Protect yourself from the sun. As a side note, remember that there is no shade on a tennis court, so wear sunscreen with a high SPF, a hat, and sunglasses

WRIST FLEXORS

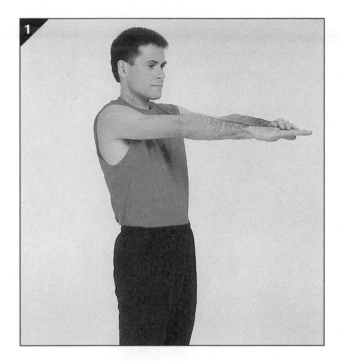

Active Muscles You Contract: Muscles on the outsides of your forearms

Isolated Muscles You Stretch: Muscles on the insides of your forearms

Hold Each Stretch: 2 seconds

Reps: 10 on the right, 10 on the left

1. Stand at the edge of a table with your feet a few inches apart and slightly bend your knees. This exercise also can be done while sitting in a chair. Either turn around so your opponent can't see you or do it right in front of him to intimidate him. Hold the exercising arm straight in front of you and lock your elbow. With your palm facing down, extend your fingers.

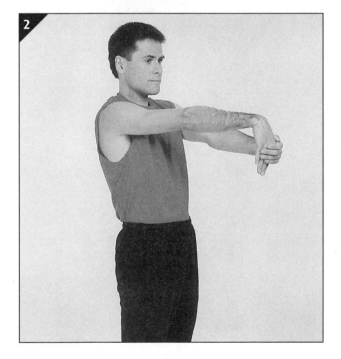

2. Lead with your fingers to the floor, until your palm is facing your body and your fingers are down. With the nonexercising hand, reach around the fronts of the fingers of the exercising hand and gently assist with a little pull toward the body.

WRIST EXTENSORS

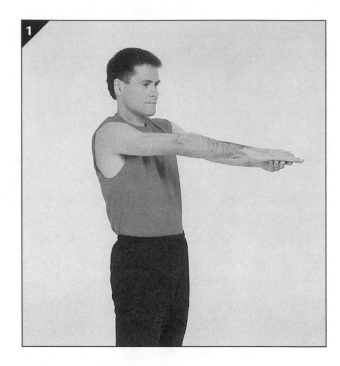

Active Muscles You Contract: Wrist flexor muscles

Isolated Muscles You Stretch: Wrists and the outsides of the forearms

Hold Each Stretch: 2 seconds

Reps: 10 on the right, 10 on the left

1. Still standing at the edge of the table with your feet a few inches apart and your knees slightly bent, or seated in a chair, continue. Hold the exercising arm straight in front of you and lock your elbow. With your palm still facing down, extend your fingers.

2. Bring your palm back toward your body as far as possible. With the nonexercising hand, reach around the tops of the fingers of the exercising hand and gently assist with a little pull back toward the body.

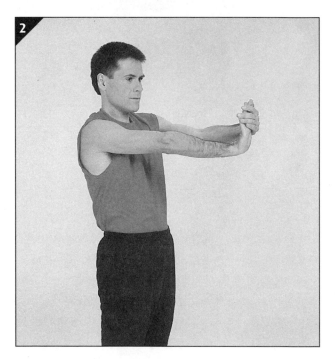

that are shatter-proof. Also, drink plenty of water before, during, and after play. Put a large bottle of water at the edge of your court and use every opportunity to swing by for a sip—like when your opponent is busy trying to locate the ball you just rocketed straight past him.

Make the most of pauses in play. As you are strolling to the side, use that time to stretch out your shoulders and shake off some tension. If anything hurts, stop the game.

Know your secret-weapon stretch: hip abductors. Before you hit the court, try this stretch to warm up your back, hips, and legs and put speed and power into your ability to run, pivot, jump, and back up.

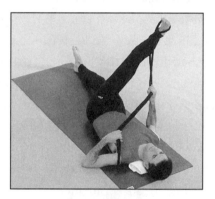

HIP ABDUCTORS
See complete instructions on page 44.

TRIATHLON

The triathlon is the love child of injured and bored endurance athletes. When a runner was injured and couldn't run but needed to keep up cardio fitness levels, she took to the pool. When the swimmer was waterlogged, he hopped on his bike. When the cyclist's bike was in the shop, he strapped on his running shoes. In the process, they thought, "Hey! This is fun!"

This switching from one endurance sport to another is called cross-training. And it's essential for maintaining cardiovascular fitness when one's chosen sport is out of reach. It's not at all uncommon for an endurance athlete to be good at more than one sport. In fact, it's necessary, because injury can side-line a one-sided competitor and erode fitness levels fast.

The triathlon today is identified as a single sport, but it is, in fact, a combination of three distinct endurance sports: swimming, cycling, and running. For individual discussions on swimming, cycling, and running, we refer you to the sections on these sports. (See "Swimming" on page 351, "Cycling" on page 326, and "Running" on page 340.)

The difficulty in triathlons is not necessarily in the components of the separate sports, but in the transitions between them. Moving rapidly from one to another is no easy task, but these tricky transitions are among the most fun and challenging of all the demands the triathlon makes on its athletes.

The race can be won or lost in the struggle to change clothes or get a bike off a rack. Not only are the logistics of clothing and equipment difficult, but the human body is not at all impressed by moving from swimming to cycling and from cycling to running. The ability to quiet screaming muscles and repattern them for entirely different movement separates the champions from the bedraggled masses with numbers drawn on their thighs in Magic Marker.

Most triathlons start with a swim. Your body is horizontal, your neck is flexed and rotated to keep your head above water, your arms are pulling as your shoulders rotate, your legs are kicking from your hips, your back is holding your body in a stabilized position, and your heart is pounding. In fact, swimming at this level takes you to the anaerobic threshold and perhaps beyond. Your body is losing heat in the cold water.

Once the swim is over, you're probably tired, but you dash barefoot out of the water. Lactic acid and other metabolic waste products from muscles firing begin to build, but you wrestle your wet, crinkly, bare feet into rock-hard cycling shoes, perch your fanny on the bike seat, and rocket out of the parking lot.

You might be warmed up from the swim, but

you're not actually warmed up for pedaling and hunching over your grips. As far as your muscles are concerned, you've prepared not at all. Ah, challenge! The fun is only just starting. Now your arms, tired and pumped from swimming, are extended down as your hands clamp onto your grips and bear the weight of your torso flexed forward. Legs that were extended and kicking in the water are now constricted by the circumference of the pedals and are required to flex and pump in a very limited range. And feet that were relaxed in the water to serve as flippers are now bearing down on the pedals. A back that was straight and slightly extended to lift your face out of the water is now flexed forward. A body that was cold and shivering in the water now begins to heat up. Cycling is hard, fast work, so it heats up a lot. Lactic acid and other waste products from muscles firing continue to build, and fatigue is beginning to be a major factor, but at the end of the ride, you're only two-thirds of the way to the finish line.

The physical demands of the run are the most shocking of the three events to your body. You leap off your bike, shove it into the rack, hurl yourself to the ground, rip off your cycling shoes, change into running shoes, leap up, and explode out onto the course. Your body might be warmed up from the cycling, but running is another matter altogether. A back that has been bent forward and fatigued is now straight up and getting hammered with every step. Legs that have been constricted with bent knee in spinning must now extend and bear weight—and lots of it—for the first time all day.

The forces of running slam 1.5 to 5 times your body weight down to your feet. A 150-pounder can exert 750 pounds of force with each footstrike. Arms that have been frozen in a bent-elbow position on the handlebar grips of your bike and are fatigued from supporting the weight of your torso must now pump to help balance, amplify your energy, and propel you forward. Lactic acid and other metabolic waste make your legs feel as if your shoes are filled with concrete.

Muscles strain. Everything hurts. (Is this a great sport, or what?)

One caution: Do your best to resist overtraining. It's easy to do when you have three sports to cover and a race on the horizon. Scott Thompson is a triathlete and friend who has competed well in five Ironman Triathlons. At some point, he changed a successful training program and managed to venture into overtraining, a dark and dangerous place. As his friends watched in horror, he crossed the finish line of the SOS Triathlon here in New York in terrible pain with one leg out of control, flailing out to the side and then crossing the midline of his body. It looked as though his leg was broken.

Scott had been all right running down hills, but when he hit the flats, he lost control. He had to lean back to stabilize his body to keep from falling. His friends rushed him to the hospital. After testing, when physicians couldn't explain this loss of control, they considered the diagnosis of multiple sclerosis.

He didn't have MS, thankfully—he had shorted out his body by overtraining with some minor imbalances that didn't reveal themselves until that day. This confusing, frightening incident taught him well. He still trains, but he goes at it a little easier.

As far as most injuries are concerned, sports medicine statisticians cite the component sports as being the culprits, but add that the combination can traumatize even the most fit body. Back problems in the triathlon are common, particularly in the running phase. But don't blame the running. It's actually the cycling's fault. Hamstrings get shortened and tightened in pedaling, so when it's time to run, the back is brutalized. Here are a few ways to avoid that abuse.

Mirror race day in your training. You can avoid some of the problems by making sure you're fit in all three sports before you compete. Training for all three events is radically different from competing in all three in rapid succession. Athletes rarely do that in training. Most often, different sports are highlighted on different days—a sort of mix and match of training regimens designed to develop high levels of skill in each on a limited schedule. To train for the transitions, we coach our triathletes to do "bricks," training frequently with two of the three sports back-to-back in one workout. You can work up to all three.

Be smart. The key to success is to train intelligently—don't overtrain—and pay attention to transitions and the stresses they place on your body. Each sport is demanding; in concert, they are three times as demanding. Knowing how to mesh them makes a huge difference. Practice gently and pay attention to the tiny details and subtle cues that direct you to the small problems that don't have to become big ones if they're managed well.

Pour on the water. In competition, hydrate adequately. In fact, try to overdo it. It's especially important that you not be deceived by the swim. You sweat. Being wet masks dehydration. You still need to drink.

Practice fueling for the long haul. Your energy expenditure is enormous in a long-distance triathlon, so plan on getting some extra calories for energy with supplement bars, replacement fluids, or fruit. But don't do anything in competition that you've not tried in training—throwing up can really slow you down.

Know your secret-weapon stretch: neck extensors. This baby busts the tension that begins in the swim as you bring your head up to breathe, the tension that intensifies as you cycle with your back down and your head up, and the tension that results from the pounding of the run (especially at the end when you're straining and craning your neck to see the finish line). Although we prefer that you do this stretch sitting, unless the rules have changed, "sitting" isn't one of the three component events in the triathlon. You can do this standing in the water while waiting for the gun to go off, perched on your bike seat (if you're really balanced and careful), or on the run.

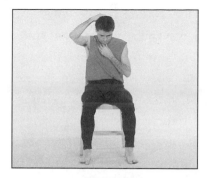

NECK EXTENSORS
See complete instructions on page 61.

WALKING

Steve Umbring is an accountant and about as intense and focused a man as we've ever met. His exercise of choice is walking, which, we were pleased to note, kept him in very good shape. One evening when we were working together at his home in Oregon, he invited us to shake out the cobwebs of our long flight to the coast by joining him on his walk on the beach. We're both marathon runners, so we assumed that this stroll would be a piece of cake. He set a blistering pace, and, although he didn't wear us out, he definitely got our attention. As proud marathoners, we experienced one of those humbling moments when one has to admit that an accountant walking through the sand could very nearly kick one's butt.

Humans, by all reckoning, have been walking for at least 3 million years. Almost everyone can do it, from toddlers right on up to the eldest among us. It's an inexpensive, low-impact, tension-busting, cardiovascular exercise that gets your heart rate up and burns off excess calories. In 30 minutes of walking at a fast pace up hills, you can burn up to 300 calories. We believe in it so much that we made it a large part of our program. (See "Your Cardio Program" on page 92.)

We describe the biomechanics of walking in chapter 2, but we want to point out that another fascinating aspect of walking is the action of your arms. The opposite arm will swing in perfect cadence with the swinging leg: right arm with left leg and left arm with right leg. Nature has designed it this way to counterbalance you as your weight shifts from foot to foot and to amplify the momentum of your gait. The faster you go, the more energetic and higher the arm swing. If you have never noticed it, try swinging your left arm forward when you swing your left leg forward—it's nearly impossible.

Injuries in walking are few and far between. To make it even safer, just take it easy, increase your distance and difficulty slowly, and keep these pointers in mind.

Don't forget to stretch and strengthen. Much as we extol the virtues of walking, we must admit that it is not the perfect exercise. You still need Active-Isolated Stretching and Strengthening to keep your muscles strong and flexible. Follow all three facets of the program for total fitness.

Walk unencumbered. We want to caution you about carrying handheld weights or strapping on shot-filled ankle and wrist weights as you walk. They change the dynamics of your stride and add stress to the arm muscle attachments at the shoulder joints.

Know your secret-weapon stretch: tibialis anteriors. Walking plants your heel flat on the ground over and over. If you're not used to it, it can strain the front of your shin, maybe even causing the dreaded, painful "shin splints." It's all easily avoided by making sure your shin can support the lift of your forefoot and the strike of your heel.

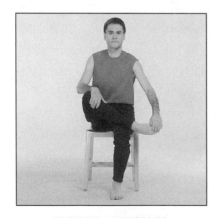

TIBIALIS ANTERIORS
See complete instructions on page 314.

WEIGHT TRAINING

We think of time spent in the gym lifting weights as a means to an end, but for many, lifting weights is not only the means but also the end. Bodybuilders are a sort of amalgamation between athlete and sculptor. While strength is the inevitable by-product of lifting, a bodybuilder is just as concerned about the shape, size, balance, and definition of each muscle. Like molding clay, a bodybuilder works muscle by muscle to form a perfect physique.

We have worked with weight lifters and bodybuilders over the years, and we are going to let you in on a little secret. Although they might be ripped, cut, strong, and well-muscled, they aren't necessarily "fit" as we define it. To be truly fit, one has to be healthy, strong, and flexible, and have stamina through cardio work.

Bodybuilding is more than lifting. It's also maintaining lean body mass so that subcutaneous fat doesn't obstruct the visible definitions and striations of the muscles. Dieting to lose weight can make it difficult to get all the nutrients you need. Fortunately, the community of body builders, particularly those who work out in gyms, seem to share information regarding appropriate supplements.

If you're going to lift weights with the aim of building muscle bulk, you have to watch out for elevated blood pressure. During dynamic resistive exercises like lifting, both the systolic and diastolic pressures rise rapidly. The good news is that normal or even slightly lower blood pressure might result from prolonged training.

Back injuries in lifting usually strike the lumbar spine, when it is asked to support heavy weight in one spectacular (and foolish) lift or cumulatively over a period of training sessions. Injuries can also result from muscular imbalance: abdominals that are weaker than the back, or tight hamstrings. And they can be the result of an accident, when the weight is suddenly unbalanced or the lifter turns quickly for

PAIN-FREE SOLUTIONS FOR EVERYDAY SITUATIONS

some reason. Sprains, strains, and soft tissue injuries are most common.

Flexibility is critical. As a bonus, muscles that are elongated tend to show off the muscle striations and cuts. Also, a flexible muscle allows better movement, and as a consequence your muscles will be able to flush metabolic waste and lactic acid more quickly for recovery.

Remember, what goes up must come down. Flexing a muscle to lift a weight is only one half of the process. You have to extend and lower that same weight to get a full range of motion and work each muscle completely. Lifting and lowering use different muscles and different functions of the same muscles. If you want to be truly strong and have a balanced physique, you have to tend to both with equal care and concentration.

Injuries are divided by experts into two categories: *acute*, like sprains or strains, and *overuse*, like tendinitis. Most can be prevented with just a few simple strategies.

Warm up and stretch. In most other sports, you can warm up your muscles and prepare them for performance by starting slowly and increasing load and demand gradually—but not so with lifting. You can't start your lift of a 25-pound weight with a lighter 25-pound weight! Your muscles are on full duty from the start. Without proper warmup, an unprepared muscle can be injured. A little preparation goes a long way toward making sure that the muscle fibers are lined up and properly oxygenated so they can fire efficiently to power the lift.

Get some good advice. The worst thing you could do is just jump into a gym and wing it. Look for a trainer who can help you gently ease into using proper techniques and advise you on how to intelligently pace your training. Ask for tricks for maintaining concentration in the crowded, loud gym, since focus is vital to perfect form.

Slow and steady. The way to make the greatest improvements with the least amount of risk is to work out consistently, gradually building weight and time. You can't cram for this—it's a slow burn.

Don't push it. You need your full strength and wits about you when you're weight training. Work out only when you're uninjured—your body needs time to rest and heal.

Remember to drink. In competition, some bodybuilders enhance muscle visibility by dehydrating—cutting down water and sweating in a sauna. This is never a great idea. In fact, it can impair performance and endanger your health.

Female bodybuilders, be aware. Estrogen is stored in body fat. Dieting and working out to drop fat content below 16 percent in order to achieve a "cut" look may cause your estrogen levels to diminish, possibly resulting in your losing estrogen's cardioprotective properties, developing amenorrhea, and running an increased risk of osteoporosis. Every woman is different, so you and your physician will want to decide what's best for you.

Know your secret-weapon stretch: pectoralis majors. So much of bodybuilding relies on using your upper body. Lifts will go better and be more complete if the muscles in your chest and shoulders are flexible and you can move through your complete range of motion. In competition, developing little muscles and crisp definition mean a lot, so you want as much range as you can get. This is an easy stretch to do, but it makes a subtle, yet important difference in your lifts.

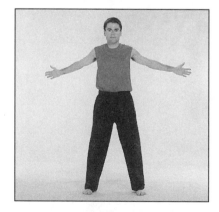

PECTORALIS MAJORS
See complete instructions on page 53.

For More Information: Internet Resources for the Back

While we hope to have answered a lot of your initial questions, you may have some concerns or interests that we couldn't cover here. All good athletes seem to enjoy doing a bit of their own investigative work, so we've collected a few of our favorite sources of solid, unassailable research on the topics included in this book. Always work with your doctor or health practitioner to formulate the best plan for you.

ACUPUNCTURE

American Academy of Medical Acupuncture

The American Academy of Medical Acupuncture offers information regarding state laws governing acupuncture, a newsletter, general information and patient education, links, a reference library, and a practitioner locator.

- www.medicalacupuncture.org

British Acupuncture Council

The British Acupuncture Council in London is the United Kingdom's main regulatory body for the practice of acupuncture by more than 2,200 professionally qualified acupuncturists. There's an online library, patient education regarding acupuncture, and a practitioner locator.

- www.acupuncture.org.uk

British Medical Acupuncture Society

The British Medical Acupuncture Society in Warrington, Cheshire, enhances the education and training of qualified practitioners in the United Kingdom and promotes high standards of practice. Their Web site has information for patients, an introduction to the London Teaching Clinic, links to other sites, updated press releases, and a practitioner locator.

- www.medical-acupuncture.co.uk

ARTHRITIS

American College of Rheumatology

For simple information regarding specific conditions such as ankylosing spondylitis, arthritis, and osteoporosis, visit the American College of Rheumatology, the professional association of rheumatologists. A geographic directory of rheumatologists will help you locate a qualified physician in your area.

- www.rheumatology.org/patients/factsheets.html

Arthritis.com

The Pharmacia Corporation produces an interactive, easy-to-use Web site for simple education regarding arthritis.

- www.arthritis.com

National Institute of Arthritis and Musculoskeletal and Skin Diseases (NIAMS)

The National Institute of Arthritis and Musculoskeletal and Skin Diseases keeps an active Web site with news, events, updates in research, and information. NIAMS is part of the U.S. National Institutes of Health.

■ www.niams.nih.gov

CHIROPRACTORS

American Chiropractic Association

The American Chiropractic Association in Arlington, Virginia, is the professional association of chiropractors in the United States. Although their Web site is oriented toward professional members, the "Patient Information" link will lead you directly to a chiropractor locator, research, education, information on back pain, health tips, frequently asked questions, news releases, health links, and news releases.

■ www.amerchiro.org

COMPLEMENTARY AND ALTERNATIVE MEDICINE

National Center for Complementary and Alternative Medicine (NCCAM)

If you step away from conventional medicine, to sort fact from fiction, visit the Web site of the National Center for Complementary and Alternative Medicine (NCCAM). As this is a division of the National Institutes of Health, the information you'll get here is credible and the advice intelligent. You'll find information on understanding complementary and alternative medicine, alerts and advisories, treatment, resources, research, and press releases. You can search the site by key words.

■ www.nccam.nih.gov

GENERAL HEALTH

National Institutes of Health (NIH)

Part of the U.S. Department of Health and Human Services, the National Institutes of Health's Web site is full of publications, fact sheets, topics, and special reports. In addition, you can use this site to access MEDLINEplus, the search engine of the U.S. National Library of Medicine.

■ www.nih.gov

U.S. National Library of Medicine

You have easy access to the world's largest medical library, the U.S. National Library of Medicine, and unparalleled health information. The site even teaches you how to search easily and effectively.

■ www.nlm.nih.gov

HEALTHY NUTRITION

American Dietetic Association

The American Dietetic Association is the nation's largest organization of food and nutrition professionals. Although its Web site is directed toward professional members, you'll find an online journal, daily tips, and a dietitian locator.

■ www.eatright.org

Food and Nutrition Information Center

The Food and Nutrition Information Center is part of the U.S. Department of Agriculture (USDA). Here, you'll find everything you ever wanted to know about food, dietary supplements, and nutritional guidelines for a healthy eating plan.

■ www.nal.usda.gov/fnic

HOME SAFETY

FirstGov for Consumers: Your Home

The U.S. government has done a good job of compiling resources for home safety. Take a look at FirstGov for Consumers: Your Home. Check out the links to information on disaster, fire and emergencies, energy information, environment, and home improvements. You'll get an education that will help prevent back injuries and just about every other disaster that can sneak up on you at home.

■ www.consumer.gov/yourhome.htm

The U.K. Department of Trade and Industry—Home Safety Network

The U.K. Department of Trade and Industry—Home Safety Network site contains a wide range of information and materials on a number of home safety topics to reduce the high toll of serious home accidents in the United Kingdom. Of particular interest are general home safety, falls, and garden safety. You'll enjoy the links.

■ www.dti.gov.uk/homesafetynetwork

OSTEOPOROSIS

National Osteoporosis Foundation (NOF)

The National Osteoporosis Foundation has the most comprehensive site regarding osteoporosis on the Web. You can use the search engine to quickly navigate the site, or enjoy this beautifully designed educational site by clicking buttons. You'll get general information and the latest in research. You'll learn how to prevent osteoporosis or mitigate the effects of the disease if you already have it. In addition, you can locate physicians who specialize.

■ www.nof.org

PAIN

American Academy of Pain Management

The American Academy of Pain Management welcomes you to its site by saying, "We know you are hurting. Let us help you find some resources and professionals for pain management." The site helps patients locate a member professional, find a clinic, and familiarize themselves with their rights, and it provides patient education through links and the latest clinical articles in *The Pain Practitioner*.

■ www.aapainmanage.org/info/Patients.php

PREGNANCY

American College of Obstetricians and Gynecologists (ACOG)

The professional association of women's health-care physicians is the American College of Obstetricians and Gynecologists. Their Web site, although geared toward member physicians, has news releases for patients with a generous archive, information on women's issues, patient information, and a search engine by topic for the public.

■ www.acog.org

PRIMARY-CARE PHYSICIANS

American Medical Association (AMA)

The American Medical Association is the professional association of physicians and medical students in the United States. One click on the AMA Online Doctor Finder provides basic information on every licensed physician in the United States—more than 690,000 doctors of medicine (M.D.'s) and doctors of osteopathy (D.O.'s).

■ www.ama-assn.org/aps/amahg.htm

SCOLIOSIS

Scoliosis Research Society (SRS)

The Scoliosis Research Society in Milwaukee educates patients in understanding spinal deformity and helps them locate member orthopedic surgeons around the world.

■ www.srs.org

SENIOR HEALTH

Closing the Health Gap

The U.S. government makes research easy. Closing the Health Gap is health information for older Americans. You can explore selected publications such as "The Resource Directory for Older People," "Talking with Your Doctor: A Guide for Older People," "Prescription Medicines and You," "Exercise: A Guide from the National Institute on Aging," and "Safety for Older Consumers: Home Safety Checklist."

■ www.healthgap.omhrc.gov/older_americans.htm

Nutrition Resource List for Older Americans

The Nutrition Resource List for Older Americans is a Web site sponsored by the Food and Nutrition Information Center of the U.S. Department of Agriculture in Beltsville, Maryland. It contains many pages of relevant links pertaining to healthful diets and successful aging. If you're a researcher, allow a lot of time, because you'll be hooked by the vast assortment of magazines and newsletters, booklets and pamphlets, and resources including Web sites on the Internet.

■ www.nal.usda.gov/fnic/pubs/old.htm

Physical Activity and Older Americans

Although clinical and statistical in nature, Physical Activity and Older Americans is a fascinating study of exercise as we age. It's a great motivator with a generous bibliography, complete with links to Internet sites.

■ www.ahcpr.gov/ppip/activity.htm

Travel Tips for Older Americans

Travel Tips for Older Americans is a comprehensive, entertaining, easy-to-understand guide for older people on the go. In fact, travelers of all ages will enjoy this thorough compendium of tips for planning the perfect adventure.

■ www.travel.state.gov/olderamericans.html

U.S. Administration on Aging

The Web site of the U.S. Administration on Aging is a compendium of links for older people and their loved ones. Check out the links that run the gamut from nutrition and exercise to professionals and practitioners.

■ www.aoa.gov

SPINES AND BACKS

American Back Society

The American Back Society provides the health-care community with current information on interdiscipli-nary spinal care. Members include orthopedic and neurological surgeons, osteopathic physicians, physical therapists, chiropractors, neurologists, psychiatrists, radiologists, rheumatologists, internists, occupational therapists, nurses, and other health-care professionals.

While the site is oriented to professionals, you'll find an archive of their journal articles and a generous link to other professional organizations related to spinal care.

■ www.americanbacksoc.org

North American Spine Society (NASS)

The North American Spine Society in LaGrange, Illinois, has information on common spinal conditions and spinal injury prevention. You can use this site to locate a member physician.

■ www.spine.org

Spine-health.com

Spine-health.com is a simple, well-organized, entertaining, educational Web site with a broad range of topics. You can browse articles by subject. Procedures are not only explained but also animated for easy understanding. You'll be able to sign up for a free e-mail newsletter and use their physician locator.

■ www.spine-health.com

SpineUniverse.com

If you have to select one Web site for education regarding all issues related to the spine, SpineUniverse.com is the one for you. It's beautifully organized, easy to browse, and packed with information written for laypeople: conditions, treatment, technology, wellness, resources, and community. In addition, you'll be able to locate a spine specialist from their directory.

■ www.spineuniverse.com

SPORTS MEDICINE

American College of Sports Medicine (ACSM)

The American College of Sports Medicine promotes and integrates scientific research, education, and practical applications of sports medicine and exercise science to maintain and enhance physical performance, fitness, health, and quality of life. Click on the link to "Health and Fitness Information," search the site by topic, or use the site to link to other information.

■ www.acsm.org

American Orthopaedic Society for Sports Medicine

The American Orthopaedic Society for Sports Medicine in Rosemont, Illinois, hosts a Web site for their professional members but has generously included "The American Journal of Sports Medicine," "Sports Medicine Update," "Publications and Patient Education," "Media Room," and "Ask the Sports Doctor," for the rest of us. You can also find a sports medicine specialist in your area through their locator.

■ www.sportsmed.org

The Physician and Sportsmedicine Online

The Physician and Sportsmedicine Online is a wonderful source for primary-care sports medicine clinical and personal health articles. Click on the "Personal Health" link for articles relating to exercise, nutrition, injury prevention, and rehabilitation, all written for the active individual. Topics include allergies, chronic disease, lifestyle, mental health, personal fitness, rehabilitation, safety, skin care, sports equipment and apparel, strengthening exercises, weight control, and women's health.

■ www.physsportsmed.com

SportsMedicine.com

SportsMedicine.com is an Internet resource for fitness and exercise, health and wellness, organizations that can help you, and resources on topics such as anatomy, physiology, and sports injuries.

■ www.sportsmedicine.com

WORKPLACE SAFETY

The Information Network of the European Agency for Safety and Health at Work

Located in Bilbo, Spain, the Information Network of the European Agency for Safety and Health at Work was set up by the European Union in order to educate people with an interest in occupational health and safety. The site is clear, easy-to-navigate, and comprehensive. Of particular interest might be the links "Musculoskeletal Disorders," "Accident Prevention," and "Good Practice Online Forum."

■ http://europe.osha.eu.int

National Institute for Occupational Safety and Health

The Centers for Disease Control and Prevention manage the National Institute for Occupational Safety and Health. You'll find information on injury prevention, ergonomics, lifting, and back belts.

■ www.cdc.gov/niosh/homepage.html

Occupational Safety and Health Act

OSHA is the Occupational Safety and Health Act. It addresses occupational safety, accident prevention, work safety, and current events related to health in the United States. Look for tips for avoiding back problems under the link "Public Safety" and weight issues under the link "Public Health." The site is filled with practical information.

■ www.oshabulletin.com

Index

Underscored page references indicate boxed text and tables. **Boldface** references indicate illustrations and photographs.

difficulty, as warning sign in workout, <u>35</u>

during strength training, 239

Bruise, treating, 145, **146–49**

Bupropion (Wellbutrin), for back pain, 125

BuSpar, for sleeplessness, 282

C

Caffeine avoidance

for enhancing sleep, 273

during pregnancy, <u>204</u>

for weight loss, 200

Calcimar, for osteoporosis, 233

Calcitonin, for osteoporosis, 233, 234

Calcium

deficiency, as osteoporosis risk factor, 228

food sources of, 230

increasing absorption of, <u>230</u>

supplements

choosing, <u>230</u>

for osteoporosis prevention, 230–31

vitamin D and, <u>230</u>, 231

Calories

burning of, muscle increasing, 192

daily needs for, 196, <u>196</u>

in weight loss, 195

Calves, evaluating flexibility of, <u>261</u>

Carbohydrate snack, enhancing sleep, 275

Cardio program

guidelines for, 92–93

purpose of, 15, 35

for weight loss, 192–93

Carisoprodol (Soma), for back pain, 125

Carpal tunnel syndrome, from computer use,
294–95

preventing, 295–96, **296**

Carpet, preventing falls from, 300

Cars

back-friendly, 319

technique for getting out of, 19

Case studies, <u>23</u>, <u>27</u>, <u>29</u>, <u>198–99</u>, <u>251</u>, <u>263</u>, <u>268</u>, <u>286</u>, <u>289</u>, <u>295</u>,
<u>312</u>, <u>325</u>, <u>336–37</u>, <u>348</u>, <u>352</u>

Cauda equina, 13–14

Cauda equina syndrome, treating, 149

Celebrex, for back pain, 125

Celecoxib, for back pain, 125

Cervical spine. *See* Neck

Chair

getting out of, technique for, 19

office, choosing, 287

Chest discomfort, as heart attack symptom, <u>35</u>

Chewing slowly, for weight loss, 199–200

Chinese medicine, for treating back pain,
138–39

Chiropractors

Internet resources on, 364

referral to, 130

for treating back pain, 132

Chondroitin sulfate, for joint health, <u>243</u>

Chronic disease, as osteoporosis risk factor,
227

Cibacalcin, for osteoporosis, 233

Circadian rhythms, <u>271</u>, 315

Coccyx, 12

Complementary and alternative medicine

Internet resources on, 364

overview of, 135–36

types of

acupuncture, 136

applied kinesiology, 136–37

Ayurvedic medicine, 137–38

Chinese medicine, 138–39

faith healing, 139

homeopathic medicine, 139

hypnosis, 139–40

massage, 140

naturopathic medicine, 140

qigong, 140

Reiki, 140–41

Rolfing, 141

yoga, 141

Compression fracture, kyphosis from, 160

Computer

positioning, 287

use, carpal tunnel syndrome from, 294–96,
296

Cooking, back protection during, 302

Corset, for back pain, 127

Mom's gastrocnemius, 221, **221**

Mom's internal rotators, 211, **211**

Mom's lower-leg triple play, 224, **224**

Mom's medial hip rotators, 212, **212**

Mom's neck routine, 217–18, **217–18**

Mom's rhomboids/rotator cuffs, 216, **216**

Mom's seated thoracic-lumbar rotators, 214, **214**

Mom's seated trunk extensors, 213, **213**

Mom's soleus, 220, **220**

Mom's straight-leg hamstrings, 210, **210**

Mom's towel pulls, 225, **225**

Mom's trunk lateral flexors, 215, **215**

Muscle(s)

    calorie burning from, 192

    imbalanced, causing slouching, 17

    isolation of, in Active-Isolated work, 9

    stability and, 14

    working in pairs, 9, 24, 34, 63, 252

Muscle mass

    building, with strength training, 236–37

    loss of, with aging, 236

    protein preserving, 242–43

Muscle relaxants, for back pain, 125

Muscle soreness

    delayed-onset, 152

    exercise-induced, 152–53, **153–56**

Myelopathy, treating, 164–65

N

Napping

    benefits of, 277–79

    interfering with sleep, 273

    techniques for, 279

Narcotic medications, for back pain, 125–26

Naturopathic medicine, for back pain, 140

Neck

    anatomy of, 10

    discomfort, as heart attack symptom, <u>35</u>

    fatigued by sitting, 286

    locked (*see* Neck crick)

    problems affecting, 10–11

    quick releases for, in tension-related back pain, 254–58,
        254–58

Neck crick, 10

    cause of, 116

    exercises relieving

        neck extensors, 119, **119**

        neck flexors, 120, **120**

        neck lateral flexors, 121, **121**

        neck oblique extensors, 123, **123**

        neck oblique flexors, 124, **124**

        neck rotators, 122, **122**

        semi-circumduction of the neck, 117–18,
            117–18

Neck extensors

    in Active-Isolated Stretching routine, 61, **61**, **101**

    after gardening, **305**, **306**

    after housework, **303**

    for injury prevention in

        rugby players, 339, **339**

        triathletes, 359, **359**

    for treating

        back spasm, **145**

        neck crick, 119, **119**

        rheumatoid arthritis, **169**

        whiplash, **184**, **185**

Neck flexors, for neck crick, 120, **120**

Neck lateral flexors

    in Active-Isolated Stretching routine, 62, **62**, **101**

    as bedtime stretch, **276**

    after housework, **303**

    after pushing wheelbarrow, **305**

    for rugby players, 339, **339**

    for treating

        neck crick, 121, **121**

        rheumatoid arthritis, **169**

        whiplash, **184**, **185**

Neck oblique extensors, for neck crick, 123, **123**

Neck oblique flexors, for neck crick, 124, **124**

Neck roll, noises from, 253

Neck rotators, for neck crick, 122, **122**

Neck routine, mom's, 217–18, **217–18**

Nembutal, for sleeplessness, 282

Nerve compression, from cycling, 327

Nerves and nerve roots, 13–14

Neuroleptic medications, for back pain, 125

Neurologists, for treating back pain, 132–33

Sports injury prevention in (cont.)

    triathlon, 357–59, **359**

    walking, 359–60, **360**

    weight training, 360–61, **361**

Sports medicine, Internet resources on, 366–67

Sprain, treating, 177–78, **178**

Sprinting, injury prevention in, 347–49, **350**

Squash, injury prevention in, 349, 351, **351**

Squatting, purpose of, 21

SSRIs, for back pain, 125

Stairs, preventing falls on, 300

Standing

    managing transitions to, 19

    at work

        back protection for, 290, **290**

        effects of, 288–90

Standing gastrocnemius, for marathon runners, 337, **338**

Standing gluteals, for duathletes, 329, **330**

Standing quadriceps, for runners, 340, **341**

Standing straight-knee hamstring, for sprinters, 349, **350**

Steroids, for back pain, 125

Stimulation, for back pain, 126

Straight-leg hamstrings

    in Active-Isolated Stretching routine, 42, **42**, **99**

    for easing into stretching program, **193**

    mom's, 210, **210**

    for treating

        bruise, **148**

        exercise-induced muscle soreness, **155**

        sciatica, **170**

        spondylolisthesis, **174**

        spondylosis, **176**

        whiplash, **181**

Strain, treating, 178–79, **179**

Strength training. *See also* Active-Isolated Strengthening routine

    breathing during, 239

    for building muscle mass, 236–37

Stress

    as cause of back pain, 111

    exercise for reducing, 192

Stress fracture, treating, 180

Stretching. *See also* Active-Isolated Stretching routine

    for back spasms, 115

    before bedtime, 275, **276**

    muscle tears from, <u>38</u>

    during pregnancy, 205–7

    for senior fitness, 237–38, **238**

Subluxations, 151–52

Sugar, avoiding, for weight loss, 198–99

Sunlight, enhancing sleep, 275

Sun protection

    for cross-country skiers, 326

    for downhill skiers, 329

    for scuba divers and snorkelers, 343

    for soccer players, 345

Supplements

    antioxidant, <u>242</u>

    botanical, for sleeplessness, 281

    joint health, <u>243</u>

    vitamin/mineral

        for seniors, 243

        in weight-loss plan, 200

Surgery, back, 127

Swayback, 162

Swimming, injury prevention in, 351–53, **353**

T

Table tennis, injury prevention in, 353–54, **355**, **356**

Tailbone, 12

Taste, loss of, with aging, 241

Teas, herbal, for sleeplessness, 281

Tennis

    injury prevention in, 354, 357, **357**

    table, injury prevention in, 353–54, **355**, **356**

"Tennis ball" massage, for tension-related back pain, 262

TENS, for back pain, 126

Tense and release, for tension-related back pain, 262–63

Tension-related back pain

    causes of, 249–50

    hypoxia from, 252

    quick releases for

        principles of, 252

        promote neck rotation, 257, **257**

        relax the sides of your neck, 256, **256**

Whiplash, treating, 180–81, **181–85**

Whole back stretch, 260, **260**

Wong-Baker FACES Pain Rating Scale, for describing back pain, <u>113</u>

Workout log, 37, <u>97</u>

Workplace safety, Internet resources on, 367

Workshop, preventing falls in, 300

Work situations

    back protection in

        computer use, 294–96, **296**

        driving, 292–94, **294**

        lifting and hauling, 290–92, **292**

        for occupational athletes, 285

        sitting, 285–88

        standing, 288–90, **290**

    ergonomics and, 287

Wrist extensors, for table tennis players, 354, **356**

Wrist flexors, for table tennis players, 354, **355**

Wrist fractures, from osteoporosis, 227

X

Xanax, for sleeplessness, 282

Y

Yoga, for treating back pain, 141

Yoga Breath

    for sleeplessness, 279

    for tension-related back pain, 263–64

Yo-yo dieting, pitfalls of, 191

Z

Zoloft, for back pain, 125